SPEECH AND LANGUAGE PROBLEMS

Publication Number 1022
AMERICAN LECTURE SERIES®

A Monograph in

The BANNERSTONE DIVISION *of*
AMERICAN LECTURES IN SPECIAL EDUCATION

Edited by

MORRIS VAL JONES, Ph.D.
Professor of Speech Pathology
California State University
Sacramento, California

SPEECH AND LANGUAGE PROBLEMS
An Overview

Edited by

MORRIS VAL JONES, Ph.D.

Professor of Speech Pathology
California State University
Sacramento, California

With a Foreword by

Virgil A. Anderson, Ph.D.

Professor Emeritus, Speech Pathology
Stanford University
Stanford, California

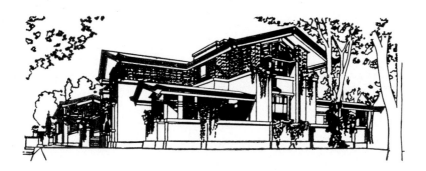

CHARLES C THOMAS · PUBLISHER
Springfield · Illinois · U.S.A.

Published and Distributed Throughout the World by
CHARLES C THOMAS • PUBLISHER
Bannerstone House
301-327 East Lawrence Avenue, Springfield, Illinois, U.S.A.

© *1979,* by CHARLES C THOMAS • PUBLISHER
ISBN 0-398-03790-6
Library of Congress Catalog Card Number: 78-1515

With THOMAS BOOKS *careful attention is given to all details of
manufacturing and design. It is the Publisher's desire to present books
that are satisfactory as to their physical qualities and artistic possibilities
and appropriate for their particular use.* THOMAS BOOKS *will be true
to those laws of quality that assure a good name and good will.*

Printed in the United States of America
W-2

Library of Congress Cataloging in Publication Data
Main entry under title:

Jones, Morris Val
Speech and language problems.

   (American lecture series; publication no. 1022)
   Includes bibliographies and index.
   1. Speech, Disorders of. I. Jones, Morris Val.
[DNLM: 1. Language disorders. 2. Speech disorders.
WM475.3 S742]
RC423.S638   616.8'55   78-1515
ISBN 0-398-03790-6

To

BREE LIANA MIDWINTER
*first grandchild who is
struggling with the major
task of speech and language
acquisition*

CONTRIBUTORS

Alan Abeson
Assistant Executive Director
Evaluation, Planning, and Development
Council for Exceptional Children
Reston, Virginia

Betty D. Anderson, R.N., M.A.
Private Practice
Speech Pathology
Sacramento, California

Evelyn Bowling, M.A.
Director
Sunrise Language, Speech, and Educational Services
Citrus Heights, California

Colette L. Coleman, Ph.D.
Associate Professor of Speech Pathology
California State University
Sacramento, California

Mary Darlow
Speech, Hearing, and Language Specialist
Sacramento Unified School District
Sacramento, California

Robert Fagella, M.D.
Plastic Surgeon
Private Practice
Sacramento, California
Clinical Assistant Professor of Spastic Surgery
University of California
Davis, California

Susan Goodrich
Graduate Assistant
Department of Speech Pathology and Audiology
California State University
Sacramento, California

Michael K. Grimes
Supervisor
Contra Costa County Schools
Pleasant Hill, California

Helen W. Harris
Speech, Hearing, and Language Specialist
San Juan Unified School District
Carmichael, California

Eileen Heaser
Librarian
California State University
Sacramento, California

Barbara Hoadley, M.A.
Clinic Supervisor
Department of Speech Pathology and Audiology
California State University
Sacramento, California

Morris Val Jones, Ph.D.
Professor of Speech Pathology
California State University
Sacramento, California

James H. McCartney, Ph.D.
Assistant Professor
Department of Speech Pathology and Audiology
California State University
Sacramento, California

Catherine McCormack
Graduate Student
Department of Speech Pathology and Audiology
California State University
Sacramento, California

Frederick Pemberton Murray, Ph.D.
Department of Communication Disorders
University of New Hampshire
Durham, New Hampshire

Richard Outland
Formerly, Consultant in the Education of Physically Handicapped Children
Department of Special Education
State of California
Sacramento, California

Miles Richmond
Principal
Special Education Center
Grant Joint Union High School District
Sacramento, California

Joan M. Smith, Ed.D.
Owner-Director
Melvin-Smith Learning Center
Sacramento, California

Pauline Stone, M.A.
Associate Professor of Speech Pathology
California State University
Sacramento, California

Jeffrey Zettel
Specialist for Policy Implementation and Governmental Relations
Council for Exceptional Children
Reston, Virginia

FOREWORD

SPECIALIZATION HAS SO dominated the areas of speech and language that it has become difficult, if not impossible, to find a single source of information that deals with the overall scope of these closely interrelated subjects that the nonspecialist can understand.

I feel that Doctor Jones has accomplished very successfully the task of providing clear and basic information on the major areas within the broad range of these two fields. He has done this on a nontechnical level that will be comprehensible and useful to the individuals who most need to be informed.

These include, in addition to laymen in general, students who may be potential majors in these fields, and specialists from a large number of related fields, including medicine, psychology, linguistics, audiology, education, counseling, and, as Doctor Jones has pointed out, many other disciplines as well.

This book is a needed addition to these fields and should prove useful to a wide range of individuals.

VIRGIL A. ANDERSON

PREFACE

T HIS BOOK IS intended to supply information about the field of Speech Pathology to individuals who have had minor or no exposure to the area. Each author was instructed to write in simple, nontechnical terms about his area of expertise. There has been no attempt to censor or modify significantly the style of writing. Hopefully, each reader will find one or more authors who appeal to his receptive appreciation. Every effort has been made to reduce duplication while allowing each chapter to remain essentially self-contained. It is assumed that this survey will whet the appetite of the reader to pursue the various sub-areas in depth. There has been a determined effort to minimize the "how-to-do-it" (therapy) aspects since, as Chapters 15 and 16 delineate, becoming a speech/language clinician is a full-time, long-term process.

The author-editor was intensely interested in the series of three articles in the August, 1977 issue of the *Journal of Speech and Hearing Disorders,* which dealt with "A critical examination of the Northwestern Syntax Screening Test." After a rather complete damning of this test instrument, the first author wrote, "Considering the already exposed inadequacies of this instrument, it seems rather futile to continue research on the NSST as it is now constituted" (p. 319). A second critic concluded, "Since the NSST shows a weak theoretical base as well as inadequate psychometric standards, we should stop using the present version" (p. 321).

The developer of the NSST, Laura L. Lee, after a four page response, replied, "Yet I want to support its continued use by clinicians who understand its purposes and know how to interpret the information they gain from it" (p. 323).

So, please temper your expectations with reason. All authors have been extremely careful to document their sources and to "stick to the truth." Enough information is available to write a volume many times the length of this one. A revised edition could include some of that material; by then, learning disabilities may have become a legitimate responsibility of the speech/ language clinician.

MORRIS VAL JONES

INTRODUCTION

I₅ 1975 THE American Speech and Hearing Association (ASHA) celebrated its fiftieth anniversary. Membership had increased from the original group of twenty-five charter members to a membership of 21,000. Growth of the organization continues and may exceed 30,000 by 1980. The national headquarters in Bethesda, Maryland have been outgrown, and plans are underway to construct new facilities nearby. Federal legislation, including Pub. L. No. 94-142, is favorable to expansion of speech therapy services, so it seems within reason to predict that the dual professions of speech pathology and audiology will have an unprecedented growth spurt for the next decade.

According to a 1975 *ASHA Facts and Figures* bulletin, the following statistics were pertinent:

Type of membership:

Regular 20,314
Graduate students 395
Spouse 325
Life 401
                                                 _____
                        Total 21,435

Employment:

Elementary or secondary schools 8,315
College or university 3,320
Clinic or center 4,172
Unknown or unemployed 5,628

The process of human communication is so complex that research is carried on by scores of interrelated professional disciplines in an attempt to unravel its intricacies. A partial list of such specialists was prepared by the Subcommittee of Human

Communication and its Disorders of the National Advisory Neurological Diseases and Stroke Council. It is as follows:

Acoustic Engineer	Neurologist
Anatomist	Neuropathologist
Anthropologist	Neurosurgeon
Audiologist	Orthodontist
Bioacoustician	Otologist
Biochemist	Otoneurologist
Biomedical Engineer	Pediatrician
Child Psychologist	Pediatric Neurologist
Comparative Psychologist	Physiologist
Cryptographer	Physiological Psychologist
Educator of the Deaf	Prosthodontist
Electroencephalographer	Psychiatrist
Embryologist	Psychoacoustician
Epidermologist	Psycholinguist
Ethnologist	Psychometrist
Experimental Phonetician	Semanticist
Experimental Psychologist	Social Psychologist
Geneticist	Speech Developmentalist
Histologist	Speech Pathologist
Information Theorist	Speech Scientist
Language Developmentalist	Structural Linguist
Laryngologist	Statistician
Learning Theorist	Zoologist
Lexicographer	

More detail will now be provided concerning those areas most closely associated with speech pathology.

I want to make it perfectly clear from the outset that becoming a speech, hearing, and language clinician is a long and tortuous journey (at least four full years) and, needless to say, should not be undertaken lightly. Why does it take so long? The answer is simple enough—there is so much to be learned. Speech Pathology overlaps many other professional fields, and the speech clinician must be conversant with all of them.

Sociology

Since man (persons) does not normally live in isolation, he must have a means of communication, a means of transmitting messages from the individual, or group of individuals, to others. The most popular method of accomplishing this necessity is through direct confrontation using oral language or speech. Although one could write a note, and often the deaf do just that, speech is more effective. The receiver, or listener, has the opportunity to make an immediate reply. Of course, the persons involved must speak the same type of language—such as English, French, Swahili—if they expect to understand each other.

It is much more difficult for large groups of people, such as nations, to communicate with each other, so they probably will need to depend upon representatives, such as ambassadors; or, they will have to depend upon another form of language, the written.

The speech clinician needs to know about group dynamics and needs to possess a facility to impart information to groups of people, such as parents or classroom teachers.

The speech clinician must realize that the basic principles of sociology also are important for the individual child who is learning to speak. Most children acquire speech and language by listening to persons in their environment and then gradually imitating what they hear. They soon learn that they can control these persons in ways that are advantageous to them by using oral language. The first person they want to influence is usually the primary caregiver, the mother, but soon this control spreads to siblings, father, and on into an ever-widening circle. If there were no home society, or if this opportunity were very restricted, the child might not learn to talk.

Physics

Speech is produced by a vibrating instrument, the vocal folds, and sound waves are set into motion. Thus, the speech clinician must know the basic principles of physics; she must know about types of vibrators, about frequency, and about resonance. For some types of voice problems, such information is essential. With the audiologist, who deals primarily with the transmission of sound, the field of physics becomes even more important. He must daily handle problems with amplification systems, including hearing aids. The vocabulary of physics—acoustic spectra, fundamental frequency, segmental vibrations, harmonic analysis, minimal perceptible differences—is a part of his professional vocabulary.

Physiology

A knowledge of anatomy and physiology is basic for the speech clinician. The production of speech is dependent upon the proper working of the muscles which are utilized in respiration, phonation, resonance, and articulation. If there is a speech or language problem, the first problem in diagnosis is determining if the etiology is organic. Does the musculature of the respiratory system—the muscles of the thoracic cavity, the abdominal cavity, or the laryngeal—provide the necessary energy to set the vocal cords into vibration? Is there some reason, such as vocal nodules, that the vocal cords produce extra noise? Or, more obviously, is there a congenital anomaly, as in the case of cleft palate, which can make speech production unintelligible? (An entire area of study, Anatomy of the Speech Mechanism, is devoted to this material.) Or, does the child have difficulty in learning speech because of an ossified oval window between the middle and inner ear?

Neurology

Both children and adults may have difficulty in speech or language because of dysfunction of the central nervous system. Again, the speech clinician must be familiar with the terminology and the methodology of this field. A problem in speech and language or in learning disability can have its basis in brain damage or a failure of the central nervous system to develop (maturate) normally. The speech clinician must be able to converse with the neurologist about the perceptual processes, the site of lesion, Broca's area, or a cerebral vascular accident. She must know about the reflex arc, the synapse, efferent and afferent nerves. As an extension of anatomy she needs to understand the functions of the various lobes of the brain, as well as the subdivisions of the brain stem. If there is a central nervous system malfunction, the speech clinician needs to determine its effect upon the various aspects of speech and language production.

Linguistics

In the past fifteen years the contributions of the field of linguistics, especially developmental psycholinguistics, to speech pathology have been extremely important. The emergence of generative transformational grammar, with Noam Chomsky of the Massachusetts Institute of Technology as its chief proponent, has revolutionized the study of the acquisition of language in childhood. This influence has been felt in all areas of speech production, phonology (the acquisition of sounds), syntax (the acquisition of vocabulary). Speech pathologists, such as those from Northwestern University and from the Institute for the Study of Aphasia in Children in San Francisco, have developed methods of obtaining and analyzing speech samples to determine the level of achievement of young children. Obviously, the speech clinician must be able to utilize these methods.

Psychology

The speech clinician will realize that the majority of children who have speech and language problems, especially of a mild or moderate degree, do not possess a faulty mechanism nor have they been subjected to a deprived environment. The etiology of their problems lies within the purview of the general field of psychology. These children do not have a cleft palate, paralyzed vocal cords, or a hearing loss. For whatever reasons, they have not been motivated to speak appropriately for their chronological age. Possibly, they have deviations in personality which have affected their speech and language development. In this area, the speech clinician needs to learn what problems he can handle himself and which ones will require the cooperation of the clinical psychologist or the psychiatrist. A useful methodology has been developed in recent years—behavior modification—which is being used by the speech clinician in selected cases.

There is also the matter of evaluation of intelligence. Some speech pathologists obtain dual majors which qualify them to administer psychometric tests, while others depend upon reports from qualified psychologists. In any event, the speech clinician must be able to interpret such reports and to know when referral for reevaluation is appropriate. There can be no doubt of a close relationship between cognitive skills and language achievement. Some experts believe the overlap is so great that both areas merge into one.

Other Fields

GENETICS. Speech clinicians are sometimes called upon to participate on teams of experts—as with the cleft lip and palate, deaf, mentally retarded, or brain damaged—in which the matter of genetic counseling becomes important. If a couple has one child who is speech and language handicapped, what are the chances (percentage of risk) that a later-born child will have the same defect?

CHEMOTHERAPY. Speech clinicians may be asked to observe the effects of drugs upon their clients. Or, they may observe significant changes and report them to the supervising medical personnel. Some knowledge of the classification of drugs and their expected effects is highly useful under these circumstances.

This list could be extended almost indefinitely, for example, into the areas of music, foreign language, statistics, legislation, special education, etc., so that the potential speech and language clinician realizes that four years, or six years, are inadequate. Indeed, life-long continued education is an absolute necessity. So, obviously, this volume or any other can present only selected information which will provide an introduction into speech pathology.

The fields of speech pathology and audiology are extensive and include numerous sub-areas. Many speech pathologists become specialists in one of these sub-areas, such as stuttering or aphasia, but the beginning clinician must be a "general practitioner." Over the past fifty years innumerable surveys have been conducted to determine the extent and variation of speech disorders; reports reflect the varying methodologies and points-of-view which have been pursued. The following statistics will give an indication of the results of some of these efforts.

Estimated prevalence of communicative disorders (National Advisory Neurological Diseases and Stroke Council, 1969):

Articulatory disorders 8,000,000
Language disorders 2,100,000
Stuttering 1,400,000
Voice disorders 1,000,000
          (*Human Communication and Its Disorders—An Overview*)

Charles Van Riper, in the fifth edition of his *Speech Correction*

(1972, p. 50), reported on the percentages of different types of cases referred to the Western Michigan University Speech Clinic in a ten-year period.

Stuttering 41%
Articulation 19%
Delayed speech 15%
Voice 9%
Cleft palate 8%
Aphasia 7%

The inflated percentage for stuttering may indicate that Van Riper's national reputation in that area attracted many referrals, possibly self-referrals, of persons with problems with dysfluency.

In ASHA, a journal of the American Speech and Hearing Association (July, 1977), Van Riper describes in some detail his attempt to prepare a stuttering specialist for the public school setting. He was able to find one graduate student who was willing to spend an additional year as a part of his Master's program as a tutorial student under Doctor Van Riper's immediate guidance. This additional training concentrated upon methods of eliminating stuttering behavior in young children. The trainee's first two years of employment, subsidized by the Speech Foundation of America, demonstrated the usefulness of employing a specialist in stuttering in the public schools. The experiment supported Van Riper's conclusion:

> Two former presidents of our association (Moll, 1974; Ainsworth, 1974) have spoken of the urgent need for continuing education for our professionals. Must that training be confined solely to preparing general practitioners, or can it also be used to train specialists in stuttering as well as other disorders? Perhaps this is an idea whose time has come. (P. 469)

ACKNOWLEDGMENTS

T HE AUTHOR WISHES to thank the typists, Eunice Naber and Laurie Val Jones, and the family whose demands for time may have diminished infinitesimally during the period of authorship.

M.V.J.

CONTENTS

SPEECH AND LANGUAGE PROBLEMS

CHAPTER 1

ACQUISITION OF LANGUAGE

MORRIS VAL JONES, PH.D.

$\mathbf{F}$ROM THE MOMENT of birth the human infant becomes an object of controversy for psycholinguists. Leaders in the behaviorist camp maintain that the neonate is a *tabula rasa* (a blank tablet). S/he* responds to the environment and learns only what s/he encounters; s/he is basically a passive instrument dependent upon the pressures of the environment; s/he has no special abilities for language acquisition, but only a general ability to learn. For further detail concerning this point of view, the reader is referred to Leonard Bloomfield (1933), B. F. Skinner (1956), O. H. Mowrer (1960), and Walburga von Raffler-Engel (1976).

An opposing school of thought is led by Noam Chomsky, who promotes transformational generative grammar. He and his followers, the most persuasive of whom was the late Eric Lenneberg, have insisted that the child is born with an innate potential for language which depends upon maturation of the nervous system (*see* Table 1-I).

Lenneberg wrote *Biological Foundations of Language* in 1967.

> The appearance of language is primarily dependent upon the maturational development of states of readiness within the child. (P. 142)
> Language cannot begin to develop until a certain level of physical maturation and growth has been attained. Between the ages of two

---

* With the relatively recent semirevolution in sex related matters has come ambiguity in the use of the pronouns. No longer can the author write "he," "him," "his" to indicate the entire human race. However, the necessity for insertion of "him/her-self," and other usages, does become burdensome, so each author has been left free to solve the problem in his and/or her own way.

TABLE 1-I

CHRONOLOGICAL DEVELOPMENT

Age in months	Vocalization and Language	Motor Development
4	Coos and chuckles	Head self-supported; tonic neck reflex subsiding; can sit with pillow on three sides.
6 to 9	Babbles; produces sounds such as *ma* or *da;* reduplication of sounds common.	Sits alone; pulls himself to standing; unilateral reaching; first thumb opposition of grasp.
12 to 18	A small number of "words"; follows simple commands and responds to "no."	Stands momentarily alone; creeps; walks sideways when holding onto a railing; takes a few steps when held by hands; grasp, prehension, and release fully developed.
18 to 21	From about 20 words at 18 months to about 200 words at 21; points to many more objects; comprehends simple questions; forms two-word phrases.	Stance fully developed; gait stiff, propulsive, and precipitated; seats himself on child's chair with only fair aim; creeps downstairs backward; has difficulty building tower of three cubes; can throw a ball, but clumsily.
22 to 27	Vocabulary of 300 to 400 words; has two-to-three-word phrases; uses prepositions and pronouns.	Runs but falls when making a sudden turn; can quickly alternate between stance, kneeling or sitting positions; walks stairs up and down, one foot forward only.
30 to 33	Fastest increase in vocabulary; three-to-four-word sentences are common; word order, phrase structure, grammatical agreement approximate language of surroundings, but many utterances are unlike anything an adult would say.	Good finger coordination; can move digits independently; manipulation of objects much improved; builds tower of six cubes.
36 to 39	Vocabulary of 1,000 or more words; well-formed sentences using complex grammatical rules, although certain rules have not yet been fully mastered; grammatical mistakes are much less frequent; about 90 percent comprehensibility.	Runs smoothly with acceleration and deceleration; negotiates sharp and fast curves without difficulty; walks stairs by alternating feet; jumps 12 inches; can operate tricycle; stands on one foot for a few seconds.

      * From Lenneberg, E., On Explaining Language, *Science, 164*:635-643, May 9, 1969. Copyright 1969 by the American Association for the Advancement of Science.

and three years language emerges by an interaction of maturation and self-programmed learning. (P. 158)

The predeterminists stress, in particular, the following:

1. There is a biological predisposition for language.
2. Universal rules of grammar and phonology emerge according to a maturation of sequence.
3. There are two levels of language—competence and performance.
4. Environmental stimulation is necessary only to trigger the biological mechanisms.

Although some psycholinguists follow one of these extreme positions, the majority tend toward a middle course and support the view expressed by Derek Sanders (1976):

It is convenient, for the purpose of discussion, to separate maturational and environmental factors. However, it is very important to realize that these two influences are not independent parallel factors. Maturation and environment are totally interdependent factors in the development of communicative behavior in the child. (P. 4)

Von Raffler-Engel (1976) has indicated a change from the either/or position:

The last five years have witnessed greater changes in the study of child language than any other period in the history of research in language acquisition. . . . The whole process of language acquisition unfolds in a delicate interplay of maturational factors, biological elements, and cultural influences. Children learn the verbal and kinesic aspects of communication while interacting with their parents, siblings, and peers. (P. 204)

After studying the development of more than 1,000 normal infants and young children, Frankenburg and Dodds (1970) published the Denver Developmental Screening Test, of which the following items illustrate the range at which 25 percent to 90 percent accomplish each item.

Personal-social:	*Range in months*
Smiles spontaneously	1½– 5
Resists toy pull	4 –10
Plays ball w/examiner	10 –16
Washes and dries hands	19 –36
Plays interactive games (tag)	20 –42

Fine motor adaptive:

Hands together	1½– 4
Regards raisin	2½– 5
Bangs two cubes held in hands	7 –12½
Tower of 8 cubes	21 –40
Draws man 3 parts	40 –66

Language:

Responds to bell	0 – 1½
Turns to voice	3½– 8½
Dada or *mama,* specific	9½–13½
Combines two different words	14 –30
Gives first and last names	24 –44

Gross motor:

Sits–head steady	1½– 4
Sits without support	5 – 8
Stands alone well	10 –14
Jumps in place	21 –36
Balances on one foot, 10 seconds	36 –72

The Prelinguistic Period

Regardless of the outcome of these theoretical battles, neonates continue to arrive in the world with limited repertoires of verbal attainment. For several weeks, they depend upon cries of varying intensity to attract the attention of caregivers, but within a month to six weeks these cries become differentiated. Spectographic analyses have indicated that they have differing structures which are associated with specific situations, such as hunger, pain, or discomfort. About this same time, babies begin to express contentment by emitting cooing sounds and indulge in smiling behavior as a response to stimulation from adults in the environment.

Paula Menyuk made the following statement in Language Perspectives—Acquisition, Retardation, and Intervention (1974):

> Communication interaction takes place between mother and child at a very early age. The pattern of this interaction seems to be one of vocalization, listening, answering, and, particularly on the part of the mother, further vocalization to elicit a response if one is not immediately forthcoming. (P. 225)

At all stages of language development, reception precedes

production. Recent research concerning the auditory reception of infants confirms that they can discriminate speech sounds when they are less than four months of age, and possibly even as young as one month. Two methods have been utilized in the laboratory to determine this ability of infants: changes in heart rate and, more recently, high amplitude sucking response. Morse (1977) was impressed with the data obtained by these methods of research:

> In sum, all of these studies in infant speech perception reveal that infants can discriminate almost every relevant acoustic cue(s) in those speech sounds that have so far been presented to them. . . . This research thus supports the position that some aspects of processing in a speech mode are either a genetically endowed capacity in infants, or they are learned within the first few weeks of life. (P. 166)

Kenneth Bzoch and Richard League (1971), after reviewing the literature about the language of infants and studying fifty babies at the University of Florida, published the REEL Scale (Receptive-Expressive Emergent Language Scale) for the measurement of language skills in infancy from birth to three years. They found that infants, for example, indicate the following language reception:

> Zero to one month: Startle response to loud, sudden noises.
> Two to three months: Regularly localizes speaker with eyes.
> Four to five months: Recognizes and responds to his (her) own name.
> Eight to nine months: Regularly stops activity in response to "no."
> Nine to ten months: Often gives toys or other objects to a parent on verbal request.

Expressive behavior is illustrated by the following actions:

> Zero to one month: Begins random vocalization other than crying.
> Two to three months: Occasionally responds to sound stimulation by vocalizing.
> Three to four months: Babbles (regularly repeats series of same sounds).
> Five to six months: May vocalize four or more different syllables at one time.
> Six to seven months: Often responds with vocalizations when called by name.

Eleven to twelve months: Frequently responds to songs and rhymes by vocalizing.

Eighteen to twenty months: Has a speaking vocabulary of ten to twenty words.

Twenty to twenty-two months: Begins combining words into simple sentences, such as "go bye-bye," "daddy come."

There has been relatively little research about speech reception during the first year because of the difficulty of obtaining reliable data. Much more research data are available concerning expressive language, especially about babbling. This spontaneous emission of speech sounds, combined with gurgling, snorts, and other assorted noises, begins about three months of age and continues as a chief means of vocalization for four to six months. Many speech pathologists have evaluated this prelinguistic period. Among them are the following:

M. M. Lewis (1963):

Babbling is a means by which the child, through repeated practice, acquires skill in making sounds. Babbling gives him the beginnings of the highly complex skills that go into the production of the sounds of speech. (P. 21)

Virgil Anderson (1973):

Pleasant states of mind facilitate that development, while unpleasant states retard it, for whenever the unpleasant states become dominant, the child will stop babbling and start to cry. Therefore, it can be said that, other things being equal, the happy child will learn to speak faster than the uphappy child, since more time will be spent in vocal play. (P. 63)

McConnell et al. (1974):

His attempts at preverbal language in these first weeks and months of life outwardly manifest his need to become a communicating member of the family unit. The child whose parents recognize this is indeed fortunate, because positive reinforcement of preverbal attempts enhances verbal language development. (P. 55)

One nationally noted pioneer in speech pathology who has emphasized the importance of babbling, both as a period in normal language development and as a method in therapy, is Charles Van Riper (1972):

When the babbling period is interrupted or delayed through illness, the appearance of true speech is often similarly retarded. (P. 57)

We know of no better way to relax than by free babbling, especially when the therapist is babbling freely, too. Perhaps we are returning to an earlier period when learning to speak was fun. (P. 59) One of the most effective methods for strengthening a new sound is to include it in babbling. (P. 223)

The value of babbling as a precursor of true speech remains controversial, but William Perkins (1971) has summarized his impressions:

Out of this period of vocal development will come three skills:
(1) a crude but effective communication system to relieve discomfort that will develop in connection with crying.
(2) a system for expressing emotion that will develop in connection with intonation.
(3) a system of coordination among mechanisms of breathing, vocalizing, articulating, and hearing that will develop with cooing and babbling and will be basic to perfecting later articulatory control of speech sound. (P. 99)

Perkins has also stressed the importance of the imitation of prosodic patterns:

The consensus of observers of vocal development is that what children imitate most in babbling is their parents' intonation patterns. The newly arrived infant apparently responds to the most salient features in the maelstrom of foreign sounds in which he grows: the melody of speech. (P. 99)

After the peaking of the babbling period around seven or eight months of age, the child moves on to the echolalic period. By this time he enters a "period of attachment" as he begins to identify with a particular person in the environment, usually the mother. Normally, this person will mediate the environment, that is, put into words the events as they happen and name items over and over for the child's benefit. Gradually, the child echoes parts of these utterances and basks in the praise s/he gets for his/her efforts. Occasionally, probably by accident, s/he will utter a word from the adult world, such as *dada* or *yum-yum*.

Andre Lecours (1975) has described the echolalic period:

In echolalic behavior, sounds are produced as specific imitative responses to specific stimuli. Prosodic components of speech may for several months be the only ones the baby endeavors to imitate; as a rule, it is during the last months of his first year of life that he begins to engage in progressively more successful attempts at reproduction of articulated speech segments. (P. 129)

The Holophrastic Period

At last, somewhere approximating the first birthday, the first real word is spoken. Philip Dale (1972) made a listing of criteria which have been proposed for this first word:

consistent use of the word by the child
spontaneity of usage (not merely imitated from adult speech)
evidence of understanding
occasionally the more stringent requirement that the word be a
    word of the adult language (P. 38)

This first word, such as *mama* or *bye-bye*, marks the dividing point between the prelinguistic period and the linguistic period. With this use of an arbitrary symbol, the child enters the human, talking world where s/he will progress in the various aspects of speech and language for the rest of his or her life.

Increase in the spoken vocabulary is slow, but infants may have a speaking vocabulary ranging from 3 to 50 words by the age of eighteen months. More rapid progress then is common, and the child may have a vocabulary of 200 words by the age of two and approximately 1,000 words by the age of three (Lenneberg, 1967, p. 128). A monumental study of expressive vocabulary size by Medorah Smith (1926) is still widely quoted (*see* Table 1-II).

For most of the period between one and two years, the average infant will remain in the holophrastic stage of language development. He will use one word to express a variety of meanings; one word is used to express a complete sentence, as David McNeill (1970) has written: "Many investigators of children's language (e.g., Stern and Stern, 1907; deLaguna, 1927; Leopold, 1949; McCarthy, 1954) have said that the single words of holophrastic speech are equivalent to the full sentences of adults (p. 20)." Around twenty months of age a child can use a single word to name an object, to give a command, and/or to express emotion. These single utterances may be nonsense, such as *dididi* or real words, such as *dada* or *more*. Bloom (1970) has questioned the interpretation by stating, "That such words are

TABLE 1-II

SIZE OF EXPRESSIVE VOCABULARY*

Age in Yrs.-Mos.	#	No. of Words	Words Gained
8	13	0	
10	17	1	1
1-0	52	3	2
1-3	19	19	16
1-6	14	22	3
1-9	14	118	96
2-0	25	272	154
2-6	14	446	174
3-0	20	896	450
3-6	26	1222	326
4-0	26	1540	318
4-6	32	1870	330
5-0	20	2072	202
5-6	27	2289	217
6-0	9	2562	273

* (From Medora Smith, *Vocabulary in Young Children*, 1926. Courtesy of University of Iowa Press.)

indeed holophrastic is open to question" (p. 10). Since the child is unable to tell us what he has in mind, we will have to put our own interpretation upon his utterances.

Greenfield and Smith (1976), two linguistically trained mothers, kept extensive notes concerning the use of one word utterances by their sons between the ages of eight months and twenty-two months. For interpretation of the child's meaning, they depended on situational context, as well as the utterance itself. The researchers found, at least in the case of these two boys, that a single word could be used to express numerous semantic relationships and that these same relationships were present in the later developing multiword sentences. They found also that semantic relationships emerged in a definite chronological order. One of the boys, Matthew, used the single word *dada* as follows—(for the first time):

Months	Days	
8	12 ...	Matthew says *dada* while looking at his father. (Here *dada* is an Indicative Object.)
11	28 ...	He says *dada* while offering a bottle to his father. (*Dada* is Dative in this situation.)
13	3 ...	He says *dada* upon hearing his father come in the door and start up the steps. (Daddy is an Agent in this context.)

17 15 ... Matthew says *Daddy*, pointing to a cup that belongs to his father.
           (*Daddy* here represents an Animate Being Associated with an Object or Location.)

18 11 ... He says *Daddy* in response to the question, "Who went bye-bye?"
           (He is responding to a verbally present situation.)

20   3 ... Matthew says *Daddy* in response to his father's question, "Who am I?"
           (An early semantic function, Indicative Object, is expressed in relation to a *wh* question.)

Thus, Matthew's word for father, the first adult word he acquired, is used successively in all semantic functions which a noun can fulfill. (P. 79)

Between the ages of two and five the child acquires the basic grammatic structures of the adult language in his environment. By the time s/he completes kindergarten, the normal child can express him- or herself fluently on an infinite number of subjects. Not only can s/he generate various sentence forms with the use of transformations, but s/he makes use of morphological changes to denote tense, possession, plurals, third person singular, and the comparative and superlative of the adjective. Berry and Talbott (1966), expanding on the work of Jean Berko with morphological changes, developed a language test, *Comprehension of Grammar*, in which they gave names to "nonsense" figures. For example,

This is a cubash.  Now there is another one. There are two of them. There are two ————.

Or

This is a tass, who knows how to gizzle. He is gizzling. He does it every day. Every day he ————.

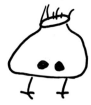

These tasks are used to test the child's understanding of the rules of morphological change.

Hubbell (1972) described the child's stages in acquiring adult forms of sentence structure by applying "rules" of generative grammar:

> A generative grammar is one that will generate all of the sentences possible in a language, and no utterances which are not permissible. Thus the generative grammarian is concerned with discovering a finite set of rules (a grammar) that will generate the infinite number of sentences possible in a language. In simplified form, this model posits three components to a grammar; the base, the output of which is called the deep structure; the syntactic component, which depends upon the mechanism of transformations for the output of surface structure; and the phonological component, which converts the surface structure into the sequence of sounds that we would use to say that sentence. (P. 96)

Hubbell, as many other experts in childhood language have done, expands the basic concept of Noam Chomsky (1969):

> I will use the term "generative grammar" to refer to a theory of language, as a system of rules that determine the deep and surface structures of the language in question, the relation between them, the semantic interpretation of the deep structures and the phonetic interpretative of the surface structures. The generative grammar of a language, then, is the system of rules which establish the relation between sound and meaning in this language. We make a fundamental distinction between *competence* (the speaker-hearer's knowledge of his language) and *performance* (the actual use of language in concrete situations). (P. 10)

Brown and Hanlon (1970), using recorded language samples of 700 to 2,100 utterances per sample, studied the emergence of certain syntactic forms in three preschool children. They transcribed at least two hours of conversation each month between mother and child at home. The period begins when the mean value (length) is 1.75 morphemes and the longest utterance is 5 morphemes; it ends when the mean is 4.00 and the longest utterance is 13 morphemes. Gathering the data took three years. The sentences seemed to emerge in the following order:

SAAD ... Simple, active, affirmative, declarative.
(We had a ball.)

Q   ... Simple, active, affirmative, interrogative.
             (Did we have a ball?)
N   ... Simple, active, negative, declarative.
             (We didn't have a ball.)
Tr   ... Simple, active, affirmative, declarative, truncated.
             (We did.)
TrN   ... Simple, active, negative, declarative, truncated.
             (We didn't.)
TrQ   ... Simple, active, affirmative, interrogative, truncated.
             (Did we?)
Tgq   ... Affirmative tag: simple, active, affirmative, interrogative, truncated.
             (We didn't have a ball, did we?)
NQ   ... Simple, active, negative, interrogative.
             (Didn't we have a ball?)
TrNQ   ... Simple, active, negative, interrogative, truncated.
             (Didn't we?)
TgNQ   ... Negative tag: simple, active, negative, interrogative, truncated.
             (We had a ball, didn't we?)*

Order of emergence seemed to be based on derivational complexity and the frequency with which the form was used in the speech of the mother.

The development of numerous modifications of the kernel sentence is essential to grammatical form which approximates the usage of adults in the environment. Among these are negation and questions, both of which emerge in a specific order. In the case of negation, Brown's group at Harvard has pinpointed four stages as follows:

Stage 1: An affirmative sentence with a *no* added.
          No wipe finger.
          More, no.
          No singing song.
          Wear mitten no.
          No a boy bed.
Stage 2: A combination of the Stage 1 form with some correct negations.
          Don't leave me.

* From Brown and Hanlon, John R. Hayes (Ed.): *Cognition and Development of Language,* 1970. Courtesy John Wiley & Sons, Inc.

I don't sit on Comer coffee.
This is a radiator no.
No pinch me.
I don't like him.

Stage 3: A closer approximation to the adult form.
I didn't did it.
Donna won't let go.
I'm not a doctor.
You don't want some supper.
This not ice cream.

Stage 4: The adult form of negation is probably accomplished by age four.

In the matter of questions there are also, according to Brown and his associates, stages of approximation to the adult form which may be subdivided into four stages.

Stage 1: Very simple, with an upward inflection.
See hole?
What doing?

Stage 2: Wh questions are used more consistently.
Where my mitten?
Why you smiling?
Why not he eat?

Stage 3: A closer approximation to the adult form.
What did he doed?
Why the kitten can't stand up?
Why he don't know how to pretend?

Stage 4: The adult form of questions takes somewhat longer than in the case of negation. Some complex forms are not accomplished until teen-age.

Trantham and Pederson (1976) made a study of eight apparently normally developing children through the critical language learning period of one and one-half to three years. Language samples were obtained from these children at three-week intervals beginning at age fifteen to eighteen months, when the children began to use two word combinations.

They summarized their findings concerning the acquisition of syntax; the following two examples give the flavor of the developmental process.

Brook:

18 months	*24 months*
Daddy's	What's that?
Daddy see	That's mine
Car	Baby crying
Daddy's car	There's sock
Snowin'	I get this box
Oh	I put it in here
Look	I can
Daddy's outside?	He's peek-a-boo
Daddy's that?	Her put a bottle in there
	Open it (imp)

30 months	*36 months*
It's not a nurse	What are these kind?
It's a Mama	We burned 'em
I watch you outside when Carla's coming	My Thane burned these candles
We going to go outside	He didn't get burned
She go downstairs	But he didn't now
Where this belong?	He did it and it was pretty
It's not going in there	He gots a knot in his tail
I don't like this washing machine	I helped her once and I couldn't turn on the water and put the water in the pan
I'm through	She worked
What is that?	Why'd you put this tail in?

Michael:

18 months	*24 months*
That baby	Kiss
This	Night-night bed
Go	In there
Want go	Daddy sit there
Kay	Night-night
Ice	Cops
Hi	Girl go night-night too
Want this	Bath
Mama	Where girl go?
Meow	Girl go?

30 months

I do there trains
See, I show you
Trains go on track
Trains go that hole like that
Choo-choos they go that hole
Trains go that hole
Trains go holes
That says "stop"
Blue light says "go"
The yellow light says, "be careful, be careful"
Where's the table?*

36 months

Where's the other one that belongs on here?
This one have clothes in it
This one have shoes in it
This one have pants in it
He has some boots on
He's at camp
Is this Lassie?
Help me put this together
I knocked it down and spilled it

One of the most detailed studies of language skills in children was published by Mildred C. Templin in 1957. Her work became the basis of several testing instruments and the authority for normal speech and language development. She tested sixty children at each of eight chronological ages, beginning with three years of age and ending with eight years of age. Her results concerning length of response are presented in Table I-III.

Templin analyzed 24,000 utterances of children from three to eight years according to length, grammatical complexity, grammatical accuracy, and the parts of speech used. A condensa-

TABLE 1-III

LENGTH OF RESPONSE†

Age in Years	Mean Length of Oral Responses	Mean: 5 Longest Responses	Median One Word Oral Responses	Mean No. of Difficult Words
3.0	4.1	7.89	4.8	92.5
3.5	4.7	9.06	3.3	104.8
4.0	5.4	10.51	2.5	120.4
4.5	5.5	10.76	2.5	127.0
5.0	5.7	11.73	2.4	132.4
6.0	6.6	12.27	0.7	147.0
7.0	7.3	13.57	0.6	157.7
8.0	7.6	14.15	0.6	166.5

† Data based on 60 cases at each age level. Basic speech of 50 responses. From Mildred Templin, *Certain Language Skills in Children*, 1957. Courtesy of University of Minnesota Press.

* From Carla Trantham and Joan Pedersen: *Normal Language Development*, 1976. Courtesy Williams & Wilkins Co.

tion of her summary statements for this portion of her study is
as follows:

1. Few significant differences in the length of responses of boys
   and girls are found. The upper socioeconomic status groups
   use longer responses at practically every age level tested, and
   in some instances the differences are statistically significant.
2. There is a consistent decrease in the proportionate use of
   structurally incomplete but functionally complete remarks with
   age; more simple sentences with phrases are used by the
   children in the present study; and there is a steady increase
   with age in the use of the more complex and elaborated forms
   of the sentence.
3. About half of the remarks of the three-year-old children are
   grammatically correct. All errors except those associated with
   the use of slang and colloquialisms decrease over the age range
   studied.
4. After the age of three the parts of speech used in both the
   total number of words and the different words uttered show
   little change. At this age the structure of adult grammar has
   already imposed the pattern of word selection upon the children.
   (Pp. 103-104)†

After reviewing the literature concerning the acquisition of
speech and language, Torres (1977) made the following summary—

0 TO 2 MONTHS: This stage lasts from the birth cry to the
beginning of babbling. During these first few weeks the infant's
vocal behavior is reflexive in nature and is made in response to
physical discomforts such as hunger, pain, or loud and sudden
noises. However, some prelanguage, noncrying sounds such as
grunts, gurgles, and sighs are heard.

2 TO 4 MONTHS: The child at this age will signal discomfort
by use of differentiated cries and will smile and laugh when
stimulated. From approximately two months on, babbling appears. These vocal utterances seem to be common to all babies
and are apparently independent of the language around them.
Babbling, a prelinguistic form of vocalization, first occurs without
direct human stimulation and appears to be self-reinforcing to
the infant through kinesthetic and auditory feedback. Receptive
capabilities are reflected in listening, and the beginning of associa-

---

† From Mildred Templin: *Certain Language Skills in Children*, 1957.
Courtesy of University of Minnesota Press.

tions with meaning and sound sources occurs. During these first four months there is progress toward integration of reflexive movements into habits and perceptions. The infant begins to listen selectively and can differentiate the moods and emotional states of the voices around him.

4 TO 12 MONTHS: From four to ten months important linguistic and intellectual development takes place. The infant still listens to himself and practices private babbling, but a new type of babbling referred to as *vocal play* now appears. Vocalization is used for getting attention and expressing demands. He frequently vocalizes in response to voice intonation of others. Syllabic repetitions begin to appear. Both imitative and nonimitative babbling occurs. Localization of sound sources and discriminatory abilities improve. In the second six months speech sounds begin to acquire meaning associated with his past experiences. The child will cease activity when his name is called or when *no-no* is said. At about eight months inflectional patterns become prominent and vocal play takes on the tonal characteristics of adult speech. Babbling and vocal play continue and the child's repertoire of sounds increases. At about twelve months the first true words will appear.

Linguistic Period

12 TO 18 MONTHS: The first words stage is variously referred to as the holophrastic stage, the linguistic developmental stage, or the paralanguage stage. This simply means that the child conveys information through single word sentences which are supplemented by intonational, situational and gestural cures. During this age period the child points to named pictures and objects, comprehends simple questions, and indicates his wants by gestures and words. A child of this age will have approximately twenty-five words in his vocabulary.

18 TO 36 MONTHS: During this period the rate of imitation predominates. Jargon (practice of adult intonation), echolalia (parrotlike imitation), and two word basal sentences appear. The two word basal sentences, or telegraphic stage of language acquisition, refers to sentences of two or more words that are used by the child, who omits articles, copulas, inflections, and

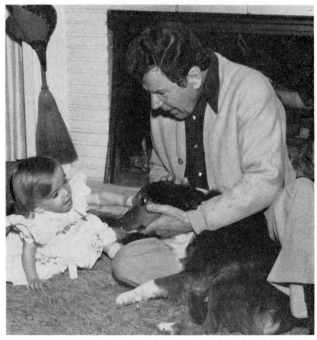

Figure 1-1.   Holophrastic phase of speech development.

auxiliary verbs. By thirty months the child is using three and four word phrases which resemble adult syntax. Jargon and echolalia have largely disappeared and simple declarative (kernal) sentences appear. Early transformations, present tense verbs, modifiers, yes/no questions, commands, prepositions, and negatives begin to appear. The child can carry out two commands, understands big and little, and points to body parts. He has a 900 to 1,000 word vocabulary at this point.

AFTER 36 MONTHS: Between the ages of three and four and one-half, further grammatical development is made through the gradual perfection of transformational rules. Kernal sentences are transformed to make other types of sentences by rearrangement, addition, and deletion of words. Linear expansions, morphological rules, past tense verbs, demonstratives, subject and object pronouns, possessive and reflexive pronouns, more negatives, some auxiliary verbs, compound nouns, contractions, and verb complements appear. Complex and compound sentences increase.

The child can verbally link past and present events, can define words by function, and spontaneously make grammatical corrections. Normally the basic foundations of spoken language are well laid by the age of four or five years. From here on, the child just increases his vocabulary, lengthens his sentence span, and refines and polishes his use of language. By age eight, a child's receptive vocabulary is 6,000 to 8,000 words, his expressive vocabulary is 2,500 words, and his speech reflects understanding of logical relationships. Words have adultlike definitions, and most of the phonemes have been mastered.

In summary, as the child passes through each stage of development, there can be significant environmental or physical changes which may alter the course of the child's normal language learning. The constructive character of the emerging linguistic knowledge of children is demonstrated by the uniqueness of most of their early sentences. Young children produce sentences which are markedly different from those of the adult speaker whom he hears. The most reasonable explanation for these novel utterances is that children construct their sentences, not as direct imitations of adult sentences, but upon the basis of their own grammar. Although the child's grammar differs from the adult's, it appears that it is constantly being modified, resulting in increasing complexity. Eventually, such increase in complexity results in an internalized grammar essentially identical to those of the adults in his language community.

Experts in language development stress the necessity of early identification of children whose acquisition of speech and language is outside the normal chronology. Bzoch and League (1971) made this summary statement at the end of the manual for the REEL Scale:

> The basic linguistic destiny of the child is essentially established by the time of his third birthday. Although modification continues in later months and years, this modification is largely a refinement and expansion of a structure that is already well defined. The linguistic process beyond the third year may be likened to the completion of a painting by the artist after he has the basic configuration of the painting already well defined. The finishing touches may continue as a process that lends character and depth to the achievement, but the earlier structure remains as the foundation of the entire creation. (P. 24)

SEQUENCE OF LANGUAGE DEVELOPMENT
Total Communication
Written language performance 1. Syntax 2. Spelling 3. Punctuation
Written language comprehension (reading)
Oral language performance 1. Vocabulary 2. Syntax 3. Phonology (articulation)
Oral language comprehension 1. Auditory 2. Visual — gesture
Experience

TABLE 1-IV

Weiss and Lillywhite (1976) have annunciated a fairly conservative statement concerning aspirations for the "normal" child:

> The eventual goal for every child who has no physical, mental, or psychological problem should be normal communication by the first grade.

REFERENCES

Anderson, Virgil A. and Newby, Hayes: *Improving the Child's Speech* 2nd ed. New York, Oxford University Press, 1973.

Berry, Mildred and Talbott, Ruth: *Berry Talbott Language Tests: Comprehension of Grammar.* 4332 Pinecrest Road, Rockford, Illinois, 1966.

Bloom, L. M.: *Language Development: Form and Function in Emerging Grammars.* Cambridge M.I.T. Press, 1970.

Bloomfield, Leonard: *Language.* New York, Holt, Rinehart & Winston, Inc., 1933.

Brown, Roger: *A First Language.* Cambridge, Harvard University Press, 1973.

Brown, Roger and Hanlon, Camilie: Derivational complexity and order of acquisition in child speech. In Hayes, John R. (Ed.): *Cognition and the Development of Language.* New York, John Wiley and Sons, Inc., 1970.

Bzoch, Kenneth and League, Richard: *Assessing Language Skills in Infancy.* Gainesville, Tree of Life Press, 1971.

Chomsky, Noam: The current scene in linguistics: Present directions. In Reibel, David A. and Schane, Sanford A. (Eds.): *Modern Studies in English.* Englewood Cliffs, Prentice-Hall, Inc., 1969.

Dale, Phillip S.: *Language Development: Structure and Function.* Hillsdale, The Dryden Press, 1972.

Frankenburg, William and Dodds, Josiah: *Denver Developmental Screening Scale.* Denver: University of Colorado Medical Center, 1970.

Greenfield, Patricia and Smith, Joshua H.: *The Structure of Communication in Early Language Development.* New York, Academic Press, 1976.

Hubbell, Robert: Children's language. In Weston, Alan J.: *Communicative Disorders.* Springfield, Charles C Thomas, Publishers, 1972.

Lecours, Andre Roth: Myelognic correlates of the development of speech and language. In Lenneberg, Eric and Lenneberg, Elizabeth (Eds.): *Foundations of Language Development, Volume I.* New York, Academic Press, 1975.

Lenneberg, Eric H.: *Biological Foundations of Language.* New York, John Wiley and Sons, Inc., 1967.

Lenneberg, Eric H.: The natural history of language. In Eliot, John (Ed.): *Human Development and Cognitive Processes.* New York, Holt, Rinehart and Winston, Inc., 1971.

Lewis, M. M.: *Language, Thought and Personality in Infancy and Childhood.* New York, Basic Books, Inc., 1963.

McConnell, Freeman; Love, Russel J., and Clark, Bertha Smith: Language remediation in children. In Dickson, Stanley (Ed.): *Communication Disorders.* Glenview, Scott, Foresman and Company, 1974.

McNeill, David: *The Acquisition of Language: The Study of Developmental Psycholinguistics.* New York, Harper and Row, 1970.

Menyuk, Paula: Early development of receptive language: From babbling to words. In Scheifelbusch, Richard and Lloyd, Lyle L. (Eds.): *Language Perspectives—Acquisition, Retardation, and Intervention.* Baltimore, University Park Press, 1974.

Morse, Philip A.: Infant speech perception. In Sanders, Derek: *Auditory Perception of Speech.* Englewood Cliffs, Prentice-Hall, Inc., 1977.

Mowrer, O. H.: *Learning Theory and the Symbolic Process.* New York, John Wiley and Sons, Inc., 1966.

Perkins, William: *Speech Pathology, an Applied Behavioral Science,* 2nd ed. St. Louis, The C. V. Mosby Company, 1977.

Piaget, Jean: *The Language and Thought of the Child.* Cleveland, Meridian Press, 1955.

Skinner, B. F.: *Verbal Behavior.* New York, Appleton-Century-Crofts, 1957.

Smith, Medorah: *Vocabulary in Young Children.* Iowa City, University of Iowa Press, 1926.

Templin, Mildred: *Certain Language Skills in Children.* Minneapolis, University of Minnesota Press, 1957.

Torres, Dorothy: A Comparison of Two Measures for Determining Language Competence. Master's thesis, California State University, Sacramento, 1977.

Trantham, Carla and Pederson, Joan K.: *Normal Language Development.* Baltimore, The Williams and Wilkins Company, 1976.

Van Riper, Charles: *Speech Correction: Principles and Methods,* 5th ed. Englewood Cliffs, Prentice-Hall, Inc., 1972.

von Raffler-Engel, Walburga: *Child Language—1975, Word* (Special Issue). London, William Crowles & Sons, Limited, 1976.

Weiss, Curtis E. and Lillywhite, Herold S.: *Communicative Disorders, a Handbook for Prevention and Early Intervention.* St. Louis, The C. V. Mosby Company, 1976.

CHAPTER 2

ARTICULATION

HELEN W. HARRIS AND MORRIS VAL JONES

SINCE THE INCEPTION of speech pathology as a profession, articulation problems have constituted the "bread and butter" basis of speech therapy departments, whether they have been in the universities, the public schools, or in private practice. In the second edition of his textbook, Virgil Anderson (1973) stated, "Articulation disorders of various kinds, including those associated with delayed speech, account for approximately 75 percent of the total speech defects among the public school population" (p. 130). Johnson et al. (1967, cited by Irwin and Weston, 1972) stated that clinicians working in the schools have reported that articulatory problems constitute as much as 85 percent of their total load (p. 161). The revolution started by the writing of Noam Chomsky (1957), with its emphasis on syntactical structures, deemphasized articulation defects to the point of neglect. Speech clinicians became speech/language clinicians, and they worked overtime to avoid the appellation of "/r/ and /s/ mechanics." More recently, there has been some swing back toward the more reasonable position that articulation problems are a legitimate responsibility of speech/language clinicians; at the present time statistics might show that 50 percent of the case load is within the category of articulation and the other 50 percent consists of language, voice, and fluency disorders.

The Sounds and How They Are Produced

The forty-three sounds (phonemes) of American English, specifically General American Speech, are produced on the exhaled air stream. The voiced sounds depend upon phonation produced by the vibration of the vocal folds, and the amplification of all the sounds is the result of resonance. For a full discussion of these three basic processes—respiration, phonation, and resonance—see Chapter 4. Discussion will now center upon the process of articulation, the breaking up of the exhaled breath stream by the articulatory mechanism. The articulators consist of the velopharyngeal port, the tongue, teeth, and lips; it is by the variation of their interrelationships that the different vowels and consonants become distinct.

Vowels

Some authorities do not consider the vowels as a part of articulation, but differentiation does depend upon the shape of the oral cavity and the position of the tongue. By definition the vowels encounter a minimum of interference as the air stream proceeds from the larynx through the oral cavity and out the mouth. However, the individual must establish a different shape of the oral cavity and relationship of the resonance chambers in order to produce an /o/ rather than an /a/; if the speaker does not do adequately in this endeavor, his speech becomes indistinct and mumbling, such as in the case of the inebriate or the victim of ataxic cerebral palsy. Tiffany and Carroll made the following statement in *Phonetics: Theory and Application* (1977):

> The three articulatory features of greatest importance in English vowel production are (1) *tongue height,* or the closeness of vocal-tract constriction; (2) *tongue fronting,* or the place of constriction within the mouth cavity; and (3) the nature of the vocal-tract opening as determined by the degree of lip *rounding* and *protrusion,* or their absence. (P. 96)

Consonants

Since the vowels and diphthongs are produced correctly by most children before the age of three unless their environment is bilingual, they are severely emotionally disturbed, or they have significant motor disabilities, the area of articulation disorders is generally restricted to the consonants, those sounds for which there is definite obstruction of the exhaled breath stream, ranging from minimal to complete. Traditionally, the consonants are divided into subgroups according to manner of production.

THE NASALS: The sphincterical gateway between the oral

and nasal cavities at the poserior end of the oral cavity is open for the emission of three sounds in General American Speech, namely /m/, /n/, and /ng/. Their differentiation depends upon the point at which the air stream is stopped as the sound vibrations travel from the larynx into the oral cavity. If the air stream is obstructed at the lips, an /m/ is heard by the listener; if it is stopped by the tongue tip at the alveolar ridge, an /n/ results, and if by lingua-velar contact, an /ng/. When the velopharyngeal port is open during the production of other phonemes, a resulting voice-articulation defect of hypernasality becomes the concern of the speech/language clinician.

THE PLOSIVES: The articulatory positions for the plosives are identical to those of the nasals; but, in addition, half of the plosives are voiceless, thus forming a series of three, voiced-voiceless pairs of stop-plosives. During the production of the plosives, the velopharyngeal port is closed rather than open as it is for the nasals.

		Plosives	
Position	*Nasals*	*Voiced*	*Voiceless*
Bilabial	/m/ (mouse)	/b/ (bounce)	/p/ (pounce)
Lingua-alveolar	/n/ (nice)	/d/ (dice)	/t/ (Tice)
Lingua-velar	/ng/ (ring)	/g/ (rig)	/k/ (Rick)

Thus, the speech pathologist realized how easy it is to substitute a /b/ for an /m/ or a /d/ for an /n/ when the nasal passages are occluded.

THE FRICATIVES: This subgroup of nine sounds is characterized by the friction noises which are produced as the air stream is forced through a somewhat more narrow cavity. In terms of articulatory position and pairing (cognates), they emerge as follows:

Position	*Voiced*	*Voiceless*
Labio-dental	/v/ (vile)	/f/ (**file**)
Lingua-dental	/th/ (either)	/th/ (ether)
Lingua-alveolar	/z/ (zoo)	/s/ (sue)
Lingua-palatal	/zh/ (measure)	/sh/ (machine)
Glottal		/h/ (history)

There is no cognate in American English for the /h/.

THE AFFRICATES: This group of two sounds, consisting of /ch/ and /j/, is a combination of one plosive and one fricative to form a voiced-voiceless pair. They begin in the position of the plosive and then merge into the position for the fricative.

Lingua-alveolar /d/ plus lingua-palatal /zh/ = /j/ (jaw)
Lingua-alveolar /t/ plus lingua-palatal /sh/ = /ch/ (chaw)

THE GLIDES: These four phonemes are characterized by movement from one position into another, and the obstruction of their passage through the oral cavity is so minimal that they are often called semivowels to indicate their proximity to the vowels. The initial position is indicated for each of the four speech sounds.

Bilabial	/w/ (water)
Lingual-alveolar	/y/ (yes)
Lateral lingua-alveolar	/l/ (lock)
Lingual-palatal	/r/ (rock)

Since these sounds are so similar, they are often difficult to discriminate auditorally; therefore, they cause considerable difficulty for young children in the early years of language usage. Young or immature children often substitute /w/ for the other glides, /y/, /l/, or /r/.

THE COMBINATIONS: These two sounds do not fit well into other categories because they are a fused emission of two separate sounds. One is /wh/, pronounced /hw/ (as in *when* or *where*), and the other is the long /ū/ (as in *use* or *music*), a combination of /y/ and /ōo/.

The author has concocted his own chart of the forty-three speech sounds, on a continuum from the most obstructed (with the air stream completely interrupted), to the least obstructed, the vowels and diphthongs (*see* Fig. 2-1).

Speech/language clinicians often use the phonetic symbols of the International Phonetic Alphabet (IPA) to assist in clarifying the differences between speech sounds or to write reports which will be intelligible to other professionals; they must be able to read the IPA in order to understand many of the articles in the professional literature. Although it is likely that the beginning speech pathology student will have limited need for such symbols, it may be of value to have them as information. Some discussion of distinctive features will be given later in the chapter.

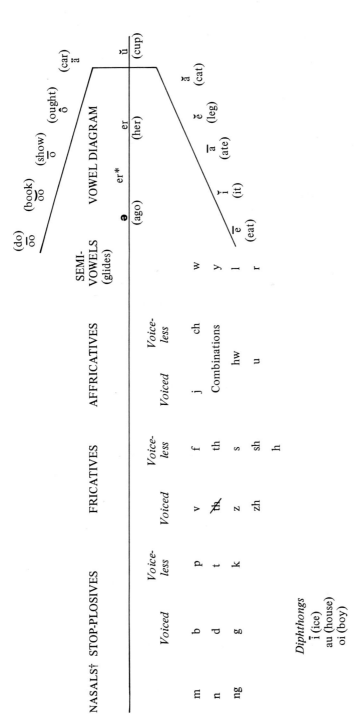

* Phoneticians make a difference between the stressed /er/ (bird) and the unstressed /er/ (mother).
† There is complete closure of the mouth with the Nasals, which are emitted through the nose.

Figure 2-1. The sounds of general American speech.

	The Phonemes	IPA Symbols	Key Word
Nasals:	/m/	[m]	me
	/n/	[n]	no
	/ng/	[ŋ]	wing
Plosives:	/b/	[b]	baby
	/p/	[p]	puppy
	/d/	[d]	daddy
	/t/	[t]	toe
	/g/	[g]	go
	/k/	[k]	kiss
Fricatives:	/v/	[v]	vote
	/f/	[f]	fish
	/th/	[ð]	that
	/th/	[θ]	thank
	/z/	[z]	zero
	/s/	[s]	son
	/zh/	[ʒ]	pleasure
	/sh/	[ʃ]	shine
	/h/	[h]	high
Affricates:	/j/	[dʒ]	joke
	/ch/	[tʃ]	choke
Glides:	/w/	[w]	win
	/y/	[j]	yell
	/l/	[l]	lost
	/r/	[r]	run
Combinations:	/hw/	[hʋ]	white
	/ū/	[ju]	you
Front vowels:	/ē/	[i]	me
	/ĭ/	[ɪ]	thin
	/ā/	[e]	ace
	/ĕ/	[ɛ]	met
	/ă/	[æ]	rat

	The Phonemes	*IPA Symbols*	*Key Word*
Back vowels:	/o͞o/	[u]	true
	/o͝o/	[ʋ]	look
	/ō/	[o]	mow
	/ô/	[ɔ]	awful
	/ä/	[a]	father
Central vowels:	/ŭ/	[ʌ]	son
	/er/	[ɚ]	dirt
	/ă/	[ə]	above
Diphthongs:	/ī/	[aɪ]	kite
	/au/	[aʋ]	mouse
	/oi/	[ɔɪ]	toy

The Acquisition of the Speech Sounds

Parents, relatives (grandmothers), and other children have always been interested in the age at which the various sounds are acquired by the individual child. Anecdotal reports, as well as professional studies, have been published since the beginning of the profession. Poole (1934), Wellman, et al. (1936), and Templin (1957) conducted studies of the articulatory acquisition of young children, beginning with age three. The results of Templin's study became the basis for standards of normal acquisition and for some of the articulation tests. Gradually, professionals began to have reservations about these criteria, and Sander (1972) published the results of his analyses of the various studies which had been done previously. As a result of his manipulation of the previously gathered data, he composed his own chronology of the acquisition of sounds; in general, his sequence tended to indicate that sounds were mastered earlier by most children than the other studies had concluded. He wrote the following:

Each sound is followed in parentheses by the percentage of children of that age correctly articulating it in the initial and final word positions. (The "before age two" percentages are, of course, for two-year-olds.)

Age	Consonant Sound and Percentage
Before 2	h(87), m(87), n(100), w(79), b(93), p(87)
2	t(80), k(66), g(57), ng(60), d(87)
3	f(88), y(70), s(70), r(58), l(67)
4	ch(72), sh(75), j(85), z(62), v(40)
5	voiceless th (67), voiced th(62)
6	zh(72)

These are assumed average ages of customary consonant production. Most of these sounds are first spoken correctly in many words at earlier average ages. Also, at years later than those indicated, the average child continues to misarticulate some of these sounds in certain contexts. (P. 61)

In 1975, Prather, Hedrick, and Kern published the results of their longitudinal studies of young children, ages two to four, and reduced the age at which sounds are acquired even further. As data are accumulated, it seems the criteria for indicating the presence of articulation problems must become more stringent. (*See* Table 2-1.) Certainly, the evidence seems to imply that normal acquisition of the speech sounds means that a child should be completely intelligible by the time he enters kindergarten and that all sounds should be mastered by the time he enters first grade.

The Etiology of Speech Defects

Why does a child not develop articulation skills normally? Van Riper (1972) has indicated that the first step in therapy is to remove or mitigate the cause; so, if the speech language clinician agrees with him, a search for the cause or causes of the difficulty becomes vital. It seems obvious that if there is interference with the movement of the muscles controlling the articulators (such as the tongue, velum, or lips), the effect upon articulation will be significant. Articulation problems caused by dysfunction of the central nervous system have been designated as dysarthria, and the therapy for articulatory errors in this category is usually quite different from that for errors of a nonorganic nature. Lack of control of the muscles may also be the result of drugs, such as alcohol or cocaine. Powers has made the relationship of articulation and muscle movement clear in

TABLE 2-I

COMPARISON OF THE AGES AT WHICH SUBJECTS CORRECTLY
PRODUCED SPECIFIC CONSONANT SOUNDS*†

Sound	SICD	Templin	Wellman	Poole
m	2	3	3	3-6
n	2	3	3	4-6
h	2	3	3	3-6
p	2	3	4	3-6
ŋ	2	3	‡	4-6
f	2-4	3	3	5-6
j	2-4	3-6	4	4-6
k	2-4	4	4	4-6
d	2-4	4	5	4-6
w	2-8	3	3	3-6
b	2-8	4	3	3-6
t	2-8	6	5	4-6
g	3	4	4	4-6
s	3§	4-6	5	7-6§
r	3-4§	4	5	7-6
l	3-4§	6	4	6-6
ʃ	3-8	4-6	‖	6-6
tʃ	3-8	4-6	5	‖
ð	4	7	‖	6-6
ʒ	4	7	6	6-6
dʒ	4§‡	7	6	‖
θ	4§‡	6	‡	7-6
v	4§‡	6	5	6-6
z	4§‡	7	5	7-6§
hw	4§‡	‡	‡	7-6

* From Elizabeth M. Prather, Articulation development in children aged two to four years, *Journal of Speech and Hearing Disorders, 40*:184, May, 1975.

† Comparison of the ages at which subjects correctly produced specific consonant sounds in the present study with those presented by Templin (1957), Wellman et al. (1931) and Poole (1934). The criterion used by SICD, Templin, and Wellman was 75 percent of the subjects; Poole used 100 percent of the subjects. In the SICD the percentage is the average of two positions, I and F; Templin, Wellman et al., and Poole averaged the percentage of three positions, I,M,F. (Templin, 1957, p. 53).

‡ Sound tested but not produced correctly by 75 percent of subjects at oldest age tested. Wellman: hw reached at 5 years but not 6. Medial at 3 years.

§ Poole: s and z appear at age 5-6, but disappear later and return at age 7-6.

‖ Sound not tested or reported.

§ Reversal: Reported at earliest age level if only one reversal occurred and percentage at all older age levels exceeded 75 percent.

her chapter in *Handbook of Speech Pathology and Audiology* (1971):

> *Articulation* can be defined as the production of speech sounds by the stopping or restriction of the vocalized or nonvocalized breath stream by movements of the lips, tongue, velum, or pharynx. *Disorders* of articulation are faulty placement, timing, direction, pressure, speed, or integration of these movements, resulting in absent or incorrect speech sounds. (P. 837)

Hearing loss as a cause of speech and language problems is discussed in Chapter 6.

The vast majority of speech sound errors, however, are probably nonorganic, usually given the categorical designation of *functional*, again discussed by Powers (1971):

> The term *functional articulation disorders* contains a wide variety of deviate speech patterns. These can all be described in terms of four possible types of acoustic deviations in the individual speech sounds; omissions, substitutions, distortions, and additions. An individual may show one or any combination of these deviations. (P. 839)

Winitz (1969) has attacked the problems of causal factors by investigating the research conducted between 1935 and 1968 concerning the variables related to articulatory development and performance. He listed the categories into which he divided his detailed analysis as follows:

chronological age
intelligence
cultural variables: socioeconomic status, sex, and sibling status
general motor skills
oral and facial motor skills
laterality
kinesthetic sensibility
dentition
oral structure
tongue thrust
development and physical health
auditory memory span
speech sound discrimination
discrimination of pitch, intensity, and rhythm
personality and adjustment
lexical and grammatical measures

fluency

educational achievement: reading, spelling, and academic evaluations
(P. 141)

He stated in most cases that an insufficient amount of well-controlled research had been conducted to warrant definite conclusions. It would seem that multicausation more often is the case; the individual, for instance, has some motor incoordination, some lack of intelligence, and some faulty development of the oral structures. For one causal factor to result in misarticulation, the condition, such as malocclusion or tongue thrust (abnormal swallow pattern), would have to be severe. Even in the area of speech sound discrimination, which is the basis of the ear-training method of therapy, the research studies brought conflicting results, with four of fifteen cited studies reporting that there is no significant difference between the speech sound discrimination skills of the control and experimental groups. Undoubtedly, there is need for additional, well-planned studies into the causes of articulation problems.

Eisenson and Ogilvie (1971) indicated that faulty learning is a major cause of articulation problems. "The child may have had no good models to imitate" (p. 221). Examples would include bilingual home environments, association with siblings and peers who have faulty articulation, and excessive "babytalk." Anderson and Newby (1972) discuss adverse environmental factors:

Many of their bad speech habits are simply the result of imitating the bad speech of their elders, who are often unaware of their own communicative shortcomings and the effect such poor models may have on the speech of their children. (P. 148)

The relation of emotional problems to articulation errors is a complex one, and authorities vary in their emphasis upon this area of potential causation. Most research in this area has been rather vague, and investigations have fluctuated from investigating the personality problems of the individual with the articulation problems to interviewing or testing his parents, grandparents, and siblings. One school of thought with a more definite position is represented by Rousey (1971), who gave an elaborate explanation of the effect of emotional problems upon articulation. After a lengthy explanation of the applicability of psychoanalytic theory to articulation, Rousey stated a number of hypotheses related to consonants. Among these are the following:

> The substitution of the /f/ for the voiceless /th/ sound is related to a disturbance in the early and significant relationships with the child's father.
> Deprivation disturbances in mother-child relationships are reflected through difficulties with the /l/ phoneme.
> The substitution of the /d/ for the voiced /th/ sound is related to an oral expression of aggression.
>
> The occurrence of a lateral lisp is a manifestation of difficulty in psychosexual development occurring earlier during the anal period than in the case of the front lisp.
> A whistle which accompanies the articulation of the /s/ phoneme is felt to reflect anxiety. (Pp. 825-826)

If one were to conduct articulation therapy in keeping with these hypotheses, he would, of course, need to have training as a psychoanalyst; he would be working on underlying etiology and not upon the speech sounds.

Nation and Aram (1977) have indicated the present status of speech therapy in relation to etiology:

> Different positions are taken about the need to understand the causes of speech and language disorders. Probably the least emphasis is given to causation by those who profess to be interested in behavioral symptoms only, as in behavior modification. At the other end of the continuum are those whose orientation justifies working only with the "underlying" or "overriding" cause of the disordered behavior. (P. 114)

APPROACHES TO ARTICULATION

Assessment and Remediation

In the concluding sections of this chapter we shall briefly review both the traditional phonetic approach to articulation and the phonemic approach, which has developed in recent years from linguistic and speech research scientists, many of whom feel that articulation is a language process. In addition, we shall look at distinctive feature theory and its emerging relevance in the field of speech therapy. We shall also attempt to include some comments about the differing methods of analysis relative to these approaches. In the remaining discussion we shall briefly introduce the beginning speech pathology student to methods, techniques, and learning principles of remediation, with particular emphasis on the phonetic approach to therapy.

Before proceeding, a few additional comments about the term *functional* would seem to be in order. The term has become synonymous with *nonorganic;* however, it is still too often used as a "catch-all" for inadequate diagnosis. As stated previously, Nathan and Aram (1977) have indicated current divergent positions in the field of speech therapy regarding the need to understand the causes of articulation disorders. Current practice in public school therapy and elsewhere, which has moved away from the medical model to a behavioral one, would seemingly support the point of view that causative factors are unimportant. In this writer's opinion such a point of view can be extremely detrimental to an effective and prescriptive remedial plan. For example, it is well understood that various causes of articulation disorders present the same speech symptoms. However the same choice of methodology would not be appropriate to all. Traditionally in the field of speech pathology a condition has been considered functional in the absence of any demonstrable pathology. Sommers and Kane (1974) have suggested the need for a more discriminate use of the word *functional* if it is to clarify the etiology of articulation disorders (p. 106). They summarize earlier writers, Powers, Koepp-Baker, and Van Riper, as follows:

> Functional is appropriately applied to inadequate performance of the articulatory forms within a language, irrespective of etiology, when there are no obvious signs of structural and neurological deviations. (P. 106)

They continue thus:

> . . . this is not to suggest the cause is unimportant but on the contrary the more we learn about the determining factors . . . the more effective will be our remediation. (P. 106)

Phonetic Approach to Articulation Disorders

In the traditional phonetic approach to the study of articulation disorders, speech has been viewed as a physiological and acoustic phenomenon. The articulation process has been considered a separate parameter of speech, though related to phonation, respiration, prosody, and resonance. It has further been defined as a mechanical act performed by specific muscles to modify the outgoing breath stream into the sounds of the language.

The focus of study has been the sounds of speech without regard to the language in which they occur. The smallest unit of articulation which carries no meaning is a phone (sound). Therapy has been directed to the error sounds as heard by the listener, and the task has been to help the client learn new and acoustically acceptable speech patterns.

Analysis of the sound errors is determined on the basis of a phonetic inventory. Consequently, this approach requires the therapist to be thoroughly familiar with phonetics and skilled in phonetic transcriptions. In phonetic analysis the speech sounds have been classified by the manner and place of production, i.e. bilabial plosives (b, p), labio-dental fricatives (f, v).

Articulation is analyzed by listening to samples of spontaneous speech in various systematic ways and by preparing a phonetic inventory which enables the examiner to identify the most obvious articulation errors. Many phonetic inventories are available to the speech clinician. Most inventories primarily test the consonants in terms of the position in which they occur in a word. Error sounds are recorded in terms of omissions, substitutions, distortions, and additions. McDonald, however, stresses the importance of testing sounds in all phonetic contexts.

Phonemic Approach to Articulation Disorders

Another perspective of articulation disorders may be gained if one views articulation as a language function. In recent years we have seen an increasing awareness of the contributions from the field of linguistics. Linguistic theorists cite generative analysis of Chomsky (1957) and distinctive feature theory to show how phonological rules of sound can explain seemingly inconsistent misarticulations and to predict the various types of errors children have been found to make. In contrast with phonetic theory, phonemic theory considers speech sounds to have a fundamental linguistic function. The phoneme is considered to be the basic element of spoken language that differentiates meaning. Tiffany and Carrell (1977), in their discussion on the nature of spoken language, state the following:

> Broadly defined, a phoneme consists of a "family" of phonetically similar sounds which, in serving linguistic function, contrast with one another in such a way as to differentiate the meaning of spoken words. Such contrasting sound classes are said to be the *phonemes* of the language under study. (P. 31)

They further point out that, from the standpoint of linguistic theory, the phonemic system functions as a network of differences (p. 33). Language competency is considered by some to depend on a person's knowledge and perception of these phonemic contrasts. Phonemic analysis limits itself generally to identification and classification of these contrastive classes, or phonemes, known to occur in the language.

Distinctive Feature Theory

Distinctive feature theory as an approach to the description and analysis of spoken language is coming into increasing use in the field of communication disorders. Proponents of this theory believe that it is distinctive characteristics of the sounds within the phoneme that cause them to be perceived as contrastive. Tiffany and Carrell (1977) summarize the salient points of this theory as follows:

> In broadest outline, the theory holds that (1) the sounds of speech are bundles of distinctive articulatory and acoustic features, (2) that it is the feature and not the phoneme which is the ultimate discrete unit into which speech can be analyzed, and (3) that the recognition of any given speech sound depends on a set of binary (either-or) judgments as to the presence or absence of those features which are distinctive to it. (P. 11)

Although supporters of this theory believe the features are basic to perceiving the contrast between phonemes, there is as yet no consensus as to what constitutes the most valid set of distinctive features.

The concept of distinctive features does provide us with a method of speech sound analysis which goes beyond older systems, which were classified by type and place of articulation.

Procedures generally present the findings in the form of a matrix which identifies a determined list of features and the phones of the language. An agreed-upon system of symbols is used in transcription. The broad phonemic transcription generally uses the basic IPA and is concerned with recording the smallest units of sound that distinguish meaning. Feature analysis also uses allophonic symbols for closer transcription. Allophones are perceptually different from each other but do not distinguish meaning.

The general procedure following transcription is to identify a pattern of feature violations common to phonemes erroneously produced and to compare features of each error with features of the target phonemes. Some feature theorists hold that error phonemes are usually wrong only in a particular characteristic, e.g. bees for peas; and that it is easier to make a change when it is only necessary to change one feature. For example in the substitution b/p, only the voicing feature is in error. Therefore, note where the child is making the same feature error, e.g. d/t, g/k, and then teach him specifically relative to the feature error. Feature theorists believe this enables the child to generalize and reduces the time necessary for therapy. Sommers and Kane (1974) indicate that studies on response generalization seem to support this hypothesis (p. 127).

Although phonetic analysis and feature analysis proceed from different points of view, they have a common goal. Both also require sophisticated listening skills and techniques of recording of the standard sounds of the language and being able to perceive and transcribe deviations and nonstandard forms.

Phonetic analysis and feature analysis are considered to be complimentary and overlapping approaches. According to Sommers and Kane (1974) both types can contribute to our knowledge of the etiology, maintenance, and remediation of articulatory disorders (p. 111).

APPROACHES TO THERAPY

The choice of articulation approach is not easy for the therapist and will often depend to some extent on his training. We have little information in the literature concerning the comparative effectiveness of various therapy methods. Research in this area is certainly needed. For the present, choosing the method for therapy must still depend on the clinician's judgment as to what will best serve the needs of the client.

Inasmuch as the purpose of this discussion is to introduce the beginning student of speech pathology to an overview of functional articulation disorders and speech therapy, it is beyond the scope of this chapter to present a comprehensive review of all the methodologies in the field of speech pathology. For the student who is interested in pursuing this subject in more depth, Sommers and Kane (1974) have presented a comprehensive discussion of a wide range of articulation methodologies. Some of the methods which they discuss and their proponents are as follows:

1. Scripture (Phonetic Placement)
2. Stinchfield-Hawk and Young (Motokinesthesis)
3. Van Riper (Ear-training: Progressive Approximation)
4. Backus Beasley (Group Therapy)
5. McDonald (Sensorimotor Skills)
6. Mysak (Feedback) (P. 129)

For our purposes we shall direct our attention primarily to the traditional phonetic approach to speech therapy which has been largely based on the principles and methods formulated by Van Riper (1939-1972). Some brief discussion of a few additional methods which emphasize a different sensory perception or which are based on a different rationale will illustrate variances in methods which are available to the therapist.

Phonetic Approach to Speech Therapy

The traditional phonetic approach to functional articulation problems holds that speakers with an articulation defect accept their errors as correct due to previous faulty learning and habituation, and that speakers generally attend to the content and not to the form of their speech. Carrell (1968) points out that the client must learn to listen perceptively to his own speech in order to recognize its fine details and compare with the speech he is trying to develop (p. 95). The starting point in any remedial program therefore has been perceptual training. Training in the

perceptive processes is considered essential to the establishment
of correct motor patterns.

The major proponent of auditory discrimination training has
been Van Riper (1972). The primary emphasis of Van Riper's
"ear-training" techniques is to guide the client to recognition
and discrimination of articulation errors in both his own and the
clinician's speech. In this method sounds are presented first in
isolation, on the theory that when the error sounds are embedded
in a matrix of sounds it is more difficult for the student to acquire
the necessary perceptual skills. Van Riper groups his method
for teaching auditory perceptual skills into the following four
major categories: (1) isolation, (2) stimulation, (3) identification, and (4) discrimination.

Although the method of stimulation is primarily auditory,
Van Riper suggests that new learning is most effective if kinesthetic and tactile cues for the sound are associated with
auditory cues. The clinician guides the client from identification
(ear training) to automation of the corrected motor pattern.
The following brief outline might serve to illustrate this
progression:

1. Numerous ear training activities are presented to help the client
   learn to identify the correct and incorrect sound, beginning with
   the sound in isolation.
2. Ear training, modeling, and client imitation of isolated sound
   to develop self-monitoring and client recognition of his error
   sound.
3. Establishing correct production of the sound through various
   techniques selected by the clinician and based on the needs
   of the client.
4. Stabilizing and habituating the new sound.

As stated before, the primary sensory stimulation in both the
receptive and production phases of this approach is auditory.
Production training is based on the stimulus-response paradigm;
it is interwoven throughout the program to associate tactile-
kinesthetic cues with the auditory. In Van Riper's method the
clinician has four additional techniques which he can select to
facilitate the needs of the client: (1) progressive approximation,
(2) phonetic placement, (3) modification of sounds already
mastered, and (4) use of key words. In his current book (1972)

he points out two important considerations in the treatment plan prior to initiating ear-training, which are client motivation and correction of contributing factors. He then offers the following guideline to the training process:

1. the client must be able to identify the error sound and the standard pattern of the sound
2. the client must develop skills in scanning and comparing his own utterance with the standard sound
3. the client must vary his utterance until the correctly produced sound is achieved; and
4. the clinician must stabilize and habituate the new correct ways of speaking so they can be used automatically. (P. 207)

McDonald (1964) has stressed articulation testing of the error sounds in all phonetic contexts based on the theory of "ballistic movement." His sensorimotor approach to remediation stresses the articulatory movement patterns and the kinesthetic-tactile senses. In this approach to therapy the clinician models bisyllables and trisyllables with the error sound in various contexts. The client repeats and is asked to describe kinesthetic-tactile cues. Auditory discrimination and memory are secondary considerations.

Winitz (1969) favors the phonemic approach to articulation training. He incorporates the principles for teaching the mechanics of speech sounds from several areas of learning theory. His method also relies on "ear-training" to develop sound discrimination skills. However, he begins with maximum linguistic contrasts and later progresses to training on sounds with a number of distinctive feature similarities. Winitz points out that while studies on the relation between articulation and discrimination are somewhat equivocal, some studies suggest that discrimination was most often impaired for those sounds whose production was in error. He takes the point of view that for some children intensive speech sound discrimination training between the error sound and the correct sound will facilitate the subsequent learning of the correct. However, this training would only be appropriate for those children who have difficulty in discriminating the correct sound from their error sound (p. 276). In this approach a considerable amount of sound discrimination learning is considered essential before the child attempts to learn a new sound, and only at later stages of sound learning should discrimination and production be combined (p. 277).

In posing the question as to whether articulatory errors are a phonetic or a phonemic problem, Winitz (1969) made the following statement:

> We would like to take the point of view that when obvious physical and mental abnormalities are not present, most if not all phonetic errors are the result of incorrectly learned phonemic systems. . . . This statement may seem too general to prove to be operationally useful. Besides, we have already said that some phonemic systems may be determined by phonetic factors. Perhaps, then, the hypothesis should be qualified by suggesting that when obvious physical and mental impairments are not present, articulatory errors represent the incorrect learning of the phoneme system of the community language, which in some cases may be partially a result of incorrectly learned phonetic productions. (P. 125)

Winitz also suggests that sound discrimination training may be administered to the child by automatic programming procedures, thus freeing the clinician for other tasks, as well as providing for a systematic and continuous presentation of the stimuli selected for training.

Mowrer, Baker, and Shultz (1968) have developed a program based on successive approximation and differential reinforcement techniques. Their studies suggest that external reinforcement facilitates learning of the correct response. They also suggest that the use of teaching machines is more effective in articulation therapy.

Techniques and Principles in the Therapy Process

Despite variations in theoretical orientation, in practice there are many commonalities. Most approaches include developing the client's awareness of the nature of his problem and of the correct sounds pattern. The client is required to learn a correct sound first in isolation and then in syllables, words, and sentences. The stimulus-response paradigm prevails. Inasmuch as articulation therapy is a learning experience, the laws of learning are operative.

Articulation training includes two major processes: perceptual training to develop the receptive processes and sound production training. The degree to which these are interwoven and the major emphasis on which are the primary sensory mode and manner of production varies.

Techniques for receptive development are reinforced through provisions for utilizing the child's visual, auditory, and kinesthetic-tactile modalities in identifying and discriminating speech sounds. These techniques include ear-training, auditory and visual discrimination tasks, oral-sensory perception training, and so forth.

The major articulation production techniques that are used to help the child acquire and habituate the correct speech sound are often common to a number of methods. Sommers and Kane (1974), in their discussion of production procedures, have grouped them into the following categories:

1. feedback training, which provides the client with skills for monitoring and adjusting his articulatory errors or movements;
2. key word practice, which features words in which the error sound is correctly produced by the client;
3. minimal pairing of defective and correct utterances to which the client can attach meaning or significance, as a means of establishing linguistic contrasts;
4. motokinesthesis, or the manipulation of the articulators or related areas to help the client acquire correct sound production;
5. negative practice, or having the client deliberately practice errors that have become habitual as a way of ending their automatic occurrence;
6. phonetic placement instruction, in which verbal explanations, mirrors, or diagrams are used to inform the client about the correct positioning and movement of the articulators in the production of specific sounds;
7. progressive approximation techniques, designed to help the client make the transitory movement from the error sound to the correct sound;
8. psychotherapy, directed at helping the client understand and deal with his articulation problem; and
9. stimulus-response procedures, in which the clinician demonstrates sounds for the client to imitate. (P. 131)*

Also common to all approaches are the three basic levels of articulation change; acquisition, habituation, and response generalization. All approaches should at least focus on the first two

---

of these. Acquisition can be viewed as the first level of remediation in which the client has learned to correctly produce the
target sound in utterances of increasing length in a structured
situation. The second level of habituation has been defined by
Chisum, Shelton, and Arndt (1969) as the correct usage of a
phoneme in the absence of deliberate or conscious effort. In
practice the term has become synonymous with "carry-over."
Response generalization is more a learning concept which can be
operative at either level of therapy. Briefly, the concept holds
that response generalization occurs when a formerly incorrect
response which has been learned correctly in certain phonetic
contexts is then produced correctly in different contexts for which
there has been no therapy. This concept has also been extended
to include the situation along distinctive feature lines where
correction of some phonemic errors causes improvement in similar
phonemes without direct intervention. Research findings tend
to support this.

In summary, the beginning clinician is still faced with the
choice of rationales, methods, and techniques that will best serve
his students' needs. In selecting the methodology he should
understand which major sensorium for perception is emphasized
as well as the major emphasis in articulation production. In many
approaches perceptual training and actual production training
are interwoven. Others, however, believe that phonic analysis
skills should be perfected before moving into production. Some
hold that auditory training is secondary and the emphasis is on
developing sensorimotor patterns. The clinician should be aware
of these variations between methodologies, as to the appropriate
time to introduce production training, but in the final analysis
recognize that this, too, must be prescriptive.

And finally, the beginning student in speech pathology faces
exciting challenges which already are on the horizon: the implications of supertechnology in the field of speech correction; the
explosion of programmed materials and the use of aides in
implementing programs; recent state and federal legislation and
the factors of "rights" for the handicapped, due process, and
accountability; and, lastly, the challenges posed by increased
knowledge from research. In articulation therapy, distinctive
feature theorists are already suggesting that therapy can be

directed in some cases to the feature error and phonological rule governing it; that the problem is neither auditory nor motor, but rule governed.

REFERENCES

Anderson, Virgil A.: *Improving the Child's Speech*, 2nd ed. New York, Oxford University Press, 1973.

Carrell, J.: *Disorders of Articulation*. Englewood Cliffs, Prentice-Hall, Inc., 1968.

Chisum, L.; Shelton, R., and Arndt, W.: Relationship between remedial speech instruction activities and articulation change. *Cleft Palate J, 6*:57-64, 1969.

Chomsky, N. and Halle, M.: *The Sound Pattern of English*. New York, Harper & Row, 1968.

Chomsky, Noam: *Syntactic Structures*. The Hague, Mouton Publishers, 1957.

Eisenson, Jon and Ogilvie, Mardel: *Speech Correction in the Schools*, 3rd ed. New York, The Macmillan Company, 1971.

Irwin, John V. and Weston, Alan J.: Articulation. In Weston, Alan J. (Ed.): *Communicative Disorders*. Springfield, Charles C Thomas, Publisher, 1972.

Jakobson, R.; Fant, G., and Halle, M.: *Preliminaries to Speech Analysis: The Distinctive Features and Their Correlates*. Cambridge, The M.I.T. Press, 1951 (2nd ed., 1963).

Locke, J. L.: Oral perception and articulation learning. *Percept Mot Skills, 26*:1259-1264, 1968.

McDonald, E. T.: *Articulation Testing and Treatment: A Sensory Motor Approach*. Pittsburgh, Stanwix House, 1964.

Mowrer, D.; Baker, R. L., and Schultz, R. D.: Operant procedures in the control of speech articulation. In Sloane, H. N. and MacAulay, B. D. (Eds.): *Operant Procedures in Remedial Speech and Language Training*. Boston, Houghton Mifflin Company, 1968.

Mysak, E. D.: A servo model for speech therapy. *J Speech Hear Disord, 24*:144-149, 1959.

Mysak, E. D.: *Speech Pathology and Feedback Theory*, 2nd ed. Springfield, Charles C Thomas, 1971.

Nation, James E. and Aram, Dorothy M.: *Diagnosis of Speech and Language Disorders*. St. Louis, The C. V. Mosby Company, 1977.

Palmer, John M.: *Anatomy for Speech and Hearing*. 2nd ed. New York, Harper and Row, 1972.

Perkins, William H.: *Speech Pathology: An Applied Behavioral Science*, 2nd ed. St. Louis, The C. V. Mosby Company, 1977.

Poole, Irene: Genetic development of articulation of consonant sounds in speech. *Elementary English Review, 11*:159-161, 1934.

48 Speech and Language Problems

Powers, Margaret Hall: Functional disorders of articulation: Symptomatology and etiology. In Travis, Lee Edward (Ed.): *Handbook of Speech Pathology and Audiology.* New York, Appleton-Century-Crofts, 1971.

Prather, Elizabeth; Hedrick, Donna Lee, and Kern, Carolyn A.: Articulation development in children aged two to four years. *J Speech Hear Disord, 40:*(2), 179-191, 1975.

Rousey, Clyde: The psychopathology of articulation and voice deviations. In Travis, Lee Edward (Ed.): *Handbook of Speech Pathology and Audiology.* New York, Appleton-Century-Crofts, 1971.

Sander, Eric K.: When are speech sounds learned? *J Speech Hear Disord, 37:*1, 55-63, 1972.

Sommers, R. K. and Kane, A. R.: Nature and remediation of functional articulation disorders. In Dickson, S. (Ed.): *Communication Disorders: Remedial Principles and Practices.* Glenview, Scott, Foresman and Company, 1974.

Templin, Mildred C.: *Certain Language Skills in Children.* Minneapolis, University of Minnesota Press, 1957.

Tiffany, W. R. and Carrell, J.: *Phonetics: Theory and Application,* 2nd ed. New York, McGraw-Hill, Inc., 1977.

Van Riper, C.: *Speech Correction: Principles and Methods,* 5th ed. Englewood Cliffs, Prentice-Hall, Inc., 1972.

Van Riper, Charles and Irwin, John V.: *Voice and Articulation.* Englewood Cliffs, Prentice-Hall, Inc., 1958.

Wellman, Beth L.; Case, Ida M.; Mengert, Ida G., and Bradbury, Dorothy E.: Speech sounds of young children. *University of Iowa Studies in Child Welfare, 5:*No. 2. Iowa City, University of Iowa Press, 1936.

Winitz, H. and Billerose, B.: Sound discrimination as a function of pretraining conditions. *J Speech Hear Res, 6:*171-180, 1963.

Winitz, Harris: *Articulatory Acquisition and Behavior.* New York, Appleton-Century-Crofts, 1969.

Winitz, Harris: *From Syllable to Conversation.* Baltimore, University Park Press, 1975.

Young, E. H. and Stinchfield-Hawk, S.: *Moto-kinesthetic Speech Training.* Stanford, Stanford University Press, 1955.

Zemlin, Willard R.: *Speech and Hearing Science: Anatomy and Physiology.* Englewood Cliffs, Prentice-Hall, Inc., 1968.

CHAPTER 3

DELAYED LANGUAGE

Colette L. Coleman, Ph.D.

THE DIAGNOSIS AND remediation of a speech or language problem may be approached in any of a number of ways. The manner chosen is usually based on some theoretical framework. At one time the medical model was used as a framework. In this model the clinician attempted to find the cause of the problem and label it. A prescribed program of remediation was then provided for all individuals labeled and placed in a certain category. For example, a set program of therapy was prescribed for children who were labeled aphasic, another program for children who were labeled autistic, another for children who were labeled retarded and so on. Only minor adjustments were made for the individual child.

More recently a different theoretical framework has been employed. Each child's speech and language behavior is observed and tested in an effort to describe the child's abilities in behavioristic terms. When using this approach, a label is not important. A remedial program is designed to help in those specific areas where remediation is needed, no matter what the cause of the problem may be. This is not to say that the cause or causes are or should be ignored. Some causes, such as conductive hearing losses, can and should be remediated. Other causes, such as permanent hearing loss, must be considered in the design of therapy procedures and in the individual's long-term prognosis.

The change in emphasis from cause to description of symptoms does point to changes in philosophy and remediation in speech pathology. A particular cause is not now considered to have a specific "cure"; rather, various aspects of the problem or symptoms are treated specifically to produce speech and language more like the norm for the individual's age, sex, socioeconomic class, and so on.

A label is, however, a useful tool when talking about children with similar disorders. Although the medical model is not as commonly used as it was at one time, we still organize our thinking to some extent around a group with similar problems. In so doing, we frequently label groups such as children with cleft palates, children with cerebral palsy, and so on. The term *delayed language* has entered the vocabulary of the speech pathologist as a useful tool which labels a group of children who have at least certain characteristics in common.

Definition

We might say that the terms *developmental language disorder* and *delayed language* are umbrella terms used to cover the problems which manifest themselves as a ". . . condition in which a child's language development is significantly below his chronological age" (Hubbell, 1977, p. 216). The specific language problems manifested by children in this category may differ considerably, and the causes for the problems may also vary considerably.

Marge (Irwin and Marge, 1972) suggested that it is useful to know ". . . whether the language disability represents a developmental retardation or was acquired after the development of normal language function" (p. 86). To this end he suggested three categories: failure to acquire any language, delayed language acquisition, and acquired language disabilities. He specifically asks the following questions concerning a child's language development:

1. Has the child acquired any language by age 4 years when language should be well developed?
2. How delayed is the language usage of a child as compared with his age peers?
3. What is the status of his language after the child has acquired adequate language function? (P. 83)

In this chapter, attention will be directed mainly to delayed language; however, failure to acquire language, delayed language, and disruption of language after it is partially acquired are frequently grouped together or, at the least, they are considered to overlap somewhat in terms of cause, assessment, and remediation.

A group which is sometimes included in the category of delayed language is the group referred to as having childhood aphasia or dysphasia. The names *aphasia* and *dysphasia* may be applied to a wide variety of problems and may be defined in any number of ways. The state of California has dealt with the problem in straightforward terms using an operational definition. In brief, the California Administrative Code, Title 5, 3600 (g) (1970) makes a statement to the effect that a child is aphasic if—

1. he or she has a severe speech and language disability.
2. the dysfunction or impairment is evidenced by a written diagnosis or determination by a physician experienced in working with children with neurological defects, a psychologist, and a specialist in speech and hearing.
3. the language disability is other than that associated with deafness, mental retardation, or autism.

A question that may be of some importance in relation to delayed language or developmental language disorders is that regarding the general nature of the disorder. This question has usually been expressed in somewhat the following manner: Does the language behavior displayed by the child with delayed language represent a quantitative or qualitative deviation from the norm? In this context, the term *quantitative difference* is usually used to mean that a child of a certain age who has been identified as having delayed language will use language which is very much like that of a younger normal child. For example, a child may continue to use one word utterances while other children his age have gone on to two word utterances. Qualitative difference is used to mean that a child who has been identified as language delayed shows bizarre language behaviors unlike those encountered in the process of normal development. For example, a child might use a word order never used by children developing normal language, such as "go me" rather than "me go" to mean "I want to go."

In 1964 Menyuk compared the grammar of ten children with normal and ten with infantile (delayed) language. She matched the children using the criteria of age, sex, IQ, and socioeconomic status. The children ranged in age from 3-0 (3 years, 0 months) to 5-10. Menyuk found that the children with delayed language used fewer transformations and more restricted forms (structures which deviated from complete grammaticalness) than the children with normal language. She also compared a normal two-year-old and a three-year-old with delayed language, the youngest child in her group. She noted extensive differences in their language and drew the conclusion, "The term *infantile* seemed to be a misnomer since at no age level did the grammatical production of a child with deviant speech match or closely match that of a child with normal speech" (p. 109).

Lee (1966), in a comparison of a 3-1 year-old male with normal language and a 4-7 year-old male with delayed language, commented, "The 'language-delayed' boy was not merely slower in following a normal pattern of development but was failing to produce certain types of syntactic structures" (p. 330).

One might draw the conclusion from these studies that the child with "infantile" or "delayed" language produces bizarre, qualitatively different language from that observed in the normally developing child. In a more recent study by Morehead and Ingram (1973), this does not seem to be the case. Fifteen children with normal language and fifteen with deviant language were categorized into five linguistic levels according to their mean number of morphemes per utterance. There were three children with normal language and three children with deviant language at each of the five levels. Five aspects of their language were then analyzed and compared: phrase structure rules, transformations, construction (or sentence) types, inflectional morphology, and minor lexical categories (pronouns, demonstratives, wh forms, prepositions, and modals). The overall results indicated few significant differences when the children were matched by mean number of morphemes per utterance. There were significant differences between the two groups in infrequently occurring transformations and the number of major syntactic categories per construction type. There was also, of course, the marked delay in onset and acquisition of base syntax, which compensates for the matching procedure. Morehead and Ingram suggest that this might support a theory of quantitative difference rather than qualitative difference between children with normal and children with delayed language. More importantly, however, they point out that if a qualitative difference appears to exist it may be because qualitative differences occur in the normal development of language. One might say that a two word structure is qualitatively different from a one word utterance, and certainly that the one word utterance is qualitatively different from babbling or cooing. Morehead and Ingram note that as the child develops he or she goes through stages in cognitive growth that radically change the way the child perceives and deals with the environment (Piaget, 1970; Kohlberg, 1968). Language may merely be reflecting these more fundamental changes.

To develop some perspective on the problem of delayed language we might look at the U.S. government census figures for 1969 regarding oral language disabilities. In the total population of children ages four to seventeen years, 6.2% or 3,467,784 children had delayed language acquisition.

Causes

As noted in the first chapter, the development and use of language as a communicative device involves the acquisition of a number of complex skills. Whether authorities believe that a child acquires language through imitation, reinforcement, or by forming rules using specific innate abilities, there is agreement that the child must hear language associated with meaningful experiences in order to develop his or her own language. External factors may strongly influence the child's language development; these factors include the child's everyday environment, who talks with the child, what he sees and hears, and where he goes. What might be called *internal factors* also strongly affect the child's language development. Some of these internal factors are indirect but very important, such as attention, memory, sensation, perception, and cognitive skills.

The process of attending has been described in different ways, but it is usually defined as the ability to concentrate on one item, aspect, or action to the exclusion of others. The way in which this process occurs has been the subject of much speculation and research. Broadbent (1958) has suggested that the brain influences the senses to selectively filter incoming stimuli, accepting the desired messages and rejecting others. If an individual cannot attend, then all the stimuli in the environment impinge upon that person with equal strength, making it extremely difficult for the individual to select, remember, and use information.

Memory is needed for every aspect of language. We need to remember the appropriate order of the sounds in *eat* which, if disordered, becomes another word *tea* or nonsense *tae*. We need to remember vocabulary (lexical) items. We must remember rules, such as those needed to change a simple, active, declarative sentence, "He sees the tree" into a negative question, "Doesn't he see the tree?"

Memory is presently regarded as having encoding, storage and retrieval phases. Stimuli may be stored for a short period of time (short-term memory) and then used or forgotten. Stimuli may be stored for long periods of time (long-term memory) and be available for retrieval. It also seems that all stimuli are not stored in the same way. Small units may be stored; larger related units grouped (chunked) and stored. Some items may be completely recalled while others are not available for recall but may assist in recognition of something experienced previously as opposed to other stimuli not experienced.

Sensation may be defined as involving a consistent correlation between physical events acting as stimuli on a living organism and the experiences that they evoke when the stimulus is appropriate and intense enough to activate a receptor (*Psychology Encyclopedia*, 1973, p. 248). Sensory problems, particularly those involving hearing, may strongly influence language development. The individual with oral sensory problems may encounter speech production difficulties (Fucci and Robertson, 1971; Ringel, House, Burk, Scott and Dolinsky, 1970; Ruscello and Lass, 1972; and Sommers, Cox and West, 1972). Deficits in other senses may make the use of meaningful language related to those areas difficult. For example, the blind or color-blind do not have the same referent for color as the normally sighted individual.

Most of us are aware of the problems caused by defective receptors. Reduction or destruction of peripheral receptors for hearing and vision and their accompanying problems are familiar to all of us. Most of us are less aware of the fact that damage to certain areas of the brain may also cause reduction or destruction of hearing, vision, or other senses. In some cases the sensations are received but the individual is unable to organize or handle these sensations in a meaningful manner. This brings us to perception, ". . . the experience of objects and events in the world based upon stimulation of the sense organs" (*Psychology Encyclopedia,* 1973, p. 195). Striffler (1976, p. 78) has written that, "Perception is the process of attaching meaning to sensation and involves detection, discrimination, identification and association of incoming stimuli." We usually identify problems involving an inability to organize stimuli as "perceptual problems." Some individuals are simply unable to discriminate among things in their environment. Visually, the toy the child is holding demands no more attention than the wall, chair, rug, or floor. Auditorily, speech is given no more attention than footsteps, the roar of a lawn mower, cars on the street, or dishes clinking in the kitchen. This inability to recognize a figure versus ground relationship may create very serious problems of many kinds, including problems in language development.

Cognitive skills are the proverbial case in which everyone uses the term assuming that others have a common definition. When called upon to define cognition, most of us find ourselves at a loss and we use terms such as *thinking, knowing,* and others that are equally vague. We do know that these so-called cognitive skills are associated with the functions of the brain's cortex, although interaction with other parts of the brain is inevitable because of its constant interactive processes. We expect these skills or processes to function normally unless specific brain damage or mental retardation interferes. There do seem to be, however, individuals whose cognitive skills are within normal limits but who display a specific language problem. Lenneberg (1967, p. 248-254) suggests that this may be a hereditary characteristic which follows patterns similar to other hereditary disorders.

Problems in any of the above-mentioned areas may lead to language delay. The specific cause or causes of language delay in any particular case may be unknown or only hypothesized. The case histories of two children may appear to be exactly alike, yet one develops language normally and the other displays a marked delay. Are there hereditary factors? Does one child have a predisposition to a language disorder? Is the general or language environment significantly different? We often do not know. We can, however, speculate about possible causes in many cases. A child may be ill or hospitalized for a period of time. This reduces his or her chances of hearing and using language in a variety of meaningful situations. A child may have inter-mittent undetected ear infections which make it impossible to hear the language needed to serve as examples from which the child can develop his or her own language system. The child may have a language-impoverished environment where the care-taker does not talk to the child or where the child spends most of the time with other young children whose language skills are at the same level or lower than those of the child. These situa-tions are often difficult or impossible to identify positively as existing and/or as causing delayed language.

Language Skills

To speak a language in a normal manner the individual must be able to handle all aspects of language: phonology, morpho-logy, syntax, semantics, and pragmatics. Breakdowns may occur in any one or a combination of these aspects of language.

In the realm of phonology the individual must be able to recognize and produce the sound system of his language. Some authors (Pollack and Rees, 1972) see this aspect of language as having two components: phonetic and phonologic. These produce two quite different problems. The individual with a phonetic problem cannot produce the sounds of the language correctly. The individual may even recognize the differences, as noted in Dale (1972, p. 182), but be unable to produce them. For example, a child may have difficulty articulating sibilants, such as /s/ and /z/. Another child may tease him by saying, "Tham ith really thilly" to which Sam may respond, "You didn't thay that right." Sam has demonstrated that he recognized the error but is unable to correct it.

When the individual experiences problems in phonology, however, the sounds may be produced correctly but inconsistently or in inappropriate contexts. The speaker may randomly use [p] and [b] in contexts where only one should appear. This indicates that he or she has not yet differentiated between these two phonemes and that the speaker has a category which includes both [p] and [b] just as a normal speaker has a category which includes both [p˖] and [pʰ] as the same phoneme. The phoneme /p/ which begins and ends the word *pop* has very different characteristics in the initial and final positions of that word. The initial [pʰ] has an aspirate release. It is produced with a large explosion of air. The final [p˖] is unreleased. It is produced with little or no explosion of air. In spite of this rather large difference, speakers of English perceive these as the same phoneme. The phonemes /p/ and /b/ differ in the characteristics of voicing. The /p/ is not accompanied by voice while the /b/ is. The other characteristics of the two sounds are very similar. A child may, therefore, not note the characteristic of voice as being important; after all, aspiration was unimportant for the /p/. The child may say *ped* for *bed* yet produce *bear* or other words using /b/ correctly. This indicates that the /p/ and /b/ may be considered as the same phoneme by this child.

Competency in morphology involves the ability to understand and produce words by combining meaningful units including free morphemes (usually words) and bound morphemes (prefixes, suffixes, and so on). The bound morphemes may be used to perform various functions. Derivational suffixes change the part of speech in many cases. The verb *fail* becomes the noun *failure* when the derivational suffix *ure* is added. Inflectional suffixes serve a grammatical function, such as marking plurality—*dog, dogs*—or indicating third person singular—*walk, walks*—(Stageberg, 1971).

Syntax involves the rules which order the elements of a language and the relationships among the elements. Examples include the arrangement of words into phrases, clauses and sentences. The child learning English must learn the permissible order of the subject, verb, object and other grammatical structures in an utterance. The child must also know the rules (transformations) which add, delete, and rearrange elements from their order in a simple, active, declarative sentence to the order in questions, negatives, passives, and more sophisticated syntactical forms. This is not to say that the child carries a set of Chomsky's transformations in his head, but the child must have some system which allows him to produce grammatical utterances. The exact nature of this system is presently a source of much debate.

Semantics involves one of the most basic concepts of language, the relation between symbols and their referents or, as some suggest, the connection between features, relations, or core concepts and the symbol (Dale, 1976, p. 165-178). Before anyone can acquire language, that person must understand the arbitrary representation of one thing by another. In oral language this involves the use of a series of vocal sounds to represent things, ideas, relationships, and so on. Written symbols, hand gestures, and other nonoral methods may take the place of vocal sounds in other language forms.

Of most recent interest to students of language and language development is the field of pragmatics. Hubbell (1977, p. 216) defines pragmatics as ". . . the study of the effects of communication on behavior." Nation and Aram (1977, p. 103-106) note that the infant's first utterances serve functions of self-gratification, directiveness, and control of a listener. As meaningful speech develops, language is used to name, describe, show possession, describe qualities, direct the child's own activities, help support his own thinking and to continue to direct or control listener's behaviors. The last language uses to develop are usually poetic and metalinguistic. The speech pathologist has always been keenly aware of the need for what is usually referred to as carryover, that is, use of the principles learned in therapy in meaningful everyday communications. The current interest in and systematic study of pragmatics may produce a better understanding and more useful approaches to pragmatics. The speech pathologist may use this knowledge to facilitate his clients' use of language in meaningful communication experiences.

Informal Assessments

When language assessment is mentioned, most people think in terms of formal tests. However, a very important aspect of assessment, usually the first to be used, is careful observation. The child may be compared informally to normal criteria, such as those mentioned as developmental steps in the first chapter. Very often this is the first indication the parent or professional observer has that the child deviates from the norm. Parents may operate on an even less formal basis comparing the child to other children in the family or the neighborhood.

The language sample is another technique in common use, particularly in more recent years. There are various methods of sampling. A formalized technique may be used or a more idiosyncratic method may be developed to suit the individual clinician's needs. In a language sample, the child's spontaneous conversation is recorded and analyzed. Some analysis techniques produce an actual score which may be compared to scores of other children (Lee, 1974). Other systems are formalized, that is, a specific procedure is followed, but rather than producing a score, specific information is obtained and used as a basis for planning remediation (Tyack and Gottsleben, 1974). The area of pragmatics is also evaluated by observations rather than any formal testing procedure at the present time.

Standardized Tests

Assessment tools are commonly divided into those which evaluate receptive skills and those which evaluate expressive skills. Further divisions may be made into categories representing the various language skills, such as phonology, morphology, syntax, and semantics. One should realize, however, that all tests were not designed with these categories in mind, and some may cover a number of these categories or only portions of one category.

The number of tests presently available for measuring various language skills is extensive. The brief summary presented here is only an overview with a few representative samples in various categories. For more extensive lists and descriptions the reader is referred to Irwin and Marge (1972), Wiig and Semel (1976), and Nation and Aram (1977).

Reception

Phonology

Receptive phonology is not totally evaluated by any formal tests. To do so would require exceedingly long and tedious tasks of identification and discrimination of phonemes in various contexts. The formal tests which come closest to testing this skill are those of auditory discrimination, such as the *Goldman-Fristoe-*

Woodcock (1970). First, the tester makes sure the subject is familiar with all the words used in the test. The subject then hears the recorded stimulus and selects the picture which depicts the stimulus word. Four pictures are offered for each stimulus. The pictures represent words which are alike except for one phoneme, such as the stimulus *dig* with pictures representing *pig, wig, big,* and *dig.*

Morphology

In many tests morphology is included with syntax. The *Northwest Syntax Screening Test (NSST)* by Lee (1969), for example, contains a few items which test morphological forms; a similar test is Carrow's *Test for Auditory Comprehension of Language* (1973). In the receptive portion of the *NSST* the child will hear two sentences such as, "The boy sees the cat. The boy sees the cats." The child is presented four pictures representing "The boy sees the cats. The boy sees the cat. The cat sees the boy. The girl holds the cat." The child is then asked to point to "The boy sees the cat." The child is also asked to point to "The boy sees the cats." This gives the child the opportunity to demonstrate his or her understanding or lack of understanding of the plural morpheme. Other items are tested in the same manner.

Syntax

The two tests just mentioned, the *NSST* (Lee, 1969) and the *Test for Auditory Comprehension of Language* (Carrow, 1973), contain portions which also test receptive syntax. As just noted, in the *NSST* the child hears two utterances; they are repeated and the child is requested to select the pictures which represent the repeated sentences. In Carrow's test, the child is presented with a verbal item and must select a picture, from among three choices, which best represents the correct response. Such things as imperatives, "Don't cross;" noun-verb agreement, "sleeps;" coordination, "Look at the third picture then point to the baby of this animal;" and modification, "a large blue ball" are tested.

Semantics

It is extremely difficult to test something like semantics, since meaning is so intertwined with our own experiences on the one hand and the systems we use to talk about meaning (phonology, morphology, and syntax) on the other hand. We may touch on semantics, however, with tests such as the *Ammons and Ammons Full Range Picture Vocabulary Test* (1958) and the *Peabody Picture Vocabulary Test* (Dunn, 1965). In both tests a word is presented and the child selects from four pictures the one which best represents the meaning of the word.

Tests for older children which involve more complex verbal abstractions include those such as the *Proverbs Test* (Gorham, 1956), which requires spontaneous or multiple choice interpretations of proverbs.

Expression

Phonology

Standardized tests which come closest to testing expressive phonology are usually referred to as articulation tests. It is hoped that these will tap the deeper structure of the child's knowledge about the sound system of his language. With the test structure imposed, however, we are usually only tapping the articulation production abilities. The standardized tests used for this include ones such as the *Templin-Darley Tests of Articulation* (1969). The child is shown pictures and asked questions about them. The answers to these questions are words which contain the sounds the examiner wishes to evaluate. Older children may read sentences containing the desired words.

The *McDonald Deep Test of Articulation* (1964) provides more information by having the child produce the same sound in a variety of contexts. The samples are, however, still carefully regulated by the arbitrary juxtaposition of words and are not necessarily representative of conversational speech. For example, the child may be asked to look at two pictures and say the names as one word, such as *batpie* or *housebell*. Similar methods are used to test children in order to do a distinctive feature analysis.

Morphology

The most extensive test of morphology is probably that devised by Berko (1958) as mentioned in the first chapter. Some research has been done using this material, but it has not been normed. It still remains a valuable tool, since it tests both inflectional and derivational morphemes of English. The Berry-Talbot (Berry, 1966) is based on Berko's research. It contains thirty items suggested for use with children five to eight years of age. Inflectional suffixes are tested, but this material, like Berko's, is not normed. As mentioned in the section on receptive morphology, the *NSST* contains a few items requiring knowledge of morphology.

Syntax

The *NSST* is one of the best known tests of syntax. It tests both receptive and expressive components. In the expressive section, two sentences are spoken to the child as the tester points to accompanying pictures. The examiner then points to one and then the other of the pictures again and the child is asked to say the sentence which goes with each picture.

The *Michigan Picture Language Inventory* (Lerea, 1958) is another example of a test containing items that tap expressive syntax, but which also taps expressive vocabulary, expressive and receptive morphology, and receptive syntax. Again pictures are used as stimuli to elicit responses. The examiner describes all the pictured items in a section. The child is then tested on the expressive items, and lastly, the child is asked to show comprehension of items by identifying the pictures which represent what the examiner says. Test items include such things as the use of personal pronouns, adjectives, demonstratives, articles, adverbs, prepositions, verbs, and auxiliaries.

Semantics

The *Detroit Tests of Learning Aptitude* (Baker and Leland, 1967) are not one test but a battery of tests. This has certain advantages over other similar tests composed of various subtests. In the Detroit tests, each test is normed individually; therefore, each can be given and scored separately. The tests are also normed for people with MA's from 3-0 to 19-0. Many test norms do not go beyond 6 to 12 years of age. Detroit tests pertinent to semantic abilities include ones concerning verbal absurdities, verbal opposites, and likenesses and differences.

> Verbal absurdities—"If I am in a hurry, I get a horse because automobiles are too slow."

Verbal opposites—"front-_____, brother-_____."
Likenesses and differences—"How are the following alike and different—morning and afternoon?"

Assessment Summary

Remediation was and still is sometimes based on the cause of the speech and language problem. Most clinicians, however, now base their remediation procedures on data from formal and informal tests, like those just discussed, which identify specific areas or individual items which need to be remediated. For example, a series of tests may indicate that a child is not articulating /s/ or /r/ correctly; the child does not appropriately form the comparative and superlative (large, larger, largest); and that the child has difficulty and is not correctly forming yes-no questions, wh questions, and passives. These things are only considered a problem, however, if other children of the same age have already mastered these skills. We would not expect a two- or three-year-old child to be able to do these perfectly, but if a ten-year-old child cannot do these, we know that he or she is seriously behind the development of his or her peers. In most cases where there are norms on standardized tests, we consider it a serious delay when the child is in the lowest 10 percent for his or her age, or if the child is more than a year behind his peers' development. Lee (1974), for example, uses the criterion of 10 percent. If a child's score is below 90 percent of his peers, Lee suggests the problem is serious enough to warrant remediation.

Tests to evaluate some of the prerequisites to language development (attention, sensation, perception, cognition, etc.) have not been discussed here. Most of these are within the realm of other professionals, such as audiologists, physicians, psychologists, and teachers. Some aspects, however, such as auditory perception, are so closely allied to delayed language problems that these are frequently included in the speech pathologist's assessment.

Remediation

Actual remediation techniques may vary considerably from clinic to clinic and individual to individual. The type of materials used also varies considerably. Some programs are extremely structured. Each step of the training may be carefully programmed and each behavior carefully controlled, counted, and reinforced where appropriate (Gray and Ryan, 1973). Other programs are relatively unstructured with the children being encouraged to participate in storytelling and creative play (Lee, 1975). These programs are still carefully planned and goals are specified, but they are accomplished in a less structured environment.

Some language programs, such as that by Kent (1974), also include instructions for training language prerequisites, such as attending and imitating behaviors. This draws our attention to the fact that we have been discussing mainly language components related to oral language. The assumption has been that children are capable of producing oral language and have some language skills, but that they are delayed for their ages. As mentioned earlier, another group of children is sometimes included in the category of delayed language but might more appropriately be called nonlanguage children. These children have developed no oral language. Until recently, most of these children were given therapy in an attempt to develop oral language. These attempts often met with failure and frustration, particularly in cases of severe mental retardation or brain damage. More recently, attempts have been made to teach these children to communicate by employing sign language or a system using plastic or fiberboard symbols arranged in specified order (Carrier, 1974). This developed out of the research done by Gardner and Gardner (1969) and Premack (1970), which indicated that chimpanzees could learn language when it was presented in the form of sign language or visible, manipulable symbols. Although these systems are not as universal as oral language, they give the individual who uses them some means of communicating. In some cases of severely retarded individuals, it is certainly easier for the family or caretakers to learn the language system of the retarded individual than it is for the retarded to learn oral language.

Summary

Children whose language development is significantly below that of their peers in the areas of phonology, morphology, syntax, semantics, and/or pragmatics are considered language delayed. This delay may be caused by external factors, such as the language environment, or internal factors, such as attention, memory, sensation, perception, and cognitive skills. Present assessment procedures attempt to describe the child's abilities in all aspects of language and define them in terms of how they differ from the norm for the child's age, sex, socioeconomic group, and so on. In many areas we are sadly lacking adequate norms for such comparisons.

Remediation may be based on very stringent behaviorist policies or on less structured situations more closely resembling normal language acquisition environments. The goals for language delayed children may vary considerably depending on the children's abilities. In recent years, forms other than oral language have been introduced to nonoral children in an attempt to give them some symbol system for communication. The ability to make a few simple wants known to a caretaker may be a very ambitious goal for some of these children, while the development of normal language may not be unrealistic for others. In all cases, functional language is the ultimate goal of a remedial program.

REFERENCES

Ammons, R. and Ammons, H.: *Full Range Picture Vocabulary Test.* Missoula, Psychological Test Specialists, 1958.

Baker, H. J. and Leland, B.: *Detroit Tests of Learning Aptitude.* Indianapolis, Test Division of Bobbs-Merrill, 1959.

Berko, J.: The child's learning of English morphology. *Word, 14*:150-177, 1958.

Berry, M. F.: *Berry-Talbott Language Tests.* Rockford, 1966.

Broadbent, D. E.: *Perception and Communication.* London, Pergamon Press, 1958.

California, Title 5, California Administration Code, Section 3600 (g). Sacramento, Department of General Services, Documents Section, 1970.

Carrier, J. K., Jr.: Application of functional analysis and a nonspeech response mode to teaching language. In McReynolds, L. M. (Ed.):

ASHA Monographs Number 18, Washington, American Speech and Hearing Association, 1974.

Carrow, E.: *Test for Auditory Comprehension of Language.* Austin, Urban Research Group, 1973.

Dale, P.: *Language Development: Structure and Function.* Hinsdale, The Dryden Press, Inc., 1972.

Dale, P.: *Language Development: Structure and Function,* 2nd ed. New York, Holt, Rinehart and Winston, 1976.

Dunn, L.: *Peabody Picture Vocabulary Test.* Circle Pines, American Guidance Service, 1965.

Fucci, D. J. and Robertson, J. H.: "Functional" defective articulation: an oral sensory disturbance. *Perceptual and Motor Skills, 33:*711-714, 1971.

Gardner, R. A. and Gardner, B. T.: Teaching sign language to a chimpanzee. *Science, 165:*664-672, 1969.

Goldman, R.; Fristoe, M., and Woodcock, R. W.: *The Goldman-Fristoe-Woodcock Test of Auditory Discrimination.* Circle Pines, American Guidance Service, 1970.

Gorham, D. R.: *Proverbs Test.* Missoula, Psychological Test Specialists, 1956.

Gray, B. B. and Ryan, B. P.: *A Language Program for the Nonlanguage Child.* Champaign, Research Press, 1973.

Hubbell, R. D.: On facilitating spontaneous talking in young children. *J Speech Hearing Disord, 42:*216-231, 1977.

Irwin, J. V. and Marge, M. (Eds.): *Principles of Childhood Language Disabilities.* New York, Appleton-Century-Crofts, 1972.

Kent, L. R.: *Language Acquisition Program for the Retarded or Multiple Impaired.* Champaign, Research Press, 1974.

Kohlberg, L.: Early education: A cognitive developmental view. *Child Development, 39:*1013-1062, 1968.

Lee, L. L.: *Northwest Syntax Screening Test.* Evanston, Northwestern University Press, 1969.

————: *Developmental Sentence Analysis.* Evanston, Northwestern University Press, 1974.

————: Developmental sentence types: A method for comparing normal and deviant syntactic development. *J Speech Hear Res, 31:*311-330, 1966.

Lee, L. L.; Koenigsknecht, R. A., and Mulhern, S.: *Interactive Language Development Teaching: The Clinical Presentation of Grammatical Structure.* Evanston, Northwestern University Press, 1975.

Lenneberg, E.: *Biological Foundations of Language.* New York, John Wiley and Sons, 1967.

Lerea, L.: *The Michigan Picture Language Inventory.* Ann Arbor, The University of Michigan Speech Clinic, 1958.

McDonald, E.: *Screening Deep Test of Articulation.* Pittsburgh, Stanwix House, Inc., 1964.

Menyuk, P.: Comparison of grammar of children with functionally deviant and normal speech. *J Speech Hear Res,* 7:109-121, 1964.

Morehead, D. M. and Ingram, D.: The development of base syntax in normal and linguistically deviant children. *J Speech Hear Res, 16:*330-352, 1973.

Nation, J. E. and Aram, D. M.: *Diagnosis of Speech and Language Disorders.* St. Louis, The C. V. Mosby Co., 1977.

Piaget, J.: Piaget's Theory. In Mussen, P. H. (Ed.): *Carmichael's Manual of Child Psychology, Vol. I.* New York, John Wiley and Sons, 1970.

Pollack, E. and Rees, N.: Disorders of articulation: Some clinical applications of distinctive feature theory. *J Speech Hear Disord,* 37:451-461, 1972.

Premack, D.: A functional analysis of language. *J Exp Anal Behav, 14:*107-125, 1970.

Psychology Encyclopedia. Guilford, The Duskin Publishing Group, Inc., 1973.

Ringel, R. L.; House, A. S.; Burk, K. W.; Dolinsky, J. P., and Scott, C. M.: Some relations between orosensory discrimination and articulatory aspects of speech production. *J Speech Hearing Disord,* 35:3-11, 1970.

Ruscello, D. M. and Lass, N. J.: *Articulation Improvement and Oral Tactile Changes in Children.* Unpublished manuscript. West Virginia University, 1972.

Stageberg, N. C.: *An Introductory English Grammar.* New York, Holt, Rinehart and Winston, 1971.

Sommers, R. K.; Cox, S., and West, C.: Articulatory effectiveness, stimulability, and children's performances on perceptual and memory tasks. *J Speech Hear Res, 15:*579-589, 1972.

Striffler, N.: Language function: Normal and abnormal development. In Johnston, R. B. and Magrab, P. R. (Eds.): *Developmental Disorders: Assessment, Treatment, Education.* Baltimore, University Park Press, 1976.

Templin, M. C. and Darley, F. L.: *Templin-Darley Tests of Articulation.* Iowa City, University of Iowa, 1969.

Tyack, D. and Gottsleben, R.: *Language Sampling, Analysis and Training.* Palo Alto, Consulting Psychologists Press, 1974.

United States Government Bureau of the Census. Estimates of the population of the United States by age, race, and sex. July 1, 1964 to 1967. Population Estimates, series P-25, No. 385, February 14. Washington, United States Department of Commerce, 1969.

Wiig, E. H. and Semel, E. M.: *Language Disabilities in Children and Adolescents.* Columbus, Charles E. Merrill Publishing Co., 1976.

CHAPTER 4

VOICE PROBLEMS

BETTY D. ANDERSON, R.N., M.A.

Speaking is a complex, learned process involving the generation of an undifferentiated sound in the larynx that is modified in the pharynx, mouth, and nose. The sound production is known as *phonation,* and the modification of that sound is called *resonance* (Moore, 1971). We are aware of the voices we hear and develop favorable or unfavorable reactions to those voices, usually in some vague fashion but one that is none the less real and potent. We have been told that America is "voice conscious" as a result of the influence of radio and television, so that the spoken word has a potentiality never before realized (Anderson, 1961).

Every voice has a unique character, dependent on the sex and age of the individual, and anatomical differences so that there is no single sound that can be called normal (Greene, 1972). Certain conditions can be listed, however, as characteristic of an effective speaking voice:

1. Adequate loudness (intensity)
2. Clearness of tone (quality)
3. Appropriate pitch level
4. Ease and flexibility (variety and melody)
5. Clearness and ease of diction
6. A vibrant, sympathetic quality (Anderson, 1961)

In the adult, the voice often identifies the personality of the speaker as much as or more than the words that are spoken. The voice conveys a variety of emotional undercurrents, such as joy, excitement, irritation, tranquility, suspicion, and sympathy, using subtle variations of inflections, stress, and volume (Greene, 1971).

Production of Voice

For practical purposes here, the vocal instrument will be described as consisting of three parts: respiratory mechanism, vocal folds or glottis, and resonance (supraglottic air spaces). The term *glottis* refers to the opening between the vocal folds. Supraglottic air spaces are those areas above the glottis and include the pharynx; the mouth, including the tongue, palate, teeth, cheeks, lips, and mandible; and the nasal cavity. Although each part of the vocal instrument will be considered separately, vocal production can be achieved only by highly specialized coordination of all of the parts together. It should be noted that the primary biological function of the vocal organs is not speech production. The organs were first developed to perform other vital services such as breathing, chewing, and swallowing. It was only later that they applied to the production of speech (Denes and Pinson, 1973).

Respiratory Mechanism

The function of the respiratory tract is to move air to and from the lungs during the process of breathing. The fundamental principle of air motion that pertains to breathing is that the air flows from regions of higher pressure to areas of lower pressure. Biologically, the function of the lungs is to supply oxygen to the blood and to dispose of certain waste products such as carbon dioxide (Moore, 1971). The airway through which the air moves consists of the mouth, nose, pharynx, larynx, trachea, and lungs. The act of breathing is controlled by various sets of muscles of the abdomen, rib cage, and diaphragm.

The organs of the airway form an intricately shaped "tube" extending from the lungs to the lips. The larynx, which contains the vocal folds, is located in the neck at the level of the third and sixth cervical vertebrae (Greene, 1972). The portion of the tube that lies above the larynx (supraglottic) is called the vocal tract and consists of the pharynx, mouth, and nose. The area below the larynx (subglottic) becomes the trachea, which leads directly to the lungs.

The source of energy for speech production is the steady stream of air that comes from the lungs as we exhale. During regular breathing, the air stream is inaudible. The vocal folds are open, allowing air to move to and from the lungs. When speech is produced, the air stream is set into vibration by the action of the vocal folds. The air flow to and from the lungs is interrupted as the vocal folds open and close during vocal production (Denes and Pinson, 1973). As the air pressure increases beneath the vocal folds, it pushes the folds apart, releasing a jet of air, which lowers the pressure at the level of the glottis, allowing the folds to close again. When the breath pressure increases, the cycle is repeated and will continue as long as the alternating relationship of vocal fold resistance and air pressure build-up is maintained. The series of air pulses created by the periodic interruptions of the air stream generate a sound having *pitch* that is directly related to the frequency of the air pulses and a *loudness* that is determined by the amplitude of the sound pressure wave produced (Moore, 1971). The shape of the vocal tract is varied to modify the sound (resonance), which is generated at the level of the larynx, by moving the tongue, lips, and other parts of the vocal tract (Denes and Pinson, 1973).

The regulation of the outflow of air is basically involuntary and highly automatic during ordinary speech, but singers and public speakers learn to rely on a partial control of the breathing mechanism to increase the intensity of their voices. The everyday demands of speaking require that a sufficient amount of air be taken in to maintain adequate subglottal air pressure to set the folds into action. It appears to take very little air flow for the average speaker to phonate in his optimal pitch range at low intensities (Boone, 1971).

Vocal Folds (Glottis)

The vocal folds are located in the larynx, which lies in the anterior portion of the neck. The folds serve several functions: protection of the airway from aspiration of foreign material (fluids, food particles, objects), as a passageway for air to move to and from the lungs, to lock the air into the lungs during such activities as heavy lifting, and as the instrument of voice. The larynx, then, and specifically the vocal folds, acts as a valve between the lungs and the mouth.

The vocal folds consist of muscle and cartilage that extend, one on either side of the interior of the larynx. The anterior two-thirds of the folds are muscular and the posterior third is cartilaginous. The open position of the vocal folds, or glottis, is V-shaped. The anterior portion of the folds remains stationary, and only the posterior portion moves apart (*see* Fig. 4-1). When the larynx is at rest during quiet respiration, the vocal folds remain abducted and move up and down slightly with the outflow and inflow of air. The folds open wider to a position of full abduction during forced inspiration. In quiet whispering, the folds are slightly separated along the anterior two-thirds, and air is forced through the posterior triangle (Greene, 1973).

Phonation first requires approximation of the vocal folds (adduction). During actual sound production, the length and tension of the vocal folds is continually changing. It appears that the voice pitch level is directly related to the length and thickness of the individual's vocal folds. As the person phonates at increasingly higher pitch levels, the vocal folds lengthen, which decreases the mass of tissue of the folds. Lowering the pitch then is directly related to the relaxation and shortening of the folds. Another factor determining voice pitch is the amount of air pressure from the lungs (subglottal air pressure). Increased air pressure from below the glottis usually causes an increase in pitch level (Boone, 1971).

Intensity (loudness) of the voice also appears to be related to the subglottal air pressure, the amount of air flow, and the

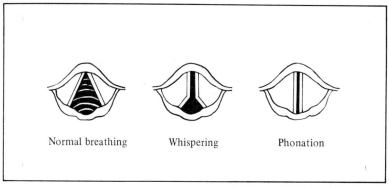

| Normal breathing | Whispering | Phonation |

Figure 4-1. Approximation of the vocal folds.

amount of glottal resistance (vocal fold adduction). Boone (1971) states that, as voice intensity is increased, the vocal folds tend to remain closed for a longer time during each vibratory cycle. The trained user of voice, such as a singer, lecturer, or actor, probably increases the intensity of the voice by increasing both the subglottal air pressure and the air flow rate rather than by increasing glottal (vocal fold) tension alone to achieve a louder voice.

Resonance (Supraglottal Air Spaces)

The supraglottic air spaces, i.e. above the vocal fold level, provide resonance for the sound generated at the level of the larynx. Without the supraglottal resonance, the sound produced by the vibrating vocal folds would be a very thin sound. The air spaces can be changed by muscular action causing widening, lengthening, or narrowing of the pharynx and mouth, and by interrupting the flow of air as speech sounds are formed. The pharynx is probably the most important resonating cavity for the voice, but the mouth, as a resonator, is capable of the greatest variation in size and shape. The tongue in particular is extremely mobile, constantly changing positions for each consonant, vowel, and diphthong of the language. The walls of the nasal cavity are very rigid, so the quality of the sound can be changed only by adjusting adjacent structures. A noticeable change in vocal quality can be noted, however, if the nasal cavities are congested or swollen as in the case of a "cold," allergies, or other pathologies.

The previous discussion has briefly described vocal production as a function of three important divisions of the vocal mechanism. The *respiratory mechanism* provides the energy in the form of air pressure below the vocal folds. The *vocal folds* vibrate to produce a modulation of the air pressure to generate a tone. Variations in the frequency and manner of vocal-fold vibration determine pitch, loudness, and quality of the vocal tones. The *resonators*, which include the pharynx, mouth, and nasal cavities, provide amplification and modification of the vocal tone with additional variations in tone quality. A voice disorder can result when one or more of the vocal mechanisms function improperly or if they are extraordinarily misused or abused (Curtis, 1967).

Phonation is the process of producing vocal sound. There are many variations and many kinds of voice. A person may speak softly or loudly, at a high or low pitch level, with a clear or hoarse voice, or produce vocal sounds expressing anger, joy, exhaustion, skepticism, or any other attitudes or emotions that can be expressed by voice. There is a wide range of voices that are accepted by the general public as normal.

Types of Faulty Vocal Production

The discussion to follow will attempt to divide voice disorders into four categories: disorders of intensity, quality, pitch, and resonance.

Disorders of Intensity (Loudness)

Most voices affected by this disorder involve lack of adequate loudness during regular phonatory activities. It appears that most phonatory tasks require little more than a normal, tidal inspiration. (*Tidal* refers to the total volume of air that is inspired and expired during each normal respiratory cycle.) Some examples of faulty control of the respiratory cycle are as follows:

SPEAKING ON RESIDUAL AIR. Residual air is the volume of air that remains in the lungs at the end of a normal expiratory cycle, after most of the tidal air has been exhaled. The residual air, when used for phonation, is insufficient to maintain adequate vocal loudness and resonance. Then the individual usually increases the tension of the laryngeal musculature in an attempt to increase loudness, since breath support is inadequate to produce a louder voice. Eventually, the muscles of the larynx become fatigued from overuse, often causing discomfort and physical damage to the vocal mechanism.

SPEAKING WITH SHORTNESS OF BREATH. Generally, when a person is unable to utter more than three to four words because of an insufficient supply of air, the problem may be related to anxiety about the speaking situation. In other cases, persons suffering from certain physical conditions, such as emphysema, quadraplegia, or tuberculosis, may be unable to maintain adequate breath support for efficient phonation.

SPEAKING WITH UNNECESSARY FOCUS ON BREATHING. Some persons deliberately take in a deep breath before speaking in an attempt to overcome phonatory difficulties, followed by rapid, uncontrolled exhalation. Vocal production demonstrates inadequate breath support for phonation, probably resulting in speaking on residual air.

STRUGGLING TO TAKE IN A BREATH. Some individuals tend to elevate the shoulders and tighten the neck muscles as they inhale preparatory to phonation. Such activity demonstrates improper and excessive use of the inspiratory muscles, resulting in inadequate air intake and increased, unnecessary tension of specific muscle groups (Boone, 1971).

EXCESSIVE LOUDNESS. Most cases of excessive loudness are related to deficiencies in hearing, since the person is unable to monitor his own vocal production.

Disorders of Quality

The most frequently occurring disorder of vocal production is that of quality. The terms sometimes used to describe disorders of quality are hoarse, strident, breathy, husky, or rough, but there seems to be little agreement as to the exact meaning of each one of the terms. What one person hears as a "hoarse" voice may be called "harsh" by someone else (Curtis, 1967; Boone, 1971). The definitions used most often for these terms include the following:

The "harsh" voice is usually described as rough or unpleasant and seems to be produced with a considerable amount of strain in the area of the larynx (Curtis, 1967). The voice quality of harshness can also be attributed to the use of inappropriate pitch level, usually at the bottom of one's pitch range (Van Riper, 1963). Moore (1971) describes the harsh voice as ". . . an unpleasant, rough, rasping sound" (p. 8).

The "breathy" voice is heard as a voice which seems to have a whispered effect added to the vocal tone (Curtis, 1967). There seems to be a sound of excessive air flow combined with the vocal production. Generally, the voice is weak and low pitched because of the escape of air through poorly approximated vocal folds (Moore, 1971).

The "hoarse" voice quality is sometimes related to the temporary condition of inflammation of the vocal folds, due to a "cold" or excessive vocal abuse (shouting at a football game). A more permanent condition of "hoarseness" can result from the habitual use of a pitch level that is too low (Curtis, 1967). Moore (1971) describes three kinds of hoarseness: *dry,* characterized by loud breathiness; *wet,* similar to the voice of laryngitis; and *rough,* characterized by two pitches produced simultaneously. Darley (1965) states that hoarseness is a combination of harshness and breathiness. Van Riper (1963) also describes the "hoarse" voice as a combination of breathy and harsh with a sound indicating considerable air wastage and vocal straining, such as that heard with the strident voice. Finally, Aronson (1973) defines vocal quality as follows:

> A voice that is subjectively determined to be deviant in clarity, color or fullness due to inadequacies in complex frequency and intensity relationships. (P. 5)

Disorders of Pitch

A person with a disorder of pitch is one who habitually talks with a pitch level that is inappropriate for his sex or age. Some of the more common types of pitch disorders are (1) the monotone voice, (2) a habitual pitch level that is too high, (3) pitch breaks, (4) falsetto and, (5) a pitch that is too low, especially in children or females.

The *monotone* voice is usually capable of some pitch change, but the key characteristic is the narrow range of inflection and pitch change. These voices are sometimes described as dull, lifeless, or lacking in variety.

Habitual pitch level refers to the pitch level habitually used during general conversation. It represents an average or median pitch around which a person speaks. The habitual pitch level varies with the age and sex of the person. For example, the voice of a young child is higher in pitch than that of an adult. Major pitch changes occur at puberty, especially in boys. The size and structure of the larynx undergoes considerable change, sometimes within a short period of time (Van Riper, 1963). The larynx becomes larger and the overall mass of the vocal folds increases so the pitch level lowers (Boone, 1971). During this period, boys may experience a full octave drop in pitch from their former pitch level. The pubescent period for girls is usually longer and occurs more slowly with less structural changes of the laryngeal mechanism and with fewer obvious voice changes. The pitch level for girls may descend from one to three tones during this period.

The pitch level may also change if the individual experiences excessive stress or tension throughout the day. The voice may then become higher in pitch because the vocal folds become tighter.

Pitch breaks are heard as shifts in pitch level, usually involuntary and usually an entire octave either upward or downward. Adults sometimes experience pitch breaks when the habitual pitch level is inappropriate (Boone, 1971). Luchsinger and Arnold (1965) report the "voice break" occurring when the person feels insecure in using the voice following laryngeal surgery or during vocal rehabilitation when a better pattern of phonation is being learned.

The *falsetto* voice is produced when the glottal opening becomes very small until only a whistle or squeak is heard (Greene, 1971). This voice is often used by singers especially when they want to extend their pitch range beyond what normal vocal fold stretching will do (Boone, 1971). Sometimes the falsetto voice occurs at times of extreme emotional distress or can occur during the changes of puberty. The shift to a falsetto pitch level may occur involuntarily or it may be used as a defense against the pitch breaks which often occur during the voice changes of puberty. Other individuals attempt to avoid a hoarse or husky voice by elevating their habitual pitch to the falsetto level.

A voice pitch that is habitually *too low* sometimes occurs in children or females. In some cases, the inappropriately low pitched voice may be the result of faulty vocal habits, much the same as a person who habitually uses a higher pitched voice (Boone, 1971). In other cases, an endocrine imbalance may cause changes in the vocal pitch, such as diseases of the thyroid, parathyroid, pituitary, or gonads (Luchsinger and Arnold, 1965). Whenever additional tissue occurs on the vocal folds, the voice pitch will lower. Such instances as the presence of growths on the vocal folds (nodules, polyps) or vocal fold thickening usually change the pitch level (Boone, 1971).

The use of inappropriate pitch carries with it certain social penalties, such as in the case of a male with a pitch level that is considered "too high." The female with an inappropriately *low* pitch may be mistaken for a male when she answers the phone. Persistent use of an inappropriate pitch level places considerable strain on the laryngeal musculature and may result in the development of serious pathological conditions of the vocal mechanism (Curtis, 1967).

Disorders of Resonance

The disorders of resonance involve the area of the vocal tract located above the level of the vocal folds and include the pharynx, the mouth, and the nasal cavities.

Boone (1971) describes two of the most common behaviors affecting resonance as unnecessary pharyngeal constriction and malpositioning of the tongue during speech. Other factors affecting resonance are lack of adequate mouth opening (such as speaking through clenched teeth) and inappropriate posturing of the soft palate (such as keeping the nasal port open when it should be closed). The voice then would be considered excessively "nasal."

Further describing specific behaviors of resonance disorders, Boone (1971) gives the following examples:

Speaking with a Taut Pharynx. The best example of the sound produced by a taut pharynx is the technique used by the carnival barker or dime-store demonstrator. The muscles of the wall of the pharynx contract creating rigidity, which not only changes the size of the pharynx but affects the sounding board characteristics as well.

Cooper (1973) describes this vocal production as use of improper *tone focus* in that the voice seems to be coming from the oropharyngeal area rather than from a balanced effort of the oral, nasal, and laryngeal areas.

Greene (1972) also discusses the disorders of resonance in terms of "overtensed" muscles of the oropharynx and oral cavity which can decrease the dimensions of the oropharyngeal resonator.

SPEAKING WITH FAULTY TONGUE POSITION. The shape and size of the tongue can alter the dimensions of the pharynx as well as the interior of the mouth. For example, a forward carriage of the tongue during speech may resemble "baby-talk resonance." If the tongue body is so far back that it nearly makes contact with the pharyngeal wall, then the resulting voice is described as "cul-de-sac" resonance. This type of resonance is frequently associated with persons who have a hearing loss (Boone, 1971).

SPEAKING WITH EXCESSIVE MOUTH OPENING. Persons with certain neuromuscular disorders, e.g. athetoid cerebral palsy, sometimes tend to lower the mandible excessively as they speak, thereby distorting the quality of the sound produced.

SPEAKING WITH IMPROPER PALATAL MOVEMENT. Some disorders of resonance are related to the misuse of the velopharyngeal mechanism. If the cause is not related to structural inadequacies, such as cleft palate, then a more oral-sounding voice may be achieved with appropriate use of the soft palate (velum) (Boone, 1971).

NASAL RESONANCE. Three speech sounds of the English language, the /m/, /n/, and /ng/, are emitted through the nasal passages and are known as nasal consonants. In certain conditions (adenoids, nasal polyps, injuries to the nose, infections, allergies) the nasal cavity may become obstructed so that the air and sounds do not pass easily through the nose. Such vocal production results in what is sometimes termed *denasal* speech. In other instances, the opposite may occur in that the nasal port remains open or does not close completely as the nonnasal consonants are produced. The vocal air stream is then directed out through the nose for all speech activities. The most obvious cause is the cleft palate, in which an opening exists at the same location of the palate.

There is some disagreement as to the appropriate terminology to describe disorders of nasal resonance. Some authors use the terms *hyponasality* (indicating too little nasal air emission) and *hypernasality* (indicating too much nasal air emission). Regardless of the terminology used, the disorders of nasal resonance are usually related to one or more of the following behaviors: improper functioning of the soft palate (velum), the condition of the nasal cavity (presence of growths, inflammation), and the position of the tongue in the mouth during speech.

Causes of Vocal Dysfunction

Successful vocal production depends on the optimum blending of respiration, vocal fold function, and resonance. Most voice disorders are related to the misuse of some or all of the mechanisms, producing various alterations of phonation or resonance, with or without the development of laryngeal pathology (Boone, 1971). Disease and other organic abnormalities in the larynx can modify the functioning of the vocal folds, causing disordered vibration and phonatory defects. Similarly, disease and organic anomalies can affect the supraglottic air spaces of the vocal tract to the detriment of the quality of the voice (Moore, 1971).

Boone (1971) uses the concept of *hyperfunction,* which was introduced by E. Froeschels (1943). *Hyperfunction* is characterized by the use of too much muscular force in the wrong places. If one is to produce optimal voice, meaning relatively effortless vocal production, then undue tensions in the vocal tract during phonation must be avoided. Brodnitz (1968) discusses *hyperfunction* as one of the first stages of a voice disorder. His use of the term covers all forms of excessive muscular tension in the vocal tract. Prolonged hyperfunctional use of the vocal mechanism eventually causes fatigue of the musculature resulting in *hypo*function of the muscles. The voice becomes weak and may decline to a whisper because the laryngeal muscles can no longer function properly. Such symptoms may be reported by professional singers or speakers, such as as lecturers, ministers, teachers, and politicians, but other persons may report similar symptoms as well. At this point, investigation of daily living patterns becomes important. People in our modern day civilization are subjected to a variety of stressful, tension-provoking situations every day. We live in a highly competitive society and may be faced with problems related to employment, interpersonal relationships, family conflicts, fears, phobias, or disappointments.

Pelletier (1977) also includes environmental conditions as possible stressors, such as ". . . air and noise pollution, overcrowding . . ., deadlines . . ., constant sense of competition . . ." (p. 4). These are all called negative stressors, but positive occurrences can also be stress producing. Such occasions as a marriage, promotion, or an outstanding personal achievement all require that the person change or adapt. "Any alteration in an individual's life requires him to adjust, and when these adjustments must be made too frequently in a brief period of time, tension or stress are the results" (p. 5). Other stresses are ambiguous and undefined. When one's life is in actual danger, such as a near car accident, the stressor is easily identified. A certain physiological excitation occurs followed by relaxation once the danger is past. One can begin breathing more slowly and return to a more normal level of functioning. In daily living, the body may react in a similar way, i.e. as though life was in danger, after a particularly stressful day. In this case, there may be no readily identifiable source of the stress, and there may be no potential danger to one's life. In such a situation, there may be no "recovery" period, such as the reduced physiological excitation and slowed breathing. The body eventually adapts to the higher level of tension, but we cannot tolerate such prolonged stress to go on unabated over a long period of time. The result may be one of many stress-related disorders, one of which is vocal dysfunction.

Boone (1971) stated that stress or tension, whether externally imposed or self-generated, can contribute to the breakdown of an individual's overall effectiveness. Although the body may react in a variety of ways, excessive muscular tension is one of the possible physiological responses to stress. Tension can occur in any group of muscles, but when the tension is reflected in the muscles of the vocal tract, then the result is a voice disorder.

The persistent practice of misuse of the laryngeal musculature can result in changes of size and mass of the vocal folds, or in the lack of adequate approximation of the folds during phonation. Some of the changes in the mass of the vocal folds include the development of nodules (a benign growth at the margin of one or both folds, varying in size, similar to a callouslike formation) or thickening of the folds. Problems of approximation include inability to bring the folds together well. The cause is often a result of hypofunction or fatigue of the laryngeal musculature or, in some cases, paralysis of one of the folds. The pitch may be altered because of the lack of vocal fold vibration and the intensity decreased because of excessive escape of air during phonation. In still other cases, extreme overadduction of the folds may interfere so much with the outward escape of air that vibration of the folds is nearly impossible, resulting in what is termed *spastic dysphonia.*

Referral

The individual with a voice disorder is usually referred to the speech pathologist by an otolaryngologist. In some instances, the speech pathologist may identify a vocal dysfunction through routine screening procedures. In that case, before remediation procedures are initiated, the person must be referred to an otolaryngologist for a complete diagnostic evaluation of the laryngeal structures. No person should receive voice therapy from a speech pathologist unless the voice problem has been diagnosed by a physician competent in the area of otolaryngology. Otherwise, the therapy might have serious consequences especially if the person's symptoms are related to laryngeal papilloma or carcinoma. In some cases, voice therapy is not indicated, such as laryngeal web (a membranous partition that extends across the glottis from one fold to the other). The cause is usually congenital or resulting from surgery or injury to the vocal folds (Moore, 1971). Voice therapy may also be deferred if the individual demonstrates severe interpersonal maladjustments. In all instances, the laryngologist makes the decision for starting voice therapy. The type of therapy, however, is decided by the speech pathologist (Boone, 1977).

Voice Evaluation

The speech pathologist is usually provided with a report of the findings by the otolaryngologist before the client is seen. A thorough understanding of the report is essential before remediation procedures begin. To understand the person with a voice disorder, the voice specialist must collect background information about that individual. Descriptions of history-taking techniques for voice disorders and other communicative disorders are included in texts, *Diagnostic Methods in Speech Pathology* (Johnson, Darley, and Spriestersbach, 1963), *Organic Voice Disorders* (Moore, 1971), and *The Voice and Voice Therapy* (Boone, 1971). One of the most important sections of the case history is the person's own description of what he thinks the problem is and what he thinks is the cause. The description reveals much about his conceptualization of the problem and what insight he may have about the cause of his voice deviation. How the person describes his voice problem often can indicate the direction of the first phases of therapy.

The onset and duration of the voice problem, as described by the person, also reveal important information. If the onset is sudden and poses a threat to the person's livelihood or any other customary activities, then his motivation to overcome the problem will be high and will greatly affect the success of the remediation program. On the other hand, if the person has a long history of indifference to his dysphonia, or if the dysphonia serves as a means of avoiding social situations, or if a specific vocal production is personally and financially rewarding (stage, screen, radio, and television personalities), then the prognosis for successful remediation is usually unfavorable.

Most persons with a voice deviation describe varying degrees of severity of the problem either throughout the day or during specific situations. A person experiencing a voice deviation reports a better voice early in the day with increasing dysphonia the more the voice is used. Another person, whose dysphonia is closely related to allergies and postnasal drip during sleep, may experience hoarseness in the morning with gradual improvement throughout the day. The variation of the voice problem can provide even more specific clues. For example, a nightclub singer may report that a voice problem does not occur during the day in conversational situations or even while practicing. The hoarseness develops only at night and only on those nights of performances. Further investigation may reveal that the adverse factors are cigarette smoke and the loud noise of the crowd, which forces the person to increase loudness in order to be heard. If the person is utilizing the vocal mechanism properly during speaking and singing, then the individual may obtain relief only by changing performance sites.

The kind of daily vocal use may be still another important factor in perpetuating a voice problem. It appears that only a small amount of vocal misuse daily will keep a vocal problem "alive." Examples cited are mothers who yell after their children, lecturers, ministers, or auctioneers who use their voices in specific ways on certain occasions, or children who scream and yell on the playground (Cooper, 1973). Sometimes the most effective voice therapy is identifying the abusive situations, followed by counseling and direct instruction (Boone, 1971).

Information regarding the person's general health history should be obtained by questions concerning any past illnesses, surgeries, chronic conditions, such as diabetes, thyroid conditions, drug or hormone therapy, and whether the person indulges in excessive smoking or drinking. A more complete medical history is usually available from the person's physician.

The voice evaluation also includes the recognition and description of the individual's vocal production and a detailed analysis of how the person utilizes the respiratory, phonatory, and resonating mechanisms relative to vocal production.

Therapeutic Procedures

Therapy for voice disorders involves restoring the vocal mechanism to its maximum possible efficiency. Often this includes not only specific exercises to achieve maximum vocal function, but also modifications of the relationships between the individual and his environment and alterations of the individual's behavior, particularly habits of vocal use (Moore, 1971).

Several speech and voice pathology texts provide detailed descriptions of therapeutic procedures for vocal dysfunction. Several are included in the following description. Boone (1971, 1977) describes symptomatic voice therapy, which attempts to identify the vocal abuses practiced by the individual and then eliminate or reduce these behaviors by direct symptom modification. Examples of vocal abuse may include loud screaming or yelling on the playground, excessive throat clearing, or use of improper pitch level during prolonged periods of speaking. In many cases the individual may be using his vocal mechanism incorrectly. The mechanisms of respiration, phonation, resonance, and speech articulation demand a combination and interaction for optimal vocal production. The general philosophy is ". . . too much muscular force in the wrong places . . ." (Boone, 1971, p. 2) and is not bound to particular etiologies or pathologies. The procedures outlined by Boone are to provide a working method for those persons who misuse or abuse their vocal mechanism. Johnson (1976) has developed the Vocal Abuse Reduction Program (VARP) for a public school population, but it can be adapted for use with adults as well. The program involves counting vocal abuse behavior during the course of a communicating day. The use of a wrist counter to tabulate abusive behavior during high probability time periods, along with daily record keeping and appropriate reinforcements, has resulted in the reduction of laryngeal pathologies, i.e. nodules, polyps, contact ulcers, and thickened vocal cords, so that normal vocal quality can be reestablished. Daily phone calls to the client over a short period of time have been an essential part of the program to ask about record keeping and, more importantly, to make daily contact with the client.

Vocal misuse, if it is the result of improper use of muscular force during phonation, must first be identified, and the person must then become aware of the faulty muscular activity. Individuals may be instructed to "feel" the tension during specific speaking situations and then asked to "relax" those areas of tension, especially in the area of the neck, jaw, and possibly upper shoulders. Specific exercises can sometimes be employed to facilitate such relaxed states. In recent years, biofeedback has been used to monitor muscular tension. Studies utilizing biofeedback techniques have demonstrated that individuals can be trained to effectively monitor and regulate specific bodily processes, such as muscular tensions and activity, heart rate, blood pressure, and brain wave patterns, by providing the individual with specific representations of that activity. Usually, these representations are in the form of auditory or visual signals that vary in direct relation to muscular activity.

Studies have been reported in which various muscles of the neck, face, and laryngeal area have been monitored and in which subjects have learned to effectively reduce the muscular tension at these sites (Boone, 1977; Cross, 1977; Aten and Blanchard, 1974; Guitar, 1975). Muscles of the areas of the neck, face, and jaw are so numerous however that it should not be assumed that the feedback is attained from any specific muscle or even muscle group. The individual is merely provided with feedback within a general area of the laryngeal musculature, e.g. thyroid prominence of the larynx. Sturlaugson, in a paper presented at the American Speech and Hearing Association (Las Vegas, 1975), discussed the use of electromyographic (EMG) biofeedback training with a case of psychogenic dysphonia. With the combined use of relaxation and biofeedback training, the individual learned to reduce muscular force during phonation and produced a "clear tone" of vocal production during the third session. Lyndes discussed his experiences using biofeedback training in a paper presented to the Biofeedback Research Society (Monterey, 1975) in which similar procedures and results were realized.

Cooper (1973) emphasizes, among other procedures, the technique of locating optimal pitch level of vocal production. According to Cooper, the optimal pitch level will achieve a balance of oronasopharyngeal resonance and laryngeal resonance when using the technique of phonating "um-hum" in a natural, unforced manner resulting in a proper tone focus. The important point in producing the "um-hum" involves a "spontaneous and sincere" production of the sound as if agreeing with what was just said. Producing such a natural sound will create a vibration about the nose and lips. When such a technique is used by an experienced therapist, Cooper believes it is a simple and direct way of determining optimal pitch. In addition to locating optimal pitch level, Cooper includes vocal psychotherapy, associate therapy, illustrative therapy, and bibliotherapy.

Schumacher (1974) developed his approach from his experiences with vocal students and teachers of singing and speaking. The emphasis is on the muscles which produce the voice and not on the voice itself. Schumacher believes that if the muscles of the cheeks, nose, lips, lower jaw, tongue, soft palate, and waist are used incorrectly in speaking, then the resulting strain can cause hoarseness, discomfort, and fatigue. If the muscles of the vocal instrument are in balance, then a good voice will result. To attain this balance of the musculature, he has designed a series of exercises for each muscle group, partly to strengthen the muscles but also to insure correct usage of this musculature. He makes no attempt to change the pitch level of the speaking or singing voice but states that when the muscles are used correctly the voice will be on its own natural pitch level.

The preceding discussion regarding the remediation of voice disorders by no means exhausts the numerous publications and procedures available. This merely provides a starting point for those who wish to investigate the field in greater detail. To quote a statement from Moore (1971), "To know theory, to know in general about diagnosis and therapy for voice defects is sterile information until it is shaped to the individual" (p. 108).

Prognosis of any vocal dysfunction depends on the type and severity of the problem. Any remediation procedure is dependent upon the cooperation of the individual in following a specific program and particularly on his motivation to change. Such change may include alteration of his environment, modification of vocal behaviors, and changes in his mental attitude.

REFERENCES

Aronson, Arnold E.: *Psychogenic Voice Disorders. An Interdisciplinary Approach to Detection, Diagnosis and Therapy.* Philadelphia, W. B. Saunders Co., 1973.

Aten, J. and Blanchard, M.: *EMG Biofeedback in the Treatment of Stuttering: Selected Case Studies.* Paper presented at the American Speech and Hearing Association Convention, Las Vegas, 1974.

Boone, Daniel R.: *The Voice and Voice Therapy.* Englewood Cliffs, Prentice-Hall, Inc., 1971.

Boone, Daniel R.: *The Voice and Voice Therapy.* Englewood Cliffs, Prentice-Hall, Inc., 1977.

Brodnitz, Friedrich S.: *Vocal Rehabilitation.* Rochester, Custom Printing, Inc., 1965.

Cooper, Morton: *Modern Techniques of Vocal Rehabilitation.* Springfield, Charles C Thomas, Publishers, 1973.

Cross, Douglas E.: Effects of false increasing, decreasing, and true electromyographic biofeedback on the frequency of stuttering. *Journal of*

Fluency Disorders, 2:109-116, 1977.

Curtis, J. F.: In Johnson, W. et al.: *Speech Handicapped School Children.* New York, Harper and Row, Publishers, 1967.

Darley, F. L.: *Diagnosis and Appraisal of Communication Disorders.* Englewood Cliffs, Prentice-Hall, Inc., 1965.

Denes, Peter B. and Pinson, Elliot N.: *The Speech Chain: The Biology of Spoken Language.* Garden City, Anchor Press, 1973.

Greene, Margaret C. L.: *The Voice and the Disorders.* Toronto, The Copp Clark Publishing Company, 1972.

Guitar, B.: Reduction of stuttering frequency using analog electromyographic feedback. *J Speech Hear Res,* 18:672-685, 1975.

Johnson, Thomas S.: *Vocal Abuse Reduction Program* (VARP). Department of Communicative Disorders, Utah State University, Logan, Utah, 1976.

Johnson, W.; Darley, F. L., Spriestersbach, D. C.: *Diagnostic Methods in Speech Pathology.* New York, Harper and Row, 1963.

Luchsinger, Richard and Arnold, Godfrey E.: *Voice-Speech Language: Clinical Communicology: Its Physiology and Pathology.* Belmont, Wadsworth Publishing Co., Inc., 1965.

Lyndes, Kellogg O.: *The Application of Biofeedback to Functional Dysphonia.* Paper presented at the Sixth Annual Biofeedback Research Society, Monterey, CA, 1975.

Moore, G. Paul: *Organic Voice Disorders.* Englewood Cliffs, Prentice-Hall, Inc., 1971.

Pelletier, Kenneth R.: *Mind as Healer, Mind as Slayer.* New York, Dell Publishing Company, 1977.

Schumacher, Walter: *Voice Therapy and Voice Improvement.* Springfield, Charles C Thomas, Publisher, 1974.

Sturlaugson, William R.: *Biofeedback and Psychogenic Voice Disorders: A General Review and Case Study.* Paper presented at the American Speech and Hearing Association Convention, Washington, 1975.

Van Riper, Charles: *Speech Correction: Principles and Methods.* Englewood Cliffs, Prentice-Hall, Inc., 1963.

CHAPTER 4

SUPPLEMENT

ALARYNGEAL PHONATION
Morris Val Jones, Ph.D.

As INDIVIDUALS APPROACH the older years, there is an increase in certain types of voice problems in addition to those which may plague persons at younger age levels. According to Jones (1957), the three most common voice problems of the older population are those associated with hearing loss (*see* Chap. 6), cerebral vascular accidents (CVA or "stroke," *see* Chap. 9), and carcinoma of the larynx. This last-named condition usually necessitates the removal of part or all of the larynx as a life-saving measure. With the improvement in surgical procedures connected with laryngectomy, there has been a steady acceleration in the laryngectomized population, as Gardner (1971) has observed:

> The increase in numbers of living laryngectomees has come from two sources. The first is the increasing survival rate as a result of improvements in surgery and medicine. The other factor stems from a marked increase of cancer of the throat in recent years. The American Cancer Society has reported that 3,000 laryngectomees yearly survive surgery for cancer of the larynx. The present estimate is that over 23,000 laryngectomees are living in the United States. (Introduction, P. xii)

Pretherapy

The speech/language clinician probably will not see the laryngectomized person until he/she has been cleared for therapy by the medical personnel. In some settings, the surgeon will request a presurgical session between the speech/language

88

clinician and the prospective laryngectomee. During this session, the clinician will explain the possibilities of speech after laryngectomy and answer questions related to speech rehabilitation. In some cities where there are local branches of the International Associations of Laryngectomees (usually called Lost Chord Club), laryngectomees who have developed intelligible speech may assume this responsibility. Whether to have a presurgical interview about speech rehabilitation, even if such personnel are available, remains with the patient. In some cases, the time between the diagnosis of carcinoma of the larynx and the surgery is so brief that arrangements for counseling cannot be scheduled.

The speech/language clinician needs to be aware of the extent of surgery because persons with radical neck dissection are likely to have greater difficulty in learning esophageal speech. With the excision of the larynx the passageway from the bronchi to the oral cavity is no longer intact; the upper end of the existing trachea is turned forward and sutured to the neck muscles. Respiration must henceforth be executed through the stoma (hole), and, naturally, does not provide subglottic pressure for articulation. The phonatory mechanism is missing, and a substitute must be found if articulate speech is to be developed. In hospital settings, the laryngectomized person can be referred to the speech/language clinician as soon as the musculature has healed sufficiently to sustain some exertion in speech rehabilitation. For those patients who did not have a presurgical speech session, the medical personnel might refer them for this information with the stipulation that speech rehabilitation should be delayed for further clearance. Surgical advances may eventually eliminate the necessity for speech therapy; at Northwestern University Medical School Dr. George Sisson, utilizing surgical techniques developed in Italy and Spain, has been able to circumvent the necessity for learning esophageal speech. Sisson made the following statement in a newspaper interview:

> We still take out the larynx and vocal cords—but instead of venting the windpipe stub through the front of the neck, we pull the windpipe up and suture it to the base of the tongue. We then slit the tongue slightly to allow air to pass. When the patient wants to talk, he exhales with more force than normal breathing. The out-

ward rush of air causes the soft folds of the tongue over the windpipe to vibrate much like the vocal cords would, and he's able to
fashion sounds easily and naturally. (*National Enquirer*, 1976)

Until this method of surgery is more generally available, traditional methods of speech rehabilitation need to be part of the
armamentarium of the speech/language clinician.

Speech Rehabilitation

Two basic forms of vocalization exist as substitutes for the
excised larynx: electrolarynx and/or esophageal speech.

ELECTROLARYNX. The most popular modern electrolarynx
has been developed by Bell Telephone Laboratories and is obtained at the local commercial departments of the Bell Telephone
Company. Gardner (1971) has described it as follows:

> Its battery-contained cylinder is shaped and tapered for the hand
> at one end and is enlarged at the other end to hold a round plastic
> diaphragm which lies on a 60-degree plane from the longitudinal
> axis. A knob-type switch controls a pitch-intensity range which
> enables the speaker to vary his speech for inflection, emphasis and
> stress, and which thereby gives him a more natural and less monot-
> onous speech than the older models. Two models are available, the
> higher-pitched one giving the female a more feminine voice. (P. 57)

At one time the use of the electrolarynx was considered to
be a last resort for those laryngectomees who were unable to
learn esophageal speech; a more recent attitude is to regard the
electrolarynx as a tool to be available either before or during
the learning of esophageal speech. The important fact is to
provide intelligible speech whenever it is needed, regardless of
the source of vibration.

ESOPHAGEAL SPEECH. Levin (1942) has written that the
mechanics upon which esophageal speech is based are relatively
simple. A comparison of the mechanics of normal speech and a
laryngectomized individual's speech indicates that the basic
essentials for producing sound are the same. In both cases a
flowing column of air from below vibrates mucous membrane
surfaces that are closely approximated, and this vibration produces a sound. Esophageal speech is different from "normal"
communication essentially because of the anatomical structures

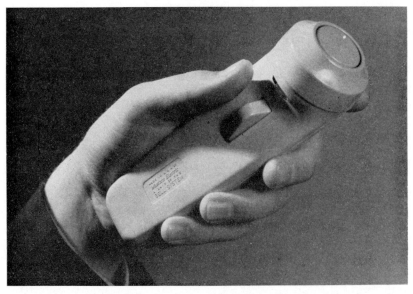

Figure 4-2a. Artificial larynx. Over 9,000 people who have lost their voices through paralysis or surgery have been aided to speak again with the help of an artificial larynx. The device is distributed on a nonprofit basis by the Bell Telephone Companies. Courtesy of the American Telephone and Telegraph Company.

that are used. Normally in exhalation, air from our lungs moves up through the narrow opening of the closely approximated and vibrating vocal folds. In the case of esophageal speech, the pocketed air in the upper esophagus moves upward through the closely approximated membranous surfaces of the vibrating cricopharyngeal sphincter, which is called the pseudoglottis, and into the hypopharynx. The produced sound is changed into speech by the articulatory structures which are left unchanged by the surgery (1952, p. 3-4).

Snidecor (1971) described briefly three methods of charging air into the esophagus: (1) the suction, "breathing," or inhalation method, (2) air injection by tongue and related structures, and (3) the glosso-pharyngeal press or plosive-injection method. Snidecor (1969) concluded that these three methods or at least two of the methods (Method 3 was not well known outside of

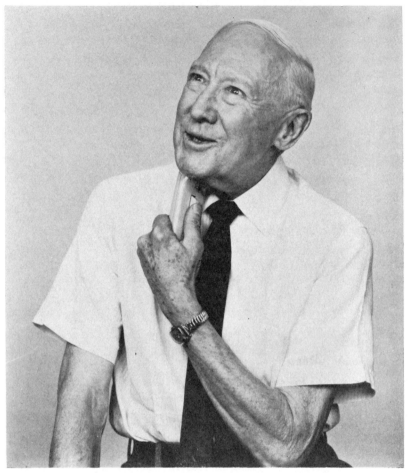

Figure 4-2b. Man with artificial larynx. Courtesy of American Telephone and Telegraph Company.

Holland until 1958) are usually used in combination and are usually used without any direct consciousness on the part of the esophageal speaker. He further noted that all three methods are valid, and he would not exclude any of them from therapy.

In his discussion of various methods of accomplishing air intake for esophageal speech, Boone (1971) described three, as follows:

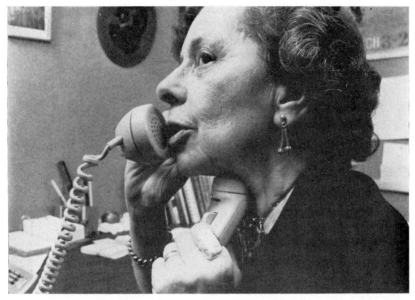

Figure 4-2c. Woman instructor. This laryngectomized instructor-patient uses esophageal speech, which is the intaking of air into the upper esophagus and forcing it up to vibrate the oral anatomy. This, coupled with normal tongue and lip movements, produces speech. The patient breathes through a stoma in the neck. The sound is low pitched and raspy, but totally intelligible. As an instructor, she prefers that the unit be held with the vibrator button at the top with the thumb near the base of the button. She is also able to show others how the lips should be used for the clearest pronunciation. Courtesy of the American Telephone and Telegraph Company.

1. The swallow method. In the swallow method the patient opens his mouth, then closes his mouth, then swallows air with his lips closed, and then quickly opens his mouth again.

2. The inhalation method. In the inhalation method, the patient is able to introduce air directly into the esophagus when he takes in a normal pulmonary inhalation.

3. The injection method. The injection method is used by the largest number of esophageal speakers. . . . This method is achieved by trapping or squeezing air between the tongue and the hard and soft palate and pharynx, forcing the compressed air mass backward into the hypopharynx. If the esophagus is open at this time, the air will rush into the esophagus and be entrapped there for phonation. (Pp. 216-217)

Boone indicated that whichever method worked best for the patient was the one the clinician should use, although he did note that the injection method worked best when used in conjunction with early training in use of the artificial larynx.

Snidecor (1969) wrote that ". . . psychological factors are in the main more important than physiological factors when it comes to acquiring a new voice" (p. 168). Stoll (1958) also recognized the psychological factors and listed postoperative fears of laryngectomees:

> (1) The fear of the recurrence of the cancer, hence the continued fear of death. (2) Fears due to the new physiological relationships resulting from the laryngectomy. (3) The fear of old age which has been aggravated by the feeling of uselessness resulting from the loss of speech. The loss of earning power further contributes to this feeling of uselessness. (4) Fear of being unable to re-establish old patterns of interpersonal relationships. (5) The fears associated with the anticipation of failing to learn a new method of speaking. (Pp. 550-551)

These fears, as noted by Snidecor (1969), could result in tension in the esophagus. The tension might inhibit the acquisition of esophageal speech which the laryngectomee is already afraid he will not be able to learn. This destructive circular process should not be allowed to start or continue, and the clinician should be responsible for controlling it.

Green (1975) recorded twenty-five common, one-syllable words as articulated by each of ten laryngectomized adults. The first trial was produced at a normal vocal intensity level, and the second trial was produced at an increased vocal intensity of at least 10 decibels. Twenty beginning students in speech pathology evaluated the taped speech samples and recorded their responses on answer sheets provided for them. According to statistical analysis of these data, increased vocal intensity provides far greater intelligibility of these one-syllable words. The significance of this finding can be translated into practical use by the clinician who plans the speech rehabilitation of laryngectomized individuals. Before discharge of the patient, emphasis can be placed on increased volume as a part of the program for improving intelligibility.

Information about the acceptability of various types of

alaryngeal speech was studied by Bennett and Weinberg (1973). Their experiment looked at the vocal attributes which differentiate good and poor esophageal speakers. They found that the following characteristics were common to all highly proficient laryngectomized speakers:

> . . . they spoke fluently and with continuity. Their speech was easily understood and naturally produced without apparent thought or effort. The esophageal speakers evidenced minimal respiratory and air intake noise and had short latencies between air intake and esophageal phonation. (P. 609)

SUMMARY. With the large laryngectomized population, methods of speech rehabilitation will continue to be vital unless advanced surgical procedures make the services of the speech/language clinician obsolete. The following listing, based on a compilation by Gardner (1971, p. 61), shows the advantages and disadvantages of electrolaryngeal speech as contrasted to esophageal speech.

Advantages
1. Permits prompt speech at any time
2. Gives early oral communication for patient
3. Prevents fatigue when conditions demand loud speech or extensive talking
4. Is free of grimaces, stoma noise, burps
5. Voice has more uniform quality; is less raucous; is more acceptable

Disadvantages
1. It is a constant reminder of a disability
2. It attracts unwanted attention and curiosity
3. Requires the use of one hand
4. Sound of instrument does not resemble natural human speech
5. Is a sign of defeat, inability to learn esophageal speech

Lauder (1970) decided to take a second look at the use of the electrolarynx. He concluded that the electrolarynx continues to be a poor substitute for the human voice, but that it can be a useful aid to the new laryngectomee. He summarizes by writing that the electrolarynx may prove effective in the following cases:

1. To provide increased volume for a patient in specific circumstances in which esophageal speech is unsatisfactory, for example, a noisy restaurant

2. To permit the patient to communicate with the clinician and with other patients during the early stages of esophageal speech instruction

3. To assist laryngectomized persons who have difficulty on the telephone (P. 64)

REFERENCES

Boone, Daniel R.: *The Voice and Voice Therapy*, 2nd ed. Englewood Cliffs, Prentice-Hall, Inc., 1977.

Gardner, Warren H.: *Laryngectomee Speech and Rehabilitation*. Springfield, Charles C Thomas, 1971.

Green, Deborah L.: *A Study of the Effect of Vocal Intensity on the Intelligibility of Esophageal Speech*. Master's thesis, California State University, Sacramento, CA, 1975.

Jones, Morris Val: Speech problems of older adults. *Newsletter of National Gerontological Society*, September, 1957.

Lauder, Edmond: The laryngectomee and the artificial larynx: A second look. *J Speech Hear Disord*, 35:(1), 62-66, 1970.

Levin, Nathaniel M.: Speech rehabilitation after total removal of larynx. *JAMA, 149*:1281-1286, 1952.

Snidecor, John C.: Speech without a larynx. In Travis, Lee Edward (Ed.): *Handbook of Speech Pathology and Audiology*. New York, Appleton-Century-Crofts, 1971.

Snidecor, John C. (Ed.): *Speech Rehabilitation of the Laryngectomized*. Springfield, Charles C Thomas, 1969.

Stoll, B.: Psychological factors determining the success or failure of the rehabilitation program of laryngectomized patients. *Ann Otol Rhinol Laryngol*, 67:550-557, 1958.

CHAPTER 5

STUTTERING

Frederick Pemberton Murray, Ph.D.

THERE ARE VARIOUS forms of dysrythmia, such as cluttering, stuttering, and bilingualism, but stuttering has always received the most emphasis. The disorder of speech flow known as stuttering is an extremely complex one. Indeed, the fact that it has been known almost as far back as recorded history indicates its long-standing tenacity.

Theories of Etiology

One cannot consider it surprising that at the present time so many divergent theories about the nature and cause of stuttering exist. This is true because any individual theorist is the product of his own particular experiences, observations, and training. A theorist whose training has been along psychological or psychoanalytical lines is likely to interpret stuttering as being a symptom of repressed conflicts, perhaps centering around such themes as oral or anal eroticism. A person with a background of training in learning theory will probably view the disorder as one involving the laws of learning and therefore will call it learned behavior. Another, indoctrinated in the area of neurology, will explain stuttering in terms of disintegration of the central nervous system (Bryngelson, 1966).

No matter what viewpoint one holds with regard to this age-old, baffling disorder, it is well to hold in mind three concepts: (1) that anatomical structure precedes physiologic function, (2) that behavior of a disintegrative type usually is not found to have one single isolated cause, and (3) that emotional reactions to one's own failure to function normally can precipitate further breakdown of such physiologic functioning.

97

Symptomotology

The distinguishing characteristics of stuttering are fixative (stoppage) and repetitive interruptions, frequently of distorted rhythm, occurring in the flow of speech during the act of speaking. These breaks in the forward-moving sequence appear intermittently, are of an involuntary nature and cannot, in the true sense, be duplicated at will. Stuttering seems, therefore, to be a difference in the *type* or *kind* of speaking rather than merely a variation in the dysfluent behaviors found at times in the speech of virtually all persons.

Further evidence that there are probably more than psychological factors involved in stuttering is suggested by the following two irrefutable facts: (1) the ratio of male to female stutterers is about five to one, (2) stuttering is often found to run in families. With regard to the latter, it should be mentioned that currently (1977) at Yale Medical School extensive research is being undertaken focusing upon the role of genetics in stuttering. It has been reported that, to date, the findings suggest a definite possibility that genetic factors are operating in many cases.

Observers have been impressed by the variability found in stuttering behavior. The symptoms often appear and disappear dramatically in different types of situations involving speech. It is obvious that the difficulty is aggravated by psychological factors and that both a theory of and a therapy for stuttering must take these into account. Certain theorists have gone so far as to say that definite proof of the totally psychic nature of the malady is demonstrated by the stutterer not stuttering when talking to himself or in talking to infants or to animals. Here let it be mentioned that a victim of epilepsy, known to be an organic abnormality, is less likely to undergo a seizure when alone or when relaxed. Emotional pressures, not unlike those present in many oral communication situations, can trigger a spasmodic response that is probably an overt sign of a deficit within the system of the person.

In light of what has been said, it is stated, as was at one time indicated by Robert West, that stuttering is seen probably to be caused by a weakness, as yet undiscovered, within the human organism. Stuttering is perpetuated and maintained by

(1) a continuation of that weakness, (2) by a morbid awareness of it, or (3) both of these factors. It is with regard to the second factor that many procedures have been developed and found to be useful in preventing the emergence of an overguarded type of "speech conscience." Some of these will be discussed later.

Investigations using hypnosis have revealed that language habits, both oral and written, change during the course of a person's lifetime. Concentrated efforts to alter them usually accelerate the process of change. However, the preexisting habits remain imbedded in the organism and are capable of being reactivated under deep hypnosis. It is very likely, therefore, that old speech/motor patterns are superseded by new ones but are never erased by them. Stutterers can learn to speak fluently, but the record of stuttering is never totally eliminated from the depths of their organism and can, under adverse and stressful conditions, occasionally reappear (Kopp, 1956).

The persistence of stuttering is often very great. This is not to be wondered at when speech is considered to be the mirror of the soul, the key item in the person's active relationship with his environment. If the disorder continues beyond adolescence, it is probable that it will be deeply entangled in the expanding web of social development. In the later stages it becomes entwined as a vine in the branches of a tree and has often become obsessive and compulsive in character. Countless cues and experiences of motor speech failure combine to create powerful forces that make it a self-reinforcing, vicious circle. It is then all but impossible to separate cause from effect, and therapy takes into account mainly those facets of the disorder that can be assessed and evaluated with some degree of accuracy.

Fortunately, however, it has been found that about three out of every four cases of stuttering in childhood recover by the age of eight. At present, factors responsible for this occurrence are not understood. When they might be known, we shall be able to be more effective in eradicating this problem. In the meantime, there is much that can be done to increase the possibilities of a young stutterer emerging with fluent speech. The following paragraphs contain information that over the years has been found to be helpful in the management of the young stutterer.

Management

Due to the fact that speech is a complicated motor act that has been superimposed upon a mechanism that was originally intended for more primitive biological functions, it is clearly apparent that a state of good overall physical condition is of prime importance. The stuttering child should receive a thorough physical examination from a physician. Any deficiencies should receive proper attention and treatment and, if possible, be corrected. In the case of the child, stuttering seems to come in waves of heightened severity. If the child is below par physically and is short on sleep, speech symptoms that otherwise might be absent or less intense may greatly increase. The stutterer usually needs more rest than the normal-speaking child.

Nutrition is another matter that deserves careful attention. The diet should be well balanced. Often a child with dysfluent speech is somewhat overactive. Certain cases may be in need of some type of sedative, which, of course, must be recommended by and prescribed by a physician.

Research has demonstrated that in some stutterers there may be a relationship between the degree of brain dominance and speech ability. It is believed that, in general, the higher the amount of dominance by one of the two cerebral hemispheres in the control of bodily motor acts, the more integrated is the speech flow. If a stutterer with high amounts of speech dysrhythm possesses any one or more of the following three conditions, it is advisable that he receive a thorough examination from a neurologist:

1. Ambidexterity
   This pertains to a highly mixed use of the body extremities to carry out motor acts; for example: The left hand is used for crayon and scissor work, while the right hand is used for eating and for opening doors.
2. Forced Shifting
   There has been a history of forced shifting from the use of one hand to the use of another.
3. Severe Incoordination
   There is much evidence of gross motor incoordination and awkwardness in performing body motor tasks.

Some childhood cases of stuttering who displayed these conditions have improved very rapidly, or have recovered, when the neurologist's recommendations for better management have been carefully followed. Sometimes this advice has called for efforts to attempt to build up a "compensatory" sidedness pattern; that is, encouraging the use of one arm to accomplish motor tasks.

One of the most vital areas to consider with regard to the child stutterer is that of environmental stress. Anything that tends to reduce stress on him is likely to have a beneficial effect on his speech. It is for this reason that mention is to be made here of some key factors that often may precipitate stuttering blocks. It is necessary to make a thorough and comprehensive study of the total environment in order to try to identify such situations. At the outset, it is wise to prepare a written list of words on which stuttering blocks occur, the communicative situation in which they arose, and the possible pressures that might be behind them. It is imperative that, once discovered, real efforts be made to reduce or minimize these situations in order to remove the pressures involved. The following are some of the frequently found speech conflicts that may need modification:

1. Hurrying the child
2. Requiring oral communication when he is excited or very tired
3. Having him "perform" in front of others
4. Interrupting him when he is talking
5. Implying disapproval of his speech by look or gestures
6. Talking for the child when he stutters
7. Suggesting other ways of talking
8. Advising that he breathe differently
9. Forcing confession of guilt
10. Using inappropriate disciplinary action. (Van Riper, 1973)

Remember—the stutterer, when stuttering, is acting according to the dictates of his organism, and even though these behaviors may not appeal to the whims of the parental or adult ego, it is imperative that interference with them be held to an absolute minimum. Many of these cited speech conflicts may not appear to be of much significance, but each one carries within it a potential force that can increase the occurrence and severity of stuttering and may hasten the development of struggle reactions and overwhelming fears of speaking. These, when full blown, present a complex, self-perpetuating disorder that is almost impossible for a normal speaker to conceive.

The speech therapist working with young cases of stuttering usually has a two-pronged task to carry out: counseling the parents of stutterers and advising the classroom teacher about management of the disorder in the school situation. With regard to the former, it is well to keep in mind the principles, already alluded to, that deal with modification of environmental pressures. Suggestions as to how to improve the atmosphere of the home in general have been found helpful. Parents and others in the home should be encouraged to use relatively slow, unhurried speech when communicating to their stuttering child. Complex vocabulary should be held to a minimum. Often, it is advisable to use self-talk, a term used to denote the adult using a slow, simple form of relaxed speech to describe what he is doing, as the child listens. Parallel talk, whereby the adult uses such speech to communicate with the child about what the child is doing at that moment, is another means of providing a model of slow and easy speech. Provided with enough models of this type of speech, the child is very likely to absorb and emulate them. Similarly, in any situations involving storytelling or oral reading, this simplified form of speech should be used. Parents should be certain that the last oral communication situation of the day, usually that one that is taking place just prior to the child's falling asleep, is of an utterly calm and unhurried nature. The child must feel loved and wanted. Such methods of simple give-and-take talk will enhance a desire to participate in communication.

In the Classroom

With regard to the classroom teacher and her role in the handling of the stutterer, some important concepts can be mentioned. First of all, one of the most terrifying of recollections in most adult stutterers is that of their humiliating experiences connected with oral recitations in the school classroom during the childhood years. It behooves the teacher, therefore, to do whatever she can to minimize the probability of significant speech failure for the stutterer. One way, of course, which many teachers are tempted to use, is not to call on him for any oral participation whatsoever. This is usually most unwise. It only serves to convince the child that he is different and engenders a habit of avoiding and giving up. Remembering the saying that "compressed metal springs carry the greatest potential for release force," we can logically speculate that inhibiting dreaded action does not eradicate future fearful expression of it. It is far better, therefore, that the stutterer be allowed to express himself, but almost always within the scope of one or more of the following limits:

1. Calling on the stutterer randomly rather than doing it in an order of sequence where he sees his turn coming
2. Requiring only short answers rather than extended discussions
3. Putting oral recitation on a voluntary basis
4. Having the stutterer recite on topics about which he feels secure
5. Encouraging the feeling that he is being allowed rather than forced to speak.

Stutterers are frequently mocked and made fun of by their young classmates and friends. It is often worthwhile to counsel the stutterer about these matters and to suggest to him various means of coping with such situations when they arise. By teaching him how to display a casual, seemingly indifferent attitude, the therapist can fortify the child against feeding the wrong kind of psychological bait to his listeners. Most teasing and ridicule cease when the perpetrators are confronted with such a nonchalant attitude.

Almost all that has been said thus far pertains to the child whose fluency breaks are such that there is little doubt about their being stuttering or, at least, noticeably different behavior capable of provoking reactions of associates. Mention should be made here of another situation which is commonly encountered between the ages of three and four. During this period, most children go through what has been termed the "normal stage of dysfluency." The breaks in speech are usually characterized by excessive rhythmical repetitions and, occasionally, some prolongations. If no attention is focused on them, they almost always cease within a short period of time. In our culture, however, with standards of speech fluency being what they are, certain parents are inclined to make an issue of these behaviors. If such practices continue and if the child is of a sensitive nature, he may interiorize the comments and suggestions made about his way of talking and may start to try hard to speak better, in fact, far too hard. It is speculated in some quarters that stuttering problems may arise and later become fixed reactions due to the overemphasis originally placed upon normal dysfluencies. Regardless of whether we are dealing with apparent true stuttering beginnings or with the often-encountered variations in fluency, it is very important for the persons in the child's environment not to react in ways which promote uneasiness, doubt, and potential fear.

In summarizing the approaches to handling the young child, it can be stated that they are almost always indirect and are aimed at eliminating or modifying those factors, particularly those of stress, that have been found to be frequently associated with increases in stuttering behavior. The outlook for the young stutterer is very good, provided that effective changes can be made in his environment and his system is not overtaxed with demands that far exceed its ability to cope with them.

The Older Stutterer

Therapy with the older stutterer, whose anomoly has been present for a long time and which has accumulated self-reinforcing strength, is a very time-consuming and challenging task. Sometimes there is not too much apparent shift in speech functioning. Nevertheless, near-recoveries and major improvements in speech have been attained in adult cases. Therapy of this type tests the qualities of the therapist to the utmost. For the confirmed adult stutterer, the major goal of therapy is that of reducing the gross abnormality and developing ways to stutter that are essentially fluent. The stutterer somehow must arrive at the conviction that he can speak with sufficient communicative fluency. This conviction, to be effective, has to be so deeply implanted that it reflects itself in the automaticity of his verbal output. The therapist acts as a catalyst in the therapy procedure, but whatever is accomplished is the result of direct efforts by the stutterer himself. In recent times, operant conditioning procedures have been incorporated into various intensive therapy programs for stuttering. Under this type of treatment, the stutterer must focus constant directed efforts on his behavior and the shaping of it.

Just as there are many roads leading to Rome, there are numerous avenues by which the goal of adequate fluency may be reached. In general, it can be said that most adult stutterers need therapeutic efforts to be directed along the following lines:

1. Familiarization with the chief habit patterns that block the flow of speech;

2. Motivation to do things to change these behaviors so that other choices of response may become possible;

3. Recognition of and alterations made in habitual patterns of avoidance of words and speaking situations;

4. Changes in self-evaluative processes that result in improved concepts of his person;

5. De-emphasis of self-punishment.

The handicapping part of stuttering consists of those aspects of the problem that have come about mainly because of the reactions of the stutterer to his condition. While it appears likely that the core roots of the disorder are firmly lodged somewhere in the neurophysiological maze of the complicated human organism, experience has shown that useful and worthwhile fluency, often approaching so-called "normal," can be achieved when most of the learned habits that have, through conditioning, been superimposed upon originally simple short stuttering interruptions are reduced or eliminated by use of one or more widely accepted therapy techniques. In extremely severe cases, the judicious use of voluntary stuttering, often involving the deliberate repetition of many initial syllables, known as "bouncing," may be indicated to break up deeply rooted struggle reactions that impair the possibility of the speech mechanism acting as a coordinated whole during speaking. It is assumed that as the case progresses in speech fluency, he will come less and less to rely on any speaking technique, per se, and eventually will be able to devote almost full attention to the content of his automatic speech.

No stutterer will make permanent gains if he is habitually avoiding many words and speaking situations. The old saying, "nothing ventured, nothing gained," applies very appropriately to this. A constant effort must be maintained to help enable the stutterer to move forward in this regard. Advances along these lines, even at the temporary price of stuttering created thereby, are to be rewarded, while the illusion of apparent fluency that is brought about by repeated use of contrived avoidance behaviors is to be discouraged. Also, distraction devices, such as arm swinging or foot stomping, have proved to be ineffective.

Psychotherapy of all types, running from simple counseling techniques to the deep analytic therapy of Freud, has been extensively used with stutterers. The results have been, for the most part, far from satisfactory. Such therapy seems to leave unaltered those cues associated with word and situation fears that typically constitute a large portion of the adult stutterer's handicap. Occasionally, a few cases are encountered where psychotherapy is indeed indicated because of deep resistances and conflicts. In these cases, it can be an effective means of preparing the way for future self-confrontation and successful speech therapy. Most cases seemingly do not need deep psychotherapy, and group therapies using mental hygiene approaches as an adjunct to ongoing speech therapy are sufficient.

It is highly doubtful that the stutterer in the advanced stages of the disorder will emerge as a highly fluent, skilled speaker. It is better, therefore, to maintain a self-concept that acknowledges, among its many varying roles, that of "stutterer" and thus not feel obliged to be defensive about any residual speech interruptions that may occur from time to time, especially in stressful oral communication situations.

As Charles Van Riper has repeatedly stated, it is possible to "stutter" a thousand times a day and still be fluent within "normal" limits. The stutterer who comes to realize this will gain a feeling of triumph and a workable solution for the problem that troubled Demosthenes!

Cluttering

A form of dysfluency that is often confused with stuttering is cluttering. Although it has been described briefly by almost every nineteenth century encyclopedist, the first complete volume devoted to cluttering appeared in 1963, written by Richard Luchsinger of the Zurich University Medical School. In 1964

Charles Van Riper edited the Prentice-Hall Foundations of Speech Pathology Series and included *Cluttering* by Deso A. Weiss, who described the condition as follows:

> Cluttering is a speech disorder characterized by the clutterer's unawareness of his disorder, by a short attention span, by disturbances in perception, articulation and formulation of speech and often by excessive speed of delivery. It is a disorder of the thought processes preparatory to speech and based on a hereditary predisposition. Cluttering is the verbal manifestation of Central Language Imbalance, which affects all channels of communication (e.g., reading, writing, rhythm, and musicality) and behavior in general. (P. 1)

Luchsinger and Arnold (1965) discussed in detail the differences between stuttering and cluttering and summarized their findings in a chart. Selected items are presented in Table 5-I.

Differential diagnosis between stuttering and cluttering became the basis of a professional controversy in the area of mental retardation. Charles Van Riper (1963) has used statistics which indicated that 20 percent of the mentally retarded population were stutterers; Martyn, Sheehan, and Slutz (1969) challenged the validity of this statement:

> Nothing we know about the social psychology of stuttering should be specially predictive of intellectual factors as major elements of the disorder. . . . If stuttering is related to retardation, then groups of stutterers should be expected to show a tendency toward the low side of IQ measurements. (P. 206-207)

They subsequently examined 500 retarded patients in Camarillo State Hospital, California. These patients ranged in age from 14 to 73 (mean of 26.4) and had levels of retardation from IQ of 6 to IQ of 79 (mean of 35.3). The researchers reached the following conclusion: "A central finding of this study was that on a cross-validity sample, the incidence of stuttering among the retarded was no different from that in the population generally" (p. 210). Van Riper (1972) hypothesized that many of the retarded individuals who had originally been classified as stutterers were probably, in fact, clutterers. Further research is needed to establish criteria for these sub-areas of dysfluency; such differential diagnosis is important because appropriate remediation techniques vary according to the diagnosis.

TABLE 5-I

DIFFERENCES BETWEEN STUTTERING AND CLUTTERING

Characteristics	Stuttering	Cluttering
Onset	Usually sudden, in childhood, or after traumatic events	Always gradual, following developmental language disorders
Aptitudes	Good to superior in most areas	Superior in sciences and mathematics but poor in languages
Musical talent	Average to superior	Usually very poor, and tone deaf
Physical findings	Normal, or vegetative dystonia, allergic tendencies	Congenital dyspraxia
Spontaneous speech	Clonic or tonic blocks, parakinesias, grimaces	Rapid, jerky, truncated, repetitive, stumbling
Consciousness of defect	Greatly concerned	Unconcerned and disinterested
Calling attention to speech	Aggravates	Improves

William Perkins (1977) has summarized the difficulties as follows: "Viewed from the behavior standpoint, to capture a difference between stuttering and cluttering is like trying to bottle fog: It evaporates when enclosed within the confines of explicit definitions" (p. 324).

REFERENCES

Beech, H. R. and Fransella, F.: *Research and Experiment in Stuttering.* New York, Pergamon, 1968.

Bloodstein, Oliver: Stuttering. *J Speech Hear Disord, 42*:(2), 148-151, 1977.

Brutten, E. J. and Shoemaker, D. J.: *The Modification of Stuttering.* Englewood Cliffs, Prentice-Hall, 1967.

Bryngelson, B.: *Clinical Group Therapy for Problem People.* Minneapolis, Denison, 1966.

Chapman, Ann Held and Cooper, Eugene B.: The nature of stuttering in a mentally retarded population. *Am J Ment Defic,* 78:153-157, 1973.

Eisenson, J. (Ed.): *Stuttering: A Second Symposium.* New York, Harper and Row, 1975.

Freeman, F. J. and Ushijima, T.: Laryngeal activity accompanying the moment of stuttering: A preliminary report of EMG investigations. *Journal of Fluency Disorders, 1*:36-45, 1975.

Gordon, T.: *Parent Effectiveness Training.* New York, Peter H. Wyden, 1970.

Gregory, H. H.: *Stuttering: Differential Evaluation and Theory.* Indianapolis, Bobbs-Merrill, 1972.

Johnson, W.: *Stuttering and What You Can Do About It.* Minneapolis, University of Minnesota Press, 1961.

Kopp, G.: In Hahn, E.: *Stuttering-Significant Theories and Therapies,* 2nd ed. Stanford, Stanford University Press, 1956.

Levy, C. M. and Bowers, D.: Hemispheric asymmetry of reaction time in a dichotic discrimination task. *Cortex, 10*:18-25, 1974.

Luchsinger, Richard and Arnold Godfrey E.: *Voice-Speech-Language.* Belmont, Wadsworth Publishing Co., 1965.

Luper, H. and Mulder, R.: *Stuttering Therapy for Children.* Englewood Cliffs, Prentice-Hall, 1965.

Martin, R. and Ingham, R.: Stuttering. In Lahey, B. (Ed.): *The Modification of Language Behavior.* Springfield, Charles C Thomas, 1973.

Martyn, M. M.; Sheehan, Joseph, and Slutz, Karen: Incidence of stuttering and other speech disorders among the retarded. *A J Ment Defic,* 74:206-211, 1969.

Murray, F. P.: Observations on therapy for stuttering in Japan. *J Speech Hear Disord,* 23:243-249, 1958.

Perkins, W. H.: *Speech Pathology,* 2nd ed. St. Louis, The C. V. Mosby Co., 1977.

Sheehan, J. F.: *Stuttering: Research and Therapy.* New York, Harper and Row, 1970.

Starkweather, C.: Analysis of a controversy in stuttering. *Journal of Fluency Disorders,* 1:10-21, 1974.

Travis, L. E. (Ed.): *Handbook of Speech Pathology and Audiology.* New York, Appleton-Century-Crofts, 1971.

Van Riper, Charles: *The Nature of Stuttering.* Englewood Cliffs, Prentice-Hall, Inc., 1971.

————: *Speech Correction,* 4th ed. Englewood Cliffs, Prentice-Hall, Inc., 1963.

————: *The Treatment of Stuttering.* Englewood Cliffs, Prentice-Hall, Inc., 1973.

Weiss, Deso A.: *Cluttering.* Englewood Cliffs, Prentice-Hall, Inc., 1964.

West, Robert: An agnostic's speculations about stuttering. In Eisenson, J. (Ed.): *Stuttering: A Symposium.* New York, Harper and Row, 1958.

Wingate, Marcel E.: *Stuttering: Theory and Treatment.* New York, Irvington Pub., Inc., 1976.

CHAPTER 6

HEARING LOSS AND DEAFNESS

JAMES H. McCARTNEY, PH.D.

T HE SPEECH AND language problems discussed in this book involve all avenues of reception, integration, and expression, but it is through hearing, more than any other sense, that one receives, comprehends, and communicates ideas. Any loss of hearing, then, would hinder the reception of language and ultimately an individual's ability to communicate. Because most of the speech and hearing clinician's therapy incorporates testing, giving directions, reinforcing appropriate behavior, modifying speech sounds, and building language, and because the usual avenue for administering or modifying each is hearing, each person in the clinician's case load must have had a hearing test.

But what is a hearing test, or a hearing loss for that matter? How significant a problem is hearing loss? What effect does the loss have on the individual and communication? Answering these questions will comprise the core of this chapter.

What Is a Hearing Loss?

Audiometrically

Hearing loss can generally be defined as any impairment in the auditory pathway affecting the sensitivity and/or perception of auditory signals. The most common signals for measuring hearing are either tones of varying pitches or speech. One measures hearing by using an audiometer (*see* Fig. 6-1) and recording the results for each ear on an audiogram (*see* Fig. 6-2).

The measurement of hearing loss for tones is recorded in decibels, abbreviated "dB," on the hearing threshold level (HL) dial on the audiometer. Zero dB on the audiometer dial is an average threshold hearing level based on normal-hearing

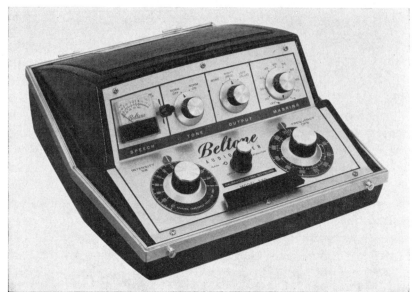

Figure 6-1a. A commercial portable audiometer. Courtesy of Beltone Electronics.

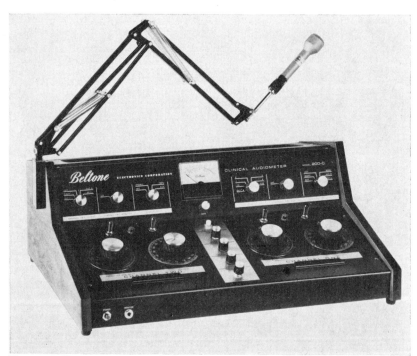

Figure 6-1b. A commercial diagnostic audiometer. Courtesy of Beltone Electronics.

SPEECH AND HEARING CENTER
CALIFORNIA STATE UNIVERSITY, SACRAMENTO

AUDIOLOGICAL EVALUATION

NAME_____ AGE_____ DATE_____

ADDRESS_____ PHONE_____

REFERRED BY_____ TESTED BY_____ AUDIOMETER_____

Audiogram
Frequency

MODALITY	RIGHT	BOTH	LEFT
Air Conduction			
Unmasked	O		X
Masked	△		◻
No Response (Unmasked)			
No Response (Masked)			
Bone Conduction			
Unmasked	<		>
Masked	C		コ
No Response (Unmasked)			
No Response (Masked)			
Sound Field		S	
No response		S	

KEY

ANSI (1969) Standards

Masking Levels	250	500	1000	2000	3000	4000	6000	8000
Air								
Bone								

White Noise_____ Live Voice_____
NB Noise _____ Tape _____
Recording _____
Speech Material_____
Reliability_____

	PTA (A/C)		SRT	MCL	T.D.
RIGHT	2 Freq.☐				
	3 Freq.☐				
LEFT	2 Freq.☐				
	3 Freq.☐				
BIN ☐	2 Freq.☐				
S.F.☐	3 Freq.☐				
Phones ☐					

	SPEECH DISCRIMINATION (PERCENT CORRECT)					
	Score%	@	Score%	@	Score%	@
RIGHT		List		List		List
MASKING						
LEFT		@		@		@
		List		List		List
MASKING						
BIN. ☐		@		@		@
S.F.☐						
PHONES ☐		List		List		List

Figure 6-2. Audiogram worksheet.

young adults. Although various audiology texts divide the severity of loss into different categories, a compromise scale for normal to profound hearing loss is presented below in dB HL.

Normal	0– 25 dB
Mild	30– 45
Moderate	50– 65
Severe	70– 85
Profound	90–110

The measurement of hearing loss for speech is recorded in percent and is usually indicative of the number of correctly perceived single syllable words a person repeats back to the examiner. For example, if a list of fifty words were administered and the patient missed ten words, then he correctly perceived forty words, or 80 percent. A general guide interpreting speech discrimination ability is as follows:

Normal	90–100%
Mild	80– 89
Moderate	70– 79
Poor	50– 69
Very Poor	0– 49

Summarizing the previous information, one can see that a hearing loss may be defined audiometrically if sensitivity is below or poorer than 25 dB HL and speech discrimination ability is below or poorer than 90 percent. Unfortunately, hearing loss is much more complicated than a few numbers or percentages describing the degree of loss. Hearing loss is also described according to anatomy (site of lesion), when the loss occurred (time of onset), and whether one or both ears are affected.

Anatomy

As seen in Figure 6-3, the ear may be grossly divided into four divisions: the outer ear, middle ear, inner ear, and central auditory system. Each division has its unique anatomy, mode of operation, and function. Although extensive description of anatomy and physiology is not warranted in an introductory

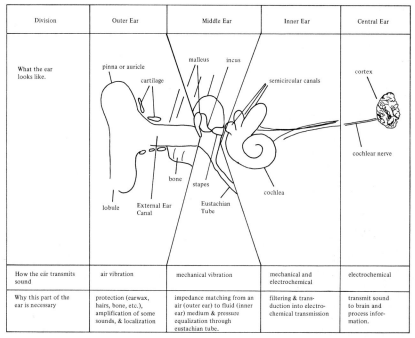

Division	Outer Ear	Middle Ear	Inner Ear	Central Ear
What the ear looks like.				
How the ear transmits sound	air vibration	mechanical vibration	mechanical and electrochemical	electrochemical
Why this part of the ear is necessary	protection (earwax, hairs, bone, etc.), amplification of some sounds, & localization	impedance matching from an air (outer ear) to fluid (inner ear) medium & pressure equalization through eustachian tube.	filtering & trans-duction into electro-chemical transmission	transmit sound to brain and process infor-mation.

Figure 6-3. Cross section of the ear showing how the ear transmits sound and the necessity of each division.

text, a simplified discussion will enable the reader to appreciate the complexity of hearing and the difficulties experienced by the hard-of-hearing and deaf.

OUTER EAR. The ear is assisted, albeit minimally, in the collection of sound waves by the pinna or auricle of the outer ear. From the pinna, the sound waves travel through the external auditory meatus, down the external auditory canal, and terminate at the tympanic membrane or eardrum. If one were to cut the ear longitudinally, as in Figure 6-3, a distinct division would be noted; about one half of the one-inch canal is composed of cartilaginous tissue and about one-half is composed of bone from the skull. Because there is no soft tissue and cartilage under the bony part, any scratch or pimple occurring on the bony canal near the eardrum would be more painful than that occurring on the cartilaginous portion.

The primary purpose of the external ear is to conduct airborne vibrations to the middle ear. Any blockage in the outer ear is therefore called a conductive hearing loss. The external ear functions to protect the middle ear from dust and bugs by hairs and earwax (cerumen); to amplify sounds in the region of 3,800 cycles per second (abbreviated Hertz or Hz), the natural resonating frequency of the ear canal; and to localize sound.

A loss in the outer ear alone usually decreases the loudness of a signal, but as soon as the sound is made loud enough it is usually heard quite distinctly and clearly. A conductive hearing impairment due to pathology in the outer ear is quite amenable to medical treatment.

MIDDLE EAR: The middle ear cavity, Figure 6-4, lies primarily between the tympanic membrane and the bony wall opposite it, behind which is the cochlea of the inner ear. From this middle ear cavity or tympanum, there are openings into the porous bone behind the pinna (mastoid process of the temporal bone), into

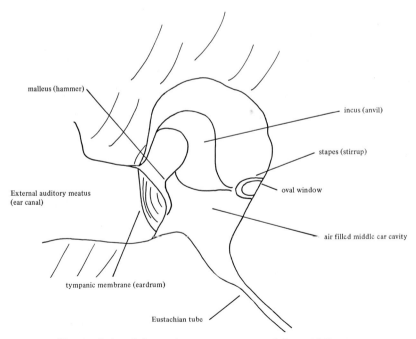

Figure 6-4. Schematic representation of the middle ear.

the inner ear via the stapes footplate in the oval window, and into the region above the nasal portion of the throat (nasopharynx) via the Eustachian or auditory tube. Through the Eustachian tube, air passes to equalize the pressure on either side of the eardrum. Equalization of air pressure is sometimes characterized by a "click" after swallowing as one's car ascends a steep mountain, or as the pressure builds in an airplane.

The middle ear cavity is traversed by the three smallest bones in the human body: the malleus, incus, and stapes. These bones are collectively called *ossicles* and are suspended in space by three means: (1) by ligaments, (2) by the attachment of the malleus to the eardrum and the stapes to the oval window, and (3) by two small muscles. The two muscles of the middle ear are the tensor tympani and the stapedius. The tensor tympani arises anteriorly near the Eustachian tube orifice and connects by means of a tendon to the maleus. The stapedius arises from the posterior part of the cavity and connects on the head of the stapes by means of a tendon. The primary purpose of the stapedius is protective in nature in that it contracts in reaction to loud sound. This contraction stiffens the ossicular chain and impedes the sound conducted from the outer to the inner ear, thus helping to prevent hearing loss caused by high intensity sounds which reach the inner ear.

Normal sound transmission causes pressure variations in air to move the tympanic membrane, and since the malleus is attached to the eardrum and each bone to one another, any movement of the eardrum causes movement of all three bones. Any blockage or obstruction in the middle ear to sound conducted in mechanical vibrations of the middle ear bones creates a conductive hearing loss. A conductive loss in the middle ear, as in the outer ear, decreases the loudness of a signal and is usually amenable to medical treatment.

The function of the middle ear is to increase the intensity of airborne sound waves so that they may stimulate the inner ear, which is filled with fluid. The necessity for such a mechanism can be explained by looking at what happens if one were to talk to a swimmer under water. The intensity of speech would be significantly decreased for the person underwater, by about

30 decibels. If one were to talk to an individual with no middle ear, the sound waves would travel directly from air to an inner ear filled with fluid, analagous to the swimming pool. The individual with no middle ear, then, has a conductive loss on the order of about 30 decibels.

The middle ear transforms the sound conducted in air into mechanical movements or vibrations of the ossicles and passes them on to a small opening (oval window) in which the footplate of the stapes rests. An analogy of the greater force exerted on the oval window to that presented to the tympanic membrane would be to equate the force exerted on the eardrum to the force the heel of the foot exerted on the "classic" spike heel of the 1950s, and the greater energy at the oval window to the increased pressure at the tip of the spike heel. Because of the increased pressure by which the stapes pushes into the oval window, little energy is lost from an air medium (at the eardrum) to a fluid medium (behind the stapes).

INNER EAR. The inner ear is completely encased in bone and has two main divisions, the vestibular mechanism, including the semicircular canals and associated structures, and the hearing mechanism, including the cochlea and associated structures. The present discussion is only concerned with the hearing mechanism.

The cochlea (Fig. 6-5) is a snail-shaped structure, spiralling about two and one-half turns around a central core (modiolus). It is through the central core that nerves pass which comprise the auditory nerve of the central auditory nervous system. A cross section of the cochlea is illustrated in Figure 6-6. To keep the drawing simple, many of the structures have not been labeled. What one sees is a structure with essentially three divisions: the scala vestibuli, scala media or cochlear duct, and scala tympani. Each is fluid filled, the scala vestibuli and scala tympani having the same but different fluid from the scala media.

When the stapes footplate moves into the inner ear, the fluid is displaced and is equalized through the movement of the round window. In this movement of the oval and round window, a depression is created along the basilar membrane which stretches the entire two and one-half turns of the snail shaped cochlea. On the basilar membrane rests the organ of hearing, the organ

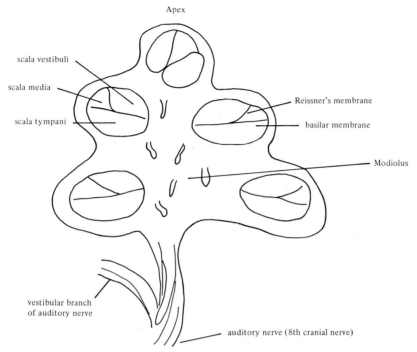

Apex

scala vestibuli

scala media

scala tympani

Reissner's membrane

basilar membrane

Modiolus

vestibular branch
of auditory nerve

auditory nerve (8th cranial nerve)

Figure 6-5. Schematic cross section of the cochlea showing modiolus and eighth cranial nerve.

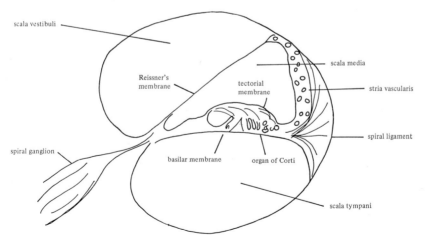

scala vestibuli

scala media

stria vascularis

Reissner's
membrane

tectorial
membrane

spiral ligament

spiral ganglion

basilar membrane

organ of Corti

scala tympani

Figure 6-6. Schematic cross section of the cochlea.

of Corti. On and adjacent to the organ of Corti rest literally thousands of moving parts and supporting cells, the actual function and purpose of each still not fully understood. The depression caused by sound stimulation travels along the length of the cochlea in a wavelike motion and stimulates the final receptor cells, the hair cells, on the organ of Corti. The hair cells and areas most receptive to high pitched sounds are located at the base of the cochlea, and low pitched sounds are located at the apical end of the cochlea. When the hair cells are finally stimulated, they exert an electrical/chemical action triggering neuronal firing that travels to the brain. Therefore, the series of events leading to nerve firing is a mechanical movement of the stapes, a hydrodynamic movement of fluid and basilar membrane deflection, and electrochemical stimulation of the hair cells leading to neuronal discharge. The purpose of the inner ear, then, is twofold: one, to transduce or change the mechanical action of the middle ear bones into an electrochemical firing compatible with nerve and cortical function; and two, to filter sound and assist in pitch and loudness perception.

Because it is difficult to differentiate between the sensory function of hair cells and the neural action of nerves adjacent to the hair cells, a loss in the inner ear is considered sensorineural. Although a loss in the inner ear may effect the intensity of a sound, as in a conductive loss, it does not necessarily become clearer when made louder, a characteristic of other conductive pathologies in the outer and middle ear. A loss in the inner ear can distort sounds so that people with sensorineural impairments report difficulty with understanding of speech even though they can hear someone talking.

CENTRAL EAR. The central auditory mechanism is comprised of the nerves and cell bodies from the cochlea to the auditory cortex (Fig. 6-7). One of the most important observations is that, although one organ of Corti is shown, neural representation appears bilaterally; that is, stimulation from one ear reaches both sides of the brain.

Neurons arising from the cochlea are arranged in an orderly fashion with the nerves carrying high frequency information on the outside of the nerve bundle and the low frequencies in the middle. This orderly arrangement is repeated in the cochlear

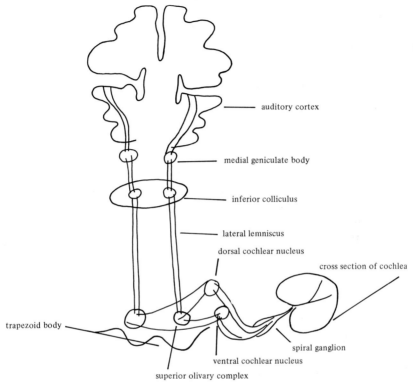

auditory cortex

medial geniculate body

inferior colliculus

lateral lemniscus

dorsal cochlear nucleus

cross section of cochlea

trapezoid body

spiral ganglion

ventral cochlear nucleus

superior olivary complex

Figure 6-7. Schematic pathway of nerve connections for hearing.

nuclei and to a lesser extent along the rest of the central pathway up to and including the auditory cortex. Although the majority of nerves are carrying information to the brain in the ascending or afferent system, a much smaller and less understood system is carrying information from central locations to the cochlea. This latter system is the descending or efferent system and seems to be mostly inhibitory in nature.

The purpose of the central auditory system is to provide complex processing of incoming nerve impulse information. This is accomplished at each major nuclear bundle along the central pathway, in addition to the cerebral cortex. Although a loss in the central auditory system may cause a loss in sensitivity to pure tones, it is commonly characterized by difficulty in understanding more complicated signals such as speech.

Obviously, a hearing loss does not have to be specific to any one of these four areas discussed: outer, middle, inner, and central auditory pathways. When a loss occurs at a combination of conductive, sensorineural and/or neural sites, it is no wonder that communication for the hearing impaired can become difficult.

How Significant a Problem Is Hearing Loss?

According to the National Advisory Council for Neurological Disease and Stroke (1969), approximately fifteen million people in the United States suffer from some degree of hearing impairment. The actual numbers in each age range will vary, however, depending upon how hearing is defined and classified. There appear to be three main factors considered in the definition and classification of hearing impairment: (1) type of loss, referring to the site of lesion (conductive, sensorineural central or mixed); (2) age of onset, leading to classifications of congenital (present at birth) or acquired (after birth) hearing loss; and (3) degree of loss, leading to classifications of hard-of-hearing and deaf.

Recognizing the inconsistent and divergent numbers that will be reported here and in other literature, the estimated number of hard-of-hearing individuals eighteen years of age and under in 1967, according to the Department of Commerce, Bureau of Census, was over one million (Table 6-I). It is quite obvious from the degree of impairment that as the severity of the hearing loss increases the number of individuals with a loss decreases. The Bureau of Education for the Handicapped, U.S. Office of Education, has reported the incidence of school-age children

TABLE 6-I

ESTIMATED NUMBER OF HARD-OF-HEARING INDIVIDUALS
18 YEARS OF AGE OR UNDER (1967)*

Difficulty with

faint speech	normal speech	loud speech	severely hard-of-hearing	TOTAL
26-40 dB	41-55 dB	56-70 dB	71-91 dB	
55%	31%	12%	1%	100%
about 637,000	about 354,000	about 141,500	about 14,200	about 1,147,000

* Modified from Department of Commerce, Bureau of Census.

(5-19) who are deaf (91 dB or higher in the better ear) as 3 in 4,000 persons and hard-of-hearing as 1 in 200 persons.

But what of the other end of the age continuum? According to the U.S. Department of Health, Education and Welfare, Social and Rehabilitation Services (1972), although persons over sixty constitute only 10 percent of the population, they constitute approximately 20 percent of those who have some degree of hearing impairment. These numbers rise dramatically in the nursing/retirement homes, where about 6 percent or 1.2 million senior citizens reside. This latter population has over an 80 percent incidence of hearing loss (Chaffee, 1967; McCartney, 1976).

Significance of a hearing loss can only partially be measured in numbers of people affected. Possibly of greater importance is what effect the loss has on the person: the person's ability to live, work and communicate.

What Effect Does the Loss Have on the Individual and Communication?

Hearing loss can be severely debilitating, and the presence of minimally useful hearing can be extremely advantageous. For this reason it is convenient to separate the effects of hearing impairment upon those in whom hearing is functional (the hard-of-hearing) and those in whom hearing is almost completely nonfunctional (the deaf). A Health, Education and Welfare Advisory Committee (1965) has differentiated the hard-of-hearing from the deaf in the following definitions:

HEW Advisory Committee

> The hard of hearing—those children with moderate hearing losses, who are still able to understand readily fluent speech through hearing whether or not amplification is used. Educationally speaking, these are the children who, with some assistance, are able to attend classes with normally hearing children.
>
> The partially hearing—those children whose loss of hearing is so severe as to require a special educational curriculum and program of training that involves full-time auditory training along with vision for developing language and communication skills; children, who because of the severity of their loss of hearing, need the full-time services of a special teacher for their education. These are

children, who, as a result of early identification of hearing loss and early auditory training, are able to progress academically at a somewhat more rapid rate than those classified as deaf by virtue of more efficient use of their residual hearing.

The deaf—those children whose principal source for learning language and communication skills is mainly visual and whose loss of hearing, with or without amplification, is so great that it is of little or no practical value in learning to understand verbal communication auditorially, and whose loss of hearing was acquired prelingually.

The preceding definitions are applicable to most of the speech and hearing clinician's case load, but they do omit the adult hearing-impaired person. What of the senior citizen who has become deaf but has good language and speech skills? A more general definition for the hearing-impaired person is: Hard-of-hearing, "those in whom the sense of hearing, although defective, is functional with or without a hearing aid"; deaf, "those in whom the sense of hearing is nonfunctional for the ordinary purposes of life" (Conference of Executives, 1938).

What is meant by "functional" or "nonfunctional" hearing for the purpose of communication? Hearing function in this sense relates to the degree and type of hearing loss. The greater the loss, the less functional is the hearing. Equal consideration should be given not only to the degree of loss but also to the frequencies or pitches at which the loss is greatest. Four points need to be made. One, of all the frequencies the normal young ear is capable of hearing, 20 to 20,000 cycles per second or Hertz (Hz), one needs to hear only the frequencies between 300 to 3,000 in order to understand speech adequately. This latter compressed range approximates the frequencies one hears on the telephone. Two, of the frequencies between 300 to 3,000 the higher pitches are the ones necessary for understanding speech, comprised mainly of consonant sounds (th, f, s, p, k, etc), while the lower pitches are comprised mainly of the vowel sounds (a, e, i, o, and u). Three, the higher pitched sounds tend to be weaker and the low pitched sounds stronger in energy. Four, the typical sensorineural hearing loss due to noise exposure and old age and to many diseases experienced by young children reveals poorer hearing in the higher pitches, the same pitches necessary for adequate understanding of speech. Knowing these four facts, then, one can see how speech could be "garbled" and misunderstood by a listener with a hearing loss; the child would be learning speech and language that was distorted by the hearing loss, and the adult would be misinterpreting information conveyed by others.

Because the problems experienced in both learning language and communicating are different for those with some hearing as compared to those with no functional hearing, the two groups will be separated for ease of discussion.

Hard-of-Hearing

If one were to define hard-of-hearing audiometrically, that is, how extensive a decibel loss was present at the better ear, it is significant to note that a wide range is encompassed. A person may be considered hard-of-hearing with a loss anywhere from 26 dB to 85 dB. Obviously, those with a milder loss tend to have better speech and language ability than those with more severe impairments. As simple a statement as that may appear, it is extremely important when developing ideas about an individual on the first visit. Two factors, the greater the number of speech and language errors and the more "different" the voice sounds, give a quick indication not only of severity of loss but also how long the individual may have had the loss.

When an individual is hard-of-hearing, he hears imperfectly and generally speaks imperfectly as a consequence. The speech discrimination loss for single syllable words compared to hearing loss categories ranges from about 73 percent with a flat loss of 70-79 dB, to 42 percent with a loss of 80-89 dB, to a minimal 14 percent with a loss around 100 dB (Ewing, 1962). This graphically illustrates the decreasing function of audition as hearing loss becomes more severe.

In speech development, if an /s/ or /sh/ is not heard because of the high pitch and low loudness, then it is not unreasonable for these sounds to be omitted. Additionally, subtle differences of nasalization (producing sounds through the nose as in /m/, /n/, and /ng/) and not nasalizing sounds may be missed. Unsurprisingly, then, an example of some errors by fifteen hard-of-hearing teen-agers, seen in Table 6-II, exhibits some of these same misarticulations (DiCarlo, 1968). The mean auditory

TABLE 6-II

PERCENTAGES OF 15 TYPES OF SPEECH ERRORS
AMOUNG 15 HARD-OF-HEARING TEEN-AGERS*

Type of Error	Percentage of Occurrence
1. Consonant omission	2.5
2. Regular consonant substitution	8.3
3. Breath-voice consonant substitution	7.9
4. Consonant blend	20.8
5. Abutting consonant	3.1
6. Releasing consonant	3.0
7. Arresting consonant	24.1
8. Nasalization of consonant	1.6
9. Substitution of vowel	9.0
10. Diphthong fractionization	8.3
11. Diphthongization of vowel	2.2
12. Neutralization of vowel	0.4
13. Nasalization of vowel	34.4
14. Abnormal rhythm (prosody)	8.0
15. Arythmic sentence	1.3

* From Frederick S. Berg and Samuel G. Fletcher (Eds.), *The Hard of Hearing Child,* 1970. Courtesy of Grune and Stratton, New York.

hearing losses for the fifteen teen-agers was about 60 dB at the better ear, and the mean discrimination loss for speech in quiet was about 34 percent. The most common errors in this group were nasalization of vowels and misarticulation of consonant blends, e.g. /str/ in strong, and of arresting consonants, e.g. /d/ in bad.

It has been a popular practice not only to describe the relation of communication difficulties to hearing loss (*see* Table 6-III), but also to classify the educational needs and methods to be used according to hearing loss (*see* Table 6-IV). Although this is a useful technique for describing the untrained and unaided child, it may be seriously misleading to the beginning reader in speech pathology. Consider what these tables do *not* tell you: how the individual will respond with a hearing aid and what the child will do with residual hearing.

Although a child may be almost deaf with a hearing loss of 70 dB in the better ear, with one or two hearing aids sounds may be brought close to normal limits. However, even though amplification may bring hearing sensitivity to within mild to moderate hearing loss ranges, no one can say how well the child

TABLE 6-III

RELATION OF AMOUNT OF HEARING LOSS TO
COMMUNICATIVE EFFICIENCY*

Amount of Hearing Loss (dB)	*Effect*
1. Less than 30	May have difficulty in hearing faint or distant speech; is likely to "get along" in school, and at work requiring listening.
2. 30 to 45 [41 to 55 I.S.O.]†	Understands conversational speech at 3 to 5 feet without too much difficulty; may have difficulty if talker's voice is faint or if face is not visible.
3. 45 to 60 [56 to 70 I.S.O.]	Conversational speech must be loud to be understood; considerable difficulty in group and classroom discussion and perhaps in telephone conversation.
4. 60 to 80 [71 to 90 I.S.O.]	May hear voice about a foot away; may identify environmental noises and may distinguish vowels, but consonants are difficult to perceive.
5. More than 80 [90 I.S.O.]	May hear only loud sounds.

* From S. R. Silverman, The education of children with hearing impairments, *Journal of Pediatrics*, 62:254-260, 1963. Used by permission.
† I.S.O.—International Standards Organization (see glossary for description).

TABLE 6-IV

EDUCATIONAL NEEDS OF CHILDREN WHO ARE HARD-OF-HEARING*

1. Hearing loss less than 30 dB
   Lip reading and favorable seating.
2. 30 to 45 dB loss [41 to 55 I.S.O.]
   Lip reading, hearing aid (if suitable) and auditory training, speech correction and conservation, favorable seating.
3. 45 to 60 dB loss [56 to 70 I.S.O.]
   Lip reading, hearing aid, and auditory training, special language work, favorable seating or special class.
4. 60 to 80 dB loss [71 to 90 I.S.O.]
   Probably special educational procedures for deaf children, with emphasis on speech, auditory training, and language with the possibility that the child may enter regular school.
5. More than 80 dB loss [90 I.S.O.]
   Special class or school for the deaf. Some of these children eventually enter regular high schools.

* From S. R. Silverman, The education of children with hearing impairments, *Journal of Pediatrics*, 62:254-260, 1963. Used by permission.

will function. Teachers will be quick to point out that a child with a mild loss may be as handicapped as a child with a severe loss, since other factors such as intelligence, home training, age of onset, and etiology are also important.

From the previous discussion one may conclude that only those children with moderate or severe sensorineural losses exhibit some difficulties in speech and language, but it is important to recognize that a seemingly "simple," potentially reversible problem, such as middle ear pathology, can also cause delay in speech and language development. Holm and Kunze (1969) studied two groups of children in order to determine the effect on language and speech development of fluctuating conductive hearing loss which accompanies chronic middle ear infection (otitis media). Sixteen children, aged five to nine years, with chronic otitis media, were matched with children with normal hearing. Various language and receptive vocabulary measures were administered to both groups. The sixteen children with chronic otitis media were delayed to a statistically significant degree in all language skills requiring the receiving or processing of auditory stimuli or the production of verbal responses. Of course, to say that chronic middle ear infection is correlated with the language delay does not necessarily provide one with a simple cause/effect relationship. However, it does suggest that the two conditions do exist together, indicating further the importance of normal hearing in the development of speech and language.

Deaf

The deaf are those in whom hearing is nonfunctional for normal communication with or without a hearing aid. The audiometric range for those classified as deaf is much more restricted than the range for hard-of-hearing. Deaf is usually defined as anything above 85 dB on the audiometer, while hard-of-hearing is 26 to 85 dB. However, the age at which the hearing loss was incurred determines to a great extent the ability of the individual to communicate in a hearing world. Although, psychologically, deafness at age fifteen or fifty-five may be more traumatic than at age one or two, certainly the effects on speech and language will be far less serious. Therefore, this section about the deaf will focus on those having or acquiring the loss early in life.

Rank ordering of phonemes from the most frequent to least frequent in need of correction has been made by teachers at the Central Institute for the Deaf (Calvert and Silverman, 1975). An example of the sounds that need correction most often are: ch, s, ng, k, m, n and h. An example of the sounds that need correction least often are: th, b, p, and w.

The rank ordering is not meant to imply necessarily that the child lacks the skill to produce an /sh/, for example, but that the correct production of the sound may either need carry-over into the classroom setting, improvement in production, or both. One should also be cognizant that many of the errors, although each is listed separately, may fall into large-class varieties. For example, many of the production errors may be a result of specific voicing versus voiceless sound confusions.

It is also interesting to note that the consonants that need more frequent correction tend to be those that are less visible on the lips, such as /s/, /sh/, /k/ and /g/, while those that need less correction tend to be those that are more visible on the lips, such as /f/, /w/, /th/, /b/ and /p/. This is understandable when one considers the increased importance of vision in communication as the severity of hearing loss becomes greater. Figure 6-8 presents a graphic display of the relationship between the dependency on vision and hearing in the reception of speech. Exceptions to correction of the sound being related to the degree of visibility do occur. For example, although the /m/ is very visible on the lips, it is one of the more frequent consonants in need of correction. This is more a function of the subtle auditory discriminations necessary in order to discriminate nasality than

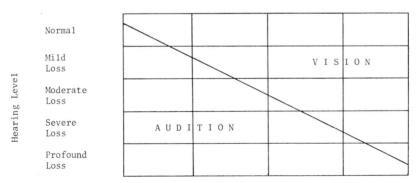

Figure 6-8.   Relationship between Relative Dependency on Vision and Audition for Reception of Speech as a Function of Hearing Level. From Kenneth W. Berger, *Speechreading*, 1972. Courtesy of Kenneth W. Berger and the National Educational Press.

it is an inability to see the lips come together when forming the /m/ sound.

That the deaf have both speech and language difficulties is rather obvious by now. But what type of language deficits are involved? To gain further knowledge of the effects of early-life deafness on verbal acquisition, the Picture Story Test was developed by Myklebust (1965). This test was administered to 800 deaf children at day and residential schools. Two hundred stories were selected from this group and compared with an equal number of matched hearing children.

Table 6-V compares the words used by the deaf and hearing

TABLE 6-V

COMPARISON OF WORD USAGE BETWEEN NORMAL AND DEAF CHILDREN ON THE PICTURE STORY TEST*

	Deaf					Hearing				
AGES	7	9	11	13	15	7	9	11	13	15
Number diff. words	147	260	422	512	548	162	472	556	640	1215
Total number words written	1251	1915	2100	2900	3204	769	2320	2540	3128	4535

* From Helmer Myklebust, Early-life deafness and mental development. In Freeman McConnell and Paul H. Ward (Eds.), *Deafness in Childhood*, 1967. Courtesy of Vanderbilt University Press, Nashville, Tennessee.

children at five age levels. The striking feature is that at age fifteen the deaf not only have increased very little from age thirteen in the number of words used, but also they only approximate the performance of the ten- to eleven-year-old, normal-hearing child. This fact correlates with their grade level in school. At age fifteen, the hearing child is usually in high school, with its increased demands on communication skills of speaking and writing; the deaf child is in the eighth grade, functioning at a fifth grade reading level.

Table 6-VI illustrates the vocabularies of the deaf children as they relate to various parts of speech. Nouns and concrete terms seem to be used consistently more often by deaf than hearing children. Although verbs seem to agree to a large extent across ages, this does not relate what kinds of verbs are

TABLE 6-VI

COMPARISON OF USAGE OF PARTS OF SPEECH BY DEAF AND HEARING CHILDREN*

	Deaf Percentage of Total Vocabulary					Hearing Percentage of Total Vocabulary				
Age	7	9	11	13	15	7	9	11	13	15
Part of speech										
Noun	55.8	29.2	36.9	32.3	31.4	38.3	28.6	27.7	27.6	25.4
Verb	12.4	23.9	25.1	26.2	26.3	19.8	24.2	22.7	24.1	28.9
Adjective	18.4	16.9	15.6	16.8	14.6	12.9	13.8	17.5	14.2	16.9
Adverb	.7	6.9	6.8	7.0	5.9	7.4	10.2	6.7	10.1	9.2
Pronoun	1.4	4.2	3.3	2.9	3.9	4.3	4.5	3.8	3.9	2.6
Preposition	2.0	4.6	3.3	3.2	3.3	6.2	3.2	3.8	3.9	2.6
Conjunction	.7	1.9	1.9	1.6	1.8	1.8	1.9	1.5	4.2	1.9
Article	2.0	.8	.5	.6	.3	1.2	.4	.5	.5	.3

* From Helmer Myklebust, Early-life deafness and mental development. In Freeman McConnell and Paul H. Ward (Eds.), *Deafness in Childhood*, 1967. Courtesy of Vanderbilt University Press, Nashville, Tennessee.

TABLE 6-VII

COMPARISON OF USE OF TENSES*

	Deaf		Hearing	
Age	No. Times Used Present Tense	No. Times Used Past Tense	No. Times Used Present Tense	No. Times Used Past Tense
7	125	29	94	36
9	327	64	103	167
11	259	74	100	234
13	273	192	148	264
15	310	153	251	339

* From Helmer Myklebust, Early-life deafness and mental development. In Freeman McConnell and Paul H. Ward (Eds.), *Deafness in Childhood*, 1967. Courtesy of Vanderbilt University Press, Nashville, Tennessee.

used. The deaf tend to use verbs describing more visible and concrete actions and tend to use the present tense much more extensively than normal-hearing children.

Table 6-VII shows a comparison of tense use between the two groups. Although the table indicates an inability of the deaf to write or speak in past and possibly future tenses, it does not necessarily indicate the inability to abstract ideas mentally or manually into past and future actions.

Even though we all know thousands of words, in everyday conversation we may call upon only a few hundred of these words and use them over and over again. An interesting comparison between deaf and hearing children, then, would be what percentage of the total words is accounted for by those most frequently used. Table 6-VIII lists the percentage for the ten, twenty and thirty most frequently used words. At all ages, the most frequently used words consistently comprised a greater percentage of the total words used by the deaf than the normal-hearing child. In addition to other speech and language problems, then, this last finding would indicate a possible lack of variety and "color" in verbal and written communication by the deaf.

Deaf and Hard-of-Hearing

It is very difficult to dichotomize hearing-impaired people into deaf and hard-of-hearing categories, even though this has been done in order to facilitate the discussion. Hearing impairment is really a continuum that spans almost insignificant losses

TABLE 6-VIII

PERCENTAGE OF TOTAL WORDS ACCOUNTED FOR BY THE
FIRST 10, 20, AND 30 MOST FREQUENTLY USED

Age	Most Frequent	Deaf	Hearing
7	10 words	59.2	54.8
	20 words	74.3	60.5
	30 words	81.9	68.9
9	10 words	44.9	34.8
	20 words	59.4	46.4
	30 words	67.3	53.9
11	10 words	40.9	30.5
	20 words	53.8	42.4
	30 words	61.8	49.5
13	10 words	35.7	32.6
	20 words	47.3	44.8
	30 words	55.2	50.8
15	10 words	38.5	26.1
	20 words	49.5	35.4
	30 words	56.5	40.7

* From Helmer Myklebust, Early-life deafness and mental development. In Freeman McConnell and Paul H. Ward (Eds.), *Deafness in Childhood*, 1967. Courtesy of Vanderbilt University Press, Nashville, Tennessee.

of auditory sensitivity and understanding to those with profound consequences on communication and education. Assuming no specific decibel hearing loss and no concomitant factors that may affect behavior, such as mental retardation, emotional disturbance, or other multiple handicaps, one can list general behaviors that tend to be characteristic of the hearing-impaired population as a whole and of children specifically. Table 6-IX attempts to summarize "typical" behaviors that the reader may observe within the younger population.

Unsurprisingly and refreshingly, the main thrust of Table 6-IX reveals how "normal" the hearing-impaired child is. The differences in behavior are due to the severity and type of loss and how the acoustic signal is changed and monitored during the perceptual process. The hearing-impaired are those with possible speech, language, and voice problems, the remediation of which will be much the same as with the normal-hearing child. Hearing loss and amplification, however, must set realistic limits upon what can be received by the hearing impaired and what can be produced. Communication problems, then, possibly become more of a problem for the therapist than the client.

TABLE 6-IX*

AUDITORY, VOCAL, VISUAL, AND SOCIAL ADAPTATION BEHAVIOR OF HEARING-IMPAIRED CHILDREN*

Auditory	Vocal	Visual	Social Adaptation
Clear-cut threshold for auditory stimuli	Uses voice to get attention and to influence environment; vocal patterns may indicate mood	Compensatory use of vision for environmental orientation; active visual scanning of environment	Behavior generally well organized, purposeful; sensitive to social environment
Responds better to high than to low intensity sound	Peculiar voice quality; pitch monotony; "deafness" more conspicuous with greater severity of hearing loss	Watches face closely, especially after speech teaching is started; alters own behavior in response to changes in facial expression of others	Quick to sense feelings of others; adjusts behavior accordingly
Usually tries to imitate sounds which he can hear	Imitates other voices when he can hear them; accuracy of imitation improves when given opportunity to lipread	Communicates by gesture; invents symbolic gesture; successfully interprets gestures of others; may use gestures to "talk" to himself	Usually likes other children; interacts with them appropriate to age
Tries to listen; gets pleasure from auditory experience; likes to play with sound toys	Articulation of speech tends to agree with predictions from threshold audiogram; articulation best with "visible" speech sounds, poorest with voiceless, high frequency consonants	Skill with visual play materials (blocks, jigsaw puzzles, etc.) appropriate to age	Heightened motor activities, but usually with definite objectives
Reasonable correspondence between threshold audiogram and other aspects of auditory behavior	Echolalic for words and short sentences in early stages of language learning, not otherwise; articulation errors of spontaneous speech are present in echoed speech		Attention span normal for age; attentiveness determined by interest value of play materials or activity
Readily shows awareness of both voice and pure tones at suprathreshold intensities			Normal emotionality for age

* Adapted from Helmer Myklebust, *Auditory Disorders in Children*, 1954. Courtesy of Grune & Stratton, New York.

The therapist must know how to send signals so that they are received by the client to generate the desired response and know how to enable the hearing impaired to monitor speech, language, and voice by using residual hearing, not the hearing loss.

How Are the Hearing Impaired Rehabilitated?

Because of the wide range of hearing losses and the different problems presented by the hearing-impaired population, many therapeutic approaches are employed. These approaches may be variously grouped under the terms *aural habilitation* or *aural rehabilitation*. Aural habilitation is a process by which an individual who has had no prior oral speech and language is taught to communicate. Aural rehabilitation is a process by which those who have had prior oral language and speech experience are either taught to retain the present ability or to improve upon their communication ability. There are three main areas and groups of hearing-impaired individuals that necessitate different techniques and strategies on the part of the speech, language, and hearing therapist: habilitating the hard-of-hearing child, habilitating the deaf, and rehabilitating the hard-of-hearing adult.

Of all the hearing-impaired groups, habilitating the hard-of-hearing child is probably the one area in which most speech and hearing therapists should feel comfortable. The surprising reaction of many beginning student clinicians, however, when first exposed to the hard-of-hearing child, is one of "disintegration." The therapy and practicuum experience dealing with speech, language, and voice problems, the work with articulation and language programs are all suddenly forgotten because this is a "hearing-impaired child," not a speech, language, and voice problem child with a hearing impairment. Often the one object that distorts the clinician's perception of the problem is the hearing aid. Once the stigma of amplification is removed, the child takes on a more realistic and manageable appearance. Analysis of articulation and language and providing a therapy plan for these areas will be much the same for the hard-of-hearing child as with the normal-hearing child, except modified to reflect the presence of a hearing aid and the type and severity of the hearing loss. No new techniques or materials should have to be developed. This is not true for the deaf, however.

Habilitating the deaf child or adult requires, first, an ability to communicate in the client's language system, if one has been developed, or the ability to communicate in a manner that is comprehensible to the child. Both of these conditions may, and probably should, include some form of manual communication. This is the main new technique that the speech and hearing therapist will have to master in order to work with the deaf. The controversy surrounding the use of manual communication is well over 100 years old. A complete understanding of the strong reservations some have against the use of sign language with children would require elaboration far beyond the scope of this chapter. Suffice it to say that some feel that using sign language with the deaf will delay or preclude the development of oral speech and language; some say that not to use sign language is denying the deaf the right to learn through their own language and is creating an overwhelming burden to learn speech and language by looking at the face and lips of the speaker, when only 20 percent of the sounds are visible on the lips. The present author takes an eclectic view and feels that speech and language are of such importance that any and all means should be utilized in the therapy and/or educational process.

Rehabilitating the hard-of-hearing adult usually requires a program of aural rehabilitation, a term generally used to denote three main areas of emphasis: speech (lip) reading, auditory training, and counseling. Because one views more activity than just the lips when trying to "read" what someone is saying, such as body language and facial expression, lipreading may more appropriately be called speech reading. Speech reading with the hard-of-hearing adult does not focus on all movements of a sound, as in articulation training of the deaf, but focuses more specifically on the actual visible sounds and those that may be confused on the lips, such as /p/, /b/, and /m/. Additionally, speech reading attempts to make the client aware of the redundancy in normal conversation and to predict what might be said in any given context. The redundancy of speech and the ability to predict statements greatly improve one's ability to speech read and to understand the "flow" of conversation. Additionally, since speech (lip) reading tests must be learned by the speech and hearing clinician, the implications of each should be recognized along with the ability to apply this information in the rehabilitative process. How specific one becomes in speech reading instruction in watching and practicing specific sound movements is a matter of contention. It is this author's opinion, however, that the adult likes some specific information provided on how sounds are made and which ones look the same on the lips. This knowledge seems to make adults more comfortable in that they leave the therapy situation with some specific information, in addition to any or all of the auditory training and counseling provided in which immediate results are not as identifiable.

Auditory training is a process through which the client learns to associate distorted sounds caused by the hearing loss and/or hearing aid to a correctly produced sound. Extensive listening of environmental sounds, words, and sentences is performed in controlled environments so that the client gains confidence in eventually listening to speech. Auditory training is especially important after receiving a hearing aid. Sounds coming from a hearing aid are not the same as heard by the normal ear or by the impaired ear without an aid. Listening with a hearing aid often takes much more time getting used to than placing a pair of glasses on for the first time. It is recommended that the new hearing aid user initially wear the aid only in quiet and gradually wear the aid in all environments over at least a two-week span. One hearing-impaired adult, who has worn hearing aids for over twenty years, commented that each time he purchased a new hearing aid it took approximately six months for him to become fully adjusted to the amplified sounds coming from the new aid. The noisy environment in which we live has probably been "fading" for the hearing-impaired adult for many years, and sudden amplification of these noises in addition to the desired speech signal may be very disconcerting.

The terms *amplification* and *hearing aid* have been used many times in this chapter. Most people know that a hearing aid amplifies sounds, that it makes them louder, but may know little else about this expensive prosthetic device. Several points should be enumerated when discussing hearing aids: (1) the hearing aid makes sounds louder, not necessarily clearer, for the client; (2) because of various pathologies which may give similar audiometric configurations, just because one person can benefit from an aid does not mean another can, and vice versa; (3) amplification in classrooms may be provided by the child's individual hearing aid, a group hearing aid, and/or one which uses signals transmitted like a miniature radio station; (4) the life span of a hearing aid is similar to that of a car, about five years, longer if it has received little abuse and has been well maintained; (5) a hearing aid fitted to a person three years ago may not be appropriate now because of changes in the person's auditory system; (6) a hearing aid is usually connected to the head by means of an earmold, and because a child's ear canal is growing along with the rest of the body, new earmolds may have to be made every six months; (7) senior citizens, because of changes in their ear canals with aging, may need new earmolds more frequently than other adults; (8) a sign of a poorly fitting earmold is the presence of a "squeal" or whistle from the aid when it is turned on. Questions regarding the child's or adult's hearing aid should immediately be directed to the audiologist or hearing aid dispenser.

Summary

Study of the theory and practical aspects of hearing loss and deafness is truly a broad and exciting area. No matter how deeply one pursues this study, however, it should always be remembered that hearing loss is first and foremost a medical problem. Appropriate medical attention is necessary for all with significant hearing impairment. Audiological intervention is necessary for assessing the hearing loss from a habilitative and rehabilitative point of view; in other words, what do the audiological tests mean in planning therapy or educating a child? The audiologist should also perform a hearing aid evaluation if necessary and maintain periodic checks to see if the aid is functioning properly. The speech, language, and hearing clinician should maintain liaison among all on the hearing health care team, the otologist (ear doctor), audiologist, and hearing aid dispenser, in order to maximize impact upon the hearing-impaired population.

REFERENCES

Ades, H. W. and Engstrom H.: Anatomy of the inner ear. In Keidel, W. D. and Neff, W. D. (Eds.): *Handbook of Sensory Physiology*, Vol. V(1). New York, Springer, 1974.

Berg, Frederick S.: *Educational Audiology: Hearing and Speech Management*. New York, Grune & Stratton, 1976.

Berg, Frederick S. and Fletcher, Samuel G. (Eds.): *The Hard of Hearing Child*. New York, Grune & Stratton, 1970.

Berger, Kenneth W.: *Speedreading: Principles and Methods*. Baltimore, National Educational Press, 1972.

Calvert, Donald and Silverman, S. R.: *Speech and Deafness*. Washington, Alexander Graham Bell Association for the Deaf, 1975.

Chafee, C.: Rehabilitation needs of nursing home patients—a report of a survey. *Rehabilitation Literature, 18*:377-389, 1967.

Committee on Nomenclature Conference of Executives, American Schools for the Deaf. *American Annals of the Deaf, 83*:1-3, 1938.

Dallos, P.: The auditory periphery. *Biophysics and Physiology*. New York, Academic, 1973.

Di Carlo, L.: Speech, language, and cognitive abilities of the hard-of-hearing. Proceedings of the Institute on Aural Rehabilitation, SRS 212-T-68. Denver, University of Denver, pp. 45-66, 1968.

Ewing, A.: Research on the educational treatment of deafness. *Teaching of the Deaf, 60*:151-168, 1962. Reprinted from *Educational Research, 4*, 1962.

Holm, Vanja A. and Kunze, LuVern H.: Effect of otitis media on language and speech development. *Pediatrics*, Vol. 43, No. 5, 833-839, May, 1969.

McCartney, James and Alexander, Donald: *Geriatric Audiology Nursing Home Project: First Year Evaluation*. Presented at ASHA Convention, Houston, Texas, 1976.

McConnell, Freeman and Ward, Paul H. (Eds.): *Deafness in Childhood*. Nashville, Vanderbilt University Press, 1967.

Neyhus, Arthur I. and Myklebust, Helmer R.: Early-life deafness and mental development.

Silverman, S. R.: The education of children with hearing impairments. *J Pediatr, 62*:254-260, 1963.

Zemlin, Willard R.: *Speech and Hearing Science: Anatomy and Physiology*. Englewood Cliffs, Prentice-Hall, Inc., 1968.

CHAPTER 7

CEREBRAL PALSY

Mary Darlow

Introduction

CEREBRAL PALSY IS A chronic condition that is manifested in motor dysfunctions. Concurrent with the motor dysfunctions, other disabilities may occur in the areas of perception, sensation, and cognition. It is imperative for the language therapist to understand the impact of the condition called cerebral palsy on the total language process.

Definitions

Cerebral palsy has been defined in many ways by authorities in the field. It has been referred to by some as an "umbrella term" for any dysfunction to the motor system which causes paralysis, weakness, incoordination, or functional deviation of that system resulting from a lesion in an immature brain. Specific definitions given by authorities in the field convey the complexity of defining cerebral palsy. Doctor Karel Bobath gave the following definition:

> Cerebral palsy is the result of a lesion from maldevelopment of the brain, nonprogressive in character and existing from earliest childhood. The motor deficit finds expression in abnormal patterns of posture and movement, in association with abnormal postural tone. The lesion which is present in the brain, when it is still immature, interferes with the normal motor development of the child. (Bobath: Clinics in Developmental Medicine)

Cruickshank offers a definition in *Cerebral Palsy*: *A Developmental Disability* (1976):

> Cerebral palsy is a problem or a series of problems far more complicated than most other types of physical disabilities. Cerebral palsy cannot just be defined in the physical terms of the disability.

It must also include the deviations that affect the functioning of the individual in the areas of behavior, cognition and learning. (P. 1)

Swartz (1951) defines cerebral palsy as follows:

Cerebral palsy should be defined as an aggregate of handicaps: emotional, neuromuscular, special sensory and peripheral sensory, caused by damage or absent brain structures. (In Cruickshank, P. 2)

Crothers and Paine (1959) give the following definition:

The term cerebral palsy does not designate a disease in any usual medical sense. It is, however, a useful administrative term which covers individuals who are handicapped by motor disorders which are due to a non-progressive abnormality of the brain. (In Cruickshank, P. 2)

In these definitions cerebral palsy is referred to as an "umbrella term." In other words, trauma has been sustained by the brain, either prior to birth, during birth, or shortly after birth. The cluster of symptoms that appears may manifest itself definitely in a motor deficit, but it may also include sensory and perceptual deficits. Not all children with cerebral palsy suffer the same cluster of symptoms.

Clinical Types of Cerebral Palsy

The clinical types of cerebral palsy have been described in terms of disordered movement. Listed in order of the most common to the least common, they are as follows:

1. Spasticity—which is characterized by the stretch reflex. These children are limited in their range of movement and have poor equilibrium responses. In short, they are stiff and lose balance easily.
2. Dyskinesia—which includes the following: athetosis, chorea, dystonia, tremor, and rigidity.
   a. Athetosis is characterized by far too much movement that is involuntary and extraneous in nature. As opposed to the spasticity which limits movement.
   b. Choreiform movements are more continuous, slower in rate, more writhing, but less tense in character than athetosis.
   c. Dystonic movements closely resemble athetosis, but the disorder of movement generally involves the trunk muscles more than the extremities.

    d. Tremor is more rhythmic and pendular in character than athetosis.

    e. Rigidity is a term used to describe increased resistance to passive movements through the entire range of movement. Rigidity resembles spasticity, but with spasticity there is a feeling of relaxation of the muscle after the stretch reflex is elicited. Rigidity may be described as continuous or "lead pipe" in character, where the feeling of resistance is constant, or as intermittent, where the resistance is interrupted at regular intervals and appears as a jerky movement.

3. Ataxia—is incoordination due to a primary disturbance of balance, sense, posture, and/or kinesthetic feedback. It is characterized by inability or awkwardness in maintaining balance with associated or gross and/or fine motor incoordination.

4. Mixed—various combinations of the above types of disordered movements. Athetosis combined with spasticity or rigidity and ataxia are frequently encountered.

5. Atonia—sometimes called hypotonia, is where the muscles fail to respond to volitional stimulation. In cerebral palsy some infants are hypotonic or "floppy" during the first year or so. (Denhoff, in Cruikshank, P. 32)

Another means of classifying cerebral palsy is by site of the neuromuscular disability. Briefly, these are as follows:

1. Hemiplegia—one-half of the body is involved. This is one-half of the body cut down through the middle; one leg, one arm, one side of the face.

2. Diplegia—here the legs are more involved than the arms, although there is involvement in the arms.

3. Quadriplegia—coming from the word *quad* meaning four, means all four *extremities* are impaired; both legs and both arms.

4. Paraplegia—the legs only are involved, both legs.

5. Monoplegia—this refers to one limb only being involved, i.e. one arm or one leg. This is very rare.

6. Triplegia—here three limbs are involved. This too is also very rare.

7. Double Hemiplegia—in other words, both halves, split lengthwise, of the body are involved. It too is rare.

A third way of classifying cerebral palsy is the severity of the involvement.

1. Mild—this involves less dramatic impairment of the fine motor movements or fine precision movements.

2. Moderate—impairment is in gross and fine movement, and speech clarity is impaired, but the functions of usual living activities can be performed.
3. Severe—this would mean the inability to perform the usual activities of daily living, the inability to use the hands, and the inability to use speech for communication. It would also mean a lack of mobility on the part of the person.

Etiology

The causes of the condition have been discussed in detail by authorities in the field of cerebral palsy. Basically, the grouping of etiological factors can be broken down for the purpose of clarification into the categories that follow:

1. Hereditary—this is a genetic abnormality and is rare.
2. Prenatal—those that are acquired *inutero,* such as maternal infections and disorders which affect the fetus. This could include rubella, maternal anoxia, prenatal cerebral hemorrhage, prenatal anoxia, and/or the effects of drugs and toxins.
3. Perinatal—those factors that occur during the latter part of pregnancy or the delivery period which would interfere with the fetus and/or maternal respiration and circulation which would then cause brain damage to the fetus. Such things as prematurity, hemorrhaging, placenta disturbance, or any condition that interferes with oxygen getting to the brain of the fetus in the latter part of pregnancy or during delivery.
4. Postnatal—trauma, such as a skull fracture, infection (encephalitis or meningitis), stroke or vascular accident, toxins, or tumors that occur in the newborn.

There are many excellent references for the etiology of cerebral palsy. They can be found in some of the books listed at the end of this chapter.

History

The early history of the condition can be found in medical writings. Splints and exercises are mentioned by Hippocrates. Braces and splints were used by many cultures such as the Chinese, Egyptians, Romans, and Greeks. The use of massage for paralysis is cited in India as early as A.D. 700. Orthopedic and medical literature traced the development of the progression of treatment of the condition.

Down through the centuries, Hippocrates, Galen, Pari, Freud, and others have expressed opinions as to the cause and treatment of cerebral palsy. In the nineteenth century, William J. Little delivered a paper outlining his observations on this condition. From his work the condition became known as Little's disease until the mid-twentieth century, when the term *cerebral palsy* came into use, mainly in the United States. Little noted in some of his cases that, along with the loss of movement of a limb or limbs, the following cluster of symptoms might occur:

> An impairment of intellectual powers, great irritability, occasional epilepsy, ungovernable temper, cunning and hebetude. The intellectual weakness appears to result less from permanent injury to the brain than from want of sufficient training and education. (Cruickshank, 1976, P. 3)

Little's contribution was twofold. He saw the physical condition as one that could be facilitated by use of appropriate movement and saw that surgery was sometimes necessary to gain more appropriate movement. Little also noted the accompanying deficits, "Cognition, appropriate behavior and learning, that were exhibited by some of his patients" (P. 3). Little then looked beyond the physical condition and noted that this lack of appropriate movement from birth could indeed affect the areas of sensory and perceptual development of the infant. He emphasized the complexity of the problem, and contemporary authorities have added to our understanding. In 1947, the American Academy for Cerebral Palsy was formed by medical specialists representing various areas involved in the treatment of cerebral palsy. More recently, the perception of the problem has expanded to view the disorder as a developmental neuromuscular disability. No longer are spastic limbs viewed as a separate identity from the individual. The child with cerebral palsy is viewed as a child first, then as one who happens to have a condition which affects his ability to walk, etc. Current legislation, public awareness, and centers such as the one in Berkeley, California for Independent Living, have helped to open up the world of everyday living for the handicapped. No longer are they shut out from society.

In brief, one can say that the condition of cerebral palsy has been known first as Little's disease, secondly as Spasticity (mainly in England), finally Phelps coined the term *cerebral palsy*, and now, since 1970, it is classified as a development disability or neuromuscular disability. The interdisciplinary approach to the nature of the problem, which has emerged within the last thirty years, has led to considering the child in his total environment. This approach looks at how the child interacts within the family structure, how he relates to others, such as his peers, and how he functions in the school setting. Many people are involved in assessing and treating these children, including the pediatrician, the orthopedist, the psychologist, the social worker, the physical therapist, the occupational therapist, the language therapist, the classroom teacher, and the teacher aide. Therefore, it is imperative that these people all relate with each other. Each one, coming from his area of expertise, can constitute knowledge to the whole team regarding the strengths or deficits that he or she finds in the child. Only with such a team approach can the child develop to the upper limits of his potential.

Speech and Language Assessments and Intervention Strategies for the Nonverbal Child with Cerebral Palsy

Much excellent material exists in the cerebral palsy literature concerning the remediation of language, speech, and hearing problems. This often concentrates on remediating those children who have some degree of verbal language potential. However, this section will be concerned only with some suggestions for working with the nonverbal child with cerebral palsy.

In assessing the child with cerebral palsy, certain conditions of atypical child development will influence the results. Misperceptions and lags in both receptive and expressive language ability may be due to the inherent disorder, not necessarily due to low mental functioning. Abnormal patterns of movement and posture appear normal to the child with cerebral palsy because that is all he knows. Gaps that are caused by the inherent disorder may occur in the learning process. Progress may be slower at each stage of development.

The development of language and speech in a normal child arises out of certain kinds of activities. These activities include breathing, body movements, sucking, chewing, lip smacking, babbling, and cooing. Physical and emotional contact with other human beings establishes a feedback pattern for further development. These activities are interrelated in preparation for later sound production and expression. Prelinguistic development during the period of infancy is the foundation for later speech and language development.

The infant with cerebral palsy is often denied the experiences necessary to develop speech and language. In normal child development, the infant responds to his environment and stimulation in more or less predictable ways, but the infant with cerebral palsy often responds in an abnormal manner. These responses are perceived as different by the parents and they, in turn, treat the infant abnormally, thereby depriving the infant with cerebral palsy of activities and stimulation which are the foundation for cognition, language, and perception.

A most challenging aspect of the language therapist's role is working with the severely involved child. To develop an alternate/nonverbal method of communication, the language therapist will utilize the expertise of many professionals. These professionals include the physical therapist, occupational therapist, the teacher, the psychologist, and the biomedical engineer. The parents, too, give valuable information to this team and are an integral part in the success of establishing and utilizing an alternate communication system. Recent developments in computers and other electronic communication devices have increased the choices available for the severely involved child to communicate. However, before the nonverbal child can utilize a device in daily living, the language therapist must do assessments and plan intervention strategies. Answers must be found to the following:

I. Assessments

A. Use of consistent motor response
   1. Does the child have a voluntary motor response?
   2. Does the child have an involuntary motor response?
B. Ability to comprehend
   1. Does the child understand?
   2. Does the child have the potential to understand cause and effect?

II. The Teaching of an Alternate System

A. Ability to master the system
1. Can the child be taught to comprehend cause and effect?
B. Ability to utilize the system
1. Does the child have a need to communicate?
2. Does the child have opportunity to communicate?
C. Practicing on the system
1. Does the child utilize system in his everyday environment?
2. Does the system meet the child's needs?

III. Evaluation of the Alternate Language System

A. Does it work for this particular child?
B. Does the child utilize the system?
C. Do others than those familiar with the child understand the system?
D. Is the system practical?
E. Is the system portable?
1. Can it be used in child's everyday environment?

The process of implementing an alternate communication language system varies from child to child. Prognosis for its success must be long-range or tentative. Gains achieved may be in small increments and not immediate. Patience and tenacity are necessary ingredients on the part of the child and the team for any degree of success.

Because the severely involved child cannot point or speak and perhaps has no consistent motor response that could be utilized for assessment purposes, most standardized language tests are inappropriate for this population. Therefore, the language therapist assesses by inference, behavioral observations, and constant monitoring of progress.

A subjective list for assessing an intact language system that the language therapist can utilize should include the following:

A. Receptive language
1. Does the child indicate recognition of *Mom*?
2. Does the child show some response to his or her name?
3. Does the child appear to recognize by name common objects in the environment? Such things might be wheelchair, therapy ball, toys, and food.
B. Expressive language
1. Does the child have any sounds?
2. Does the child attempt to imitate sounds or speech?

3. Does the child make wants and needs known by any type of movement? This could be a grunt, opening of the mouth, moving of the trunk or any extremity.

The physical therapist and language therapist can work together to assess the child for those functional motor acts that he will later utilize for operating a communication device. Such an action might be some common movement such as the shifting of eyes, foot tapping, or even the isolated movement of a small muscle group.

The classroom teacher, physical therapist, and language therapist team can share their combined observations on how they see the child functioning intellectually. The following questions are to be considered: Does the child appear aware of the environment? Does the child exhibit any response to stimuli? Does the child have a consistent response or random response that could be incorporated into a consistent response?

The parents provide information on whether the child has had the opportunity to utilize some method to express wants and needs or whether all wants and needs have been anticipated and met by the parents.

By virtue of the inherent disability, the child's need to develop an expressive language system often does not occur normally. When the language therapist starts a severely involved child on some form of an alternate method of communication, the child must learn the cause and effect relationship. In teaching this relationship, the language therapist can utilize the conditioned response method of teaching behavior. Utilizing this method, the language therapist can expand the child's expressive language by going from concrete to abstract. Common nouns are often introduced first; these can be perceived concretely by the child and utilized to serve his needs. Pronouns often follow, starting with first person. In short, the normal language acquisition pattern is followed, but one must always keep the individual child's needs and wants in mind.

Once the child has learned the cause-and-effect factor of expressive language, the language therapist must adapt the alternate means of communication so that the child can utilize it in his everyday environment. The language therapist must create a need for the child to communicate in his school and home environment. Language therapy then extends into adapting the alternate communication system so that parents, teachers, and physical and occupational therapists can afford the child opportunities to practice. At this stage, team communication is imperative to assure that the child is being stimulated, motivated, and interpreted uniformly by each of the team members. Then the alternate communication system can be expanded and refined to function as the child's method of expressive language.

Periodic evaluation and monitoring of the alternate method of communication is required by the language therapist.

It is imperative in the evaluation of this method of communication to remember the amount of time required by some of these children to be taught to express their needs. The following points should be considered in the periodic evaluations:

1. Is the method of alternate communication appropriate for the child?
2. Is the method of alternate communication at the correct level for his learning capabilities and needs?
3. Has enough time been spent trying to condition and teach the child to use an alternate method of communication?
4. Do other persons than the child understand the system? An example would be if Bliss Symbols are utilized on a language board—are the written words included so that people in the child's environment can perceive what the child is expressing?

The time spent to develop an alternate means of communication is not wasted. Studies have shown that when a severely involved child with unintelligible speech is allowed to utilize this method of communication, his verbalization increases and becomes more understandable. The language therapist is certainly aware of the frustration these children experience.

In summary, to develop an alternate method of communication, these points are to be considered:

1. Assessment of motor system to discover the child's best motor response
2. Behavioral observations to discover the child's appropriate level of functioning.
3. Trial and error in developing an alternate method of communication

4. Intensive task training of the child to use this method.

Remember any device should be dynamic, not static. The language therapist must anticipate various life experiences the child will encounter and expand his language accordingly.

Communication Devices

The field of biomedical engineering has expanded to include interest in communication devices. There are many types of communication devices, and there are many different types of interfaces (control mechanisms), from the very simple type, such as headstick, mouthpiece, joystick, to sophisticated electronically operated controls.

The language therapist can utilize the expertise of the engineers in developing the best control mechanism, which will enable a severely involved child to communicate.

It is imperative that the team of professionals consisting of the biomedical engineer, the physical and occupational therapist, the teacher, and language therapist share their combined knowledge of how the child functions in order to develop an adequate, workable device for any given child. Through this team approach, the steps for achieving the goal of an alternate means of communication can be viewed in the following areas of responsibility:

1. Assessment of motor responses by physical and occupational therapists
2. Assessment of language function by the language therapist
3. The task of developing a functional interface by the biomedical engineer
4. The task of training the child on the device by the language therapist
5. The task of utilizing the device in the educational setting by the teacher
6. Expanding the message units on the device by the child, language therapist and teacher.
7. Periodic monitoring of suitability of device by the whole team.
8. Periodic evaluations of the alternate method of communication by the whole team

In the fall of 1977 two models of the Phonic Mirror Handi-Voice became available to accommodate a wide range of non-

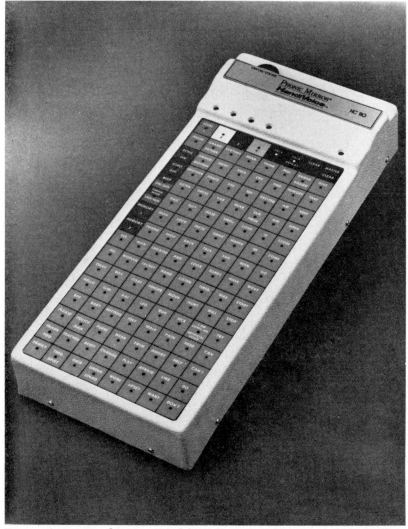

Figure 7-1a.   HandiVoice (Model H C 110).   Courtesy of H C Electronics, Inc.

vocal children and adults. Developed by VOTRAX after two years of field research, these models utilize voice synthesis technology to supply speech for individuals who have previously been separated from the mainstream of society. (*See* Figures 7-1a and 7-1b.) Model HC 110 is a lap-board style for prelanguage or developmentally disabled persons. Using selectable

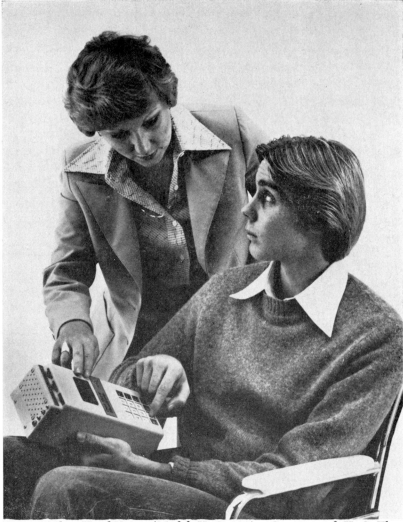

Figure 7-1b. HandiVoice (Model H C 120). Courtesy of H C Electronics, Inc.

overlays with words, graphics or symbols, it is pre-programmed with:

    ... 373 words
    ... 45 phonemes (speech sounds to create any word)
    ... 26 letters (entire English alphabet)

... 13 morphemes (word prefixes and suffixes)
... 16 short phrases (i.e. "My name is . . .")

Model HC 120 looks and operates like a calculator. All selections are accomplished through 3-digit numeric coding. It is pre-programmed with:

... 893 words
... 45 phonemes (speech sounds to create any words)
... 26 letters (entire English alphabet)
... 13 morphemes (word prefixes and suffixes)
... 16 short phrases (i.e. "I want . . .")

The Zygo Communication Device is a reasonably priced, sturdy and light-weight instrument. (*See* Figure 7-2.) Different control switches can be applied in accordance with the motoric ability of the user. The Zygo allows for flexibility since the overlays can be changed to be appropriate for each child's level of language ability. In addition to activating a light, some of the switches provide a definite "click," thus giving auditory as well as visual feedback. This instrument has been very useful to the author in her speech/language work with non-oral cerebral palsied children.

Case Study: *Anna*

Anna is a child who illustrates the development of an alternate communication system. Anna was a three-year-old child, diagnosed as severe tension athetoid when first seen by this language therapist. During her first year in the orthopedically handicapped school the following behavior was noted by her classroom teacher. On her physical therapy days she would look up at the clock and start rolling toward the doorway and down the hall towards the therapy section. Because this observed behavior indicated her understanding of cause and effect, it was decided to attempt to develop an alternate language system for Anna. The team, consisting of teacher, parent, physcial therapist, and language therapist, felt that Anna could master an alternate method of communication and could utilize it to achieve academic success.

The mother and child had independently developed a gross sign language which employed body parts. The right side of

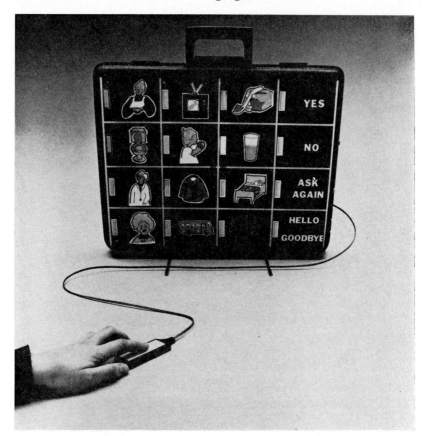

Figure 7-2. Zygo Communication Device. Courtesy of Zygo Industries, Inc.

Anna's body was *yes* and the left side was *no*. Any movement of a particular side would answer a yes-no question. A fist of either hand waving meant she had to go to the bathroom and a fist of either hand touching the nose meant desire for a drink. These signs were utilized as the starting point of a language system. The body signs were used to introduce Anna to the picture language board concept. The first items put on the picture board were a smile face with the word *yes* underneath and a frowning face with the word *no* below it. In a short time Anna was able to achieve 100 percent accuracy by hitting the appropriate picture with her hand in answer to yes-no questions. Next was added the question mark, which permitted her to express doubt.

Gradually, additional "need" items were added to the picture language board with the word printed beneath. An example of this would be *drink, potty, eat, wheelchair, toys,* and *books.* By hitting the pictured item she was able to tell what was needed.

Eventually the pictures were eliminated, leaving only words and/or phrases on a simple piece of tagboard. Some of the phrases used were "I need a————" and "Would you please get me————"; then opposite these phrases were choices of words such as, "a drink," "a book," "a pencil," "my wheelchair," "something to eat," and "help me." Using this, Anna would join phrases and corresponding words together to communicate in complete sentences.

From its humble beginning Anna's language board grew to include days of the week, the months of the year, the alphabet, numbers one through the hundreds, expressions of emotions, and current slang expressions used by her contemporaries. Anna used her board for math, spelling, reading, and communicating with her peers.

Other language boards were developed for her use in physical therapy and at home to express her food and dressing choices. For infrequent stays in the hospital a specialized language board was developed. On this board the word *ouch* was utilized the most!

Anna has now mastered the use of more sophisticated communication devices, an IBM Selectric® typewriter with a keyguard and an electric computer device. These two devices allow Anna to communicate without tutorial assistance. However, she still preferred her tagboard language boards and utilized them in all her classrooms.

Anna demonstrated that she had receptive and inner language. With the various alternate methods of communication she now has expressive language, and, at age nine, she is functioning academically at grade level. She uses this method to express her flair for creative writing. Anna learned more quickly than most such severely involved children. She is a "super star"!

List of Materials Available from   The Trace Center
922 ERB, 1500 Johnson Drive
University of Wisconsin—at Madison
Madison, Wisconsin 53706

Cost

Preliminary Edition, 1974
Annotated Bibliography of Communication Aids $3.50
(complete with photos), compiled by Mary Joe Luster and
Gregg Vanderheiden.
(Final Edition available winter, 1976)
The Bibliography was compiled in order to make available
summary information on this field. It describes some of the
communication techniques and aids for the severely physically
handicapped currently being designed, developed, or manu-
factured in the United States, Canada, or abroad.
Preliminary Edition
Master Chart and Listing of Non-Vocal Communication Aids $1.00
(Final Edition available winter, 1976)
A table of information about existing communication aids.
Preliminary Edition, 197
Annotated Bibliography of Researchers, compiled by Mary Jo
Luster and Gregg Vanderheiden. $ .50
A list and description of researchers and institutions working in
the field of communication techniques and aids for persons who
are severely physically handicapped.
Preliminary Edition
*Selected Bibliography of Articles, Brochures and Books Related
to Communication Techniques and Aids for the Severely Handi-
capped,* compiled by Mary Jo Luster.   * $ .20
(Final Edition available winter, 1976)
*A Portable Non-Vocal Communications Prosthesis for the
Severely Physically Handicapped,* by Gregg C. Vanderheiden,
Gerald A. Raitzer, David P. Kelso, and C. Daniel Geisler. $ .50
*A Portable Non-Vocal Communication Prosthesis for Severely
Handicapped Individuals—The Portable Autocom,* by Gregg C.
Vanderheiden, Gerald A. Raitzer, and David P. Kelso. $ .50
Symbol Communication for the Mentally Handicapped, by
Deborah Harris-Vanderheiden   * $ .15
This paper deals with an application of Bliss symbols as an
alternate communication mode for non-verbal mentally retarded
children. (Also available from *Mental Retardation,* Vol. 13, No.
1, February 1975.)
A "Voice" for the Non-Vocal:
A 12-minute, 16 mm film, describing the Autocom, a non-vocal

communication aid, as used by one severely physically handicapped person.

(Rental—$3.50/Wis., $7.00/outside Wis. Order #0108 Bureau of Audio-Visual Instruction, 1327 University Ave., Univ. of Wis., Madison, 53706. Phone (608) 262-1811.

State of the Art Study on Communication Aids as Aids to Education, by Gregg C. Vanderheiden and Mary Jo Luster. Available fall, 1976.

Non-Vocal Communication Techniques and Aids for the Severely Physically Handicapped, edited by Gregg C. Vanderheiden and Kate Grilley.

Based upon transcriptions of the 1975 National Workshop Series on non-vocal techniques and aids.

(Available through University Park Press, Chamber of Commerce Building, Baltimore, Maryland 21202.)

Communication techniques and aids for the non-vocal severely handicapped, by Gregg C. Vanderheiden and Deborah Harris-Vanderheiden, in the book, *Communication Assessment and Intervention Strategies,* edited by Lyle Lloyd, 1976, University Park Press, $17.50.

REFERENCES

Bobath, Karel: Clinics in Developmental Medicine, London, England.

Bobath, Karel and Bobath, Berta: *A Brief Guide for Parents.* Unpublished brochure, London, England.

Brown, Jason W.: *Aphasia, Apraxia and Agnosia.* Springfield, Charles C Thomas, Publishers, 1972.

Courville, Cyril B.: *Cerebral Palsy.* Los Angeles, San Lucas Press, 1954.

Cruickshank, William (Ed.): *Cerebral Palsy: A Developmental Disability,* 3rd revised ed. Syracuse, Syracuse University Press, 1976.

Cruickshank, William M.; Bice, Harry V.; Wallen, Norman E., and Lynch, Karen S.: *Perception and Cerebral Palsy.* Syracuse, Syracuse University Press, 1965.

Darley, Frederic L.; Aronson, Arnold E., and Brown, Joe R.: *Motor Speech Disorders.* Philadelphia, W. B. Saunders Company, 1975.

Denhoff, Eric and Robinault, Isabel: *Cerebral Palsy and Related Disorders.* New York, McGraw-Hill Book Company, Inc., 1960.

Finnie, Nancie R.: *Handling the Young Cerebral Palsied Child at Home,* 2nd ed. New York, E. P. Dutton and Company, 1975.

Kaplan, Harold M.: *Anatomy and Physiology of Speech.* New York, McGraw-Hill Book Company, 1960.

Keats, Sidney: *Cerebral Palsy.* Springfield, Charles C Thomas, Publisher, 1965.

Lloyd, Lyle L.: *Communication Assessment and Intervention Strategies.* Baltimore, University Park Press, 1976.

Magoun, H. W.: *The Waking Brain.* Springfield, Charles C Thomas, Publisher, 1963.

McDonald, Eugene T. and Chance, Burton, Jr.: *Cerebral Palsy.* Englewood Cliffs, Prentice-Hall, Inc., 1964.

Mysaak, Edward D.: *Neuroevolutional Approach to Cerebral Palsy and Speech.* New York, Teachers College Press, Columbia University, 1968.

Phelps, Winthrop M.; Hopkins, Thomas W., and Cousins, Robert: *The Cerebral-Palsied Child: A Guide for Parents.* New York, Simon and Schuster, 1958.

Sloane, Howard N., Jr. and MacAulay, Barbara D.: *Operant Procedures in Remedial Speech and Language Training.* Boston, Houghton Mifflin Company, 1968.

Wolf, James M.: *The Results of Treatment in Cerebral Palsy.* Springfield, Charles C Thomas, Publisher, 1969.

CHAPTER 7

SUPPLEMENT

WORKING WITH PARENTS
Richard Outland

Doctor Jones asked me if I would discuss working with the parents of handicapped children. Although I am not a speech specialist, I have had the basic work in speech as required of all teachers of orthopedically handicapped children.

A number of the speech therapists out in the field have made the following statement:

> I only wish I had known that I was going to work with cerebral palsied youngsters before I finished my training. When I came out to work in the field of speech pathology, I was assigned to two schools with nonhandicapped youngsters other than their speech problems and then the rest of the time they assigned me to the school for the cerebral palsied.

Cerebral palsied youngsters have some very difficult and challenging problems in speech and language. These speech/language clinicians wish they had had some experience with children with cerebral palsy before they had them as part of their case load. So, I hope that in your training experience here you will have had the opportunity some place along the line. I'm talking with you not as a speech therapist working with handicapped youngsters, but primarily as a teacher of the physically handicapped working with handicapped youngsters and their parents. I think, however, we can say that many of the principles that I share with you will probably stand you well whether you are working with the parents of speech handicapped youngsters or the parents of youngsters with other handicaps. In my particular area of specialization, the cerebral palsied, you will find that 85 percent of the athetoids, for example, have speech problems. When we are talking with the parents of cerebral palsied youngsters, we usually are talking to parents whose children have speech and language problems.

To set the stage for what I am going to say, I would like to share with you an experience that I have had over the years with a young couple. When I first came to California, special education was comparatively new and jobs were difficult to find, so I took a high school position, working with handicapped youngsters, but serving as a senior counselor for the nonhandicapped. In the senior class there was a young couple that I have followed since that time. Bill was president of the class and captain of the football team. Wonderfully well coordinated, with an outgoing personality, he was a real leader on campus. He was very much attached to the secretary of the class, a girl with a great deal of music talent—a very nice voice, sang a lead in the school operetta. Not long after they graduated, Mrs. Outland and I received an invitation to attend their wedding. I never have seen a more radiant couple than Mary and Bill on the day of their wedding. About two years later I met them on a street of a town near the area where they lived, and they were very excited to report that they were expecting their first child. I didn't see them again for three years until Mrs. Outland and I were invited to the high school class reunion. Again we went back to this community because we were very fond of so many of the young people in this class. I hadn't been there long when I saw Bill and Mary, but something had happened to them. They had aged beyond their years. They both looked as if the world were really on their shoulders. They looked sad; they looked drawn; they looked tired, and I could hardly wait for the opportunity for a chat with them.

As the evening moved along, this opportunity came, and as we talked, I discovered that their little boy was spastic cerebral palsied. He would never walk; he had fair hand usage; the prediction for some speech was fairly good, but this was developing very slowly.

I share this case with you because I want to establish four points that most parents of handicapped youngsters seem to experience in connection with dealing with their handicapped child.

First, they don't believe it when they are told that their child is handicapped. When Bill and Mary were told that they had a cerebral palsied youngster, they wouldn't believe it, and they did what so many parents do. They moved on from one doctor to another, hoping to get an answer that was better than the first one. However, the diagnosis remained essentially the same. You will often hear educators being very critical of parents. "If they'd quit shopping around and stay with one doctor, things would be better." I think this is true; things would be better. But, I think we must not be too critical of this situation because it is understandable why they shop around. They're not ready to hear what the doctor told them in the first place. Secondly, doctors are very busy these days. They may not take the time that is necessary to sit down with the parents and explain all the ramifications of what a spastic cerebral palsied youngster would face. Also, we know that some doctors use a vocabulary that a layman doesn't understand. So, there are many variables in the picture concerning why parents move around, and Bill and Mary did this.

The *second* step that many parents go through is saying, "Why did this happen to me?" Involved here is the element of self-pity. They want to know what they have done to cause this. Bill and Mary were beautiful young people, perfect physiques, and their first child was very involved with spastic cerebral palsy—not attractive at all. Bill had always dreamed of having a son who would participate in sports, but this was not the case. Bill did some of the things that other fathers do under these circumstances. He got involved in so many activities in the community that he wouldn't have to come home after work. He joined the bowling group; he joined a future farmers group in his community, the Grange. Every night he had something planned; this left Mary at home with the handicapped child, who became increasingly difficult to manage. She, too, felt a great deal of self-pity. One day she took the youngster in an elevator in his stroller. Some woman said to her, "Why don't you make that baby hold its head up, it's big enough to hold its head up," and she said, "I couldn't answer, I couldn't even bring a word out and so I got off the elevator and I went into the ladies restroom to cry." However, she said a couple of weeks ago, "I was in the supermarket carrying our boy and some lady said to me," "Why don't you let that youngster walk?" "I only wish that he could walk and I hope some day he can." In other words, you see progress is being made as far as her accepting the situation emotionally.

The *third* step that most parents go through is that of finding out what they can do for their child. Mary and Bill began to realize that this child was going to be handicapped all of his life, and their job was to help him develop to his fullest potential. So, they set out to read all they could about cerebral palsied children. They attended conferences put on by United Cerebral Palsy or by the Easter Seal Society. They also joined a parent group in the county where they lived, studying the problems of children who are handicapped.

The *fourth* step is that of helping other children. At that time, unfortunately, Bill and Mary lived in a community which did not provide a preschool program for cerebral palsied children. Although it is legal at the age of three to take these youngsters in public schools, the educational leader in that community had said that since they did not provide preschool programs for the nonhandicapped, they could not provide it for the handicapped. A group of parents went to the Board of Education, and the board members agreed to take another look at the problem if a study showed that other school districts in California were providing such programs. Bill and Mary became the co-chairpersons of the survey. They wrote to all school districts in California operating classes for orthopedically handicapped and made a report to that local school board. They were involved beyond their own youngster, and this is a good step, of course.

I think you have to be a little careful about this type of activity. In accepting this approach sometimes you will find a parent, a mother particularly, very involved in all the activities in the community related to handicapped children. Perhaps she has a cerebral palsied youngster, and she is an officer in the local cerebral palsied chapter. Also, she's out helping the epileptic league and the foundations in all other areas. She may not have gone through the other three steps. She may not have accepted the condition. She may still have a great deal of self-pity. One cannot assume that because parents are so actively involved in some of these projects that they have gone through all four steps.

Let's look at some general guidelines for working with such parents as Bill and Mary, or with parents of youngsters who are blind and deaf, or parents of youngsters who are mentally retarded, or children with severe speech and language problems.

Number one—start where the parent is. Many times the parents have overprotective attitudes and unrealistic goals for their handicapped children. When I first came on this job there was a family up in a northern county that was determined that their handicapped child be in the regular first grade of public school. He really needed to be in a special class, but the parents would not accept his limitations. He had been in the Northern School for Cerebral Palsied, where Doctor Jones was formerly on the staff, for a diagnostic work-up, and the summary report indicated that he should be in a special classroom for handicapped children, but his parents would not accept such placement. They were getting ready to sue the school district, and so I, as state consultant, was called in. I took along with me Doctor Jones and another staff member of the School for Cerebral Palsied Children. We sat down with the parents to discuss this problem. I thought I would start where it is most evident and that is that this youngster had cerebral palsy. I said to the parents, "Well of course your youngster has cerebral palsy," and before I got that out of my mouth, the mother rose from her chair, and with her fists clinched she exploded, "If I had the doctor here that put that tag on my boy I would really give him a choking." We had to do some backing up from there by mentioning the boy's hearing loss, which seemed to be more palatable to the mother. Do not be discouraged if you err in starting where the parent is, because it is not always possible to know where they are in terms of their thinking.

Number two—the parents must feel that we are not working against them, but that we are seeking solutions together. Because they often feel that other members of their family are not understanding of the problem and that neighbors are not understanding, they seem to have a "chip on their shoulder," and so we must be very careful to discuss the problems with them to convey that we are honestly interested in their problem and in helping them. We also must realize that they can tell us facts about their child that we have missed. The parents live with the youngsters twenty-four hours a day. Have you, for example, as a speech therapist, ever lived for a week on a twenty-four-hour basis with a seriously involved stutterer? It's one thing to see him in a clinic for forty-five minutes or an hour, but to live with that child around-the-clock is something else, and many times these parents—if we listen to them—can give us some clues that we would not get otherwise.

The parent must feel that we like the child and see him as an individual with a distinct personality. In other words, we see him in terms of his assets and that he does have potential. We must help the parents to realize that handicapped children are part of the general problem of human imperfections, which all parents have to face. As I look over this group today, six or seven of us are wearing glasses. We have some correction to a certain degree. Some of you have a more severe correction than others. In my case, I am wearing trifocals, so I have quite a problem. Faulty vision is part of a whole area of human imperfections. Now parents are constantly facing these situations. Some parents will want a boy and what do they get—they get a girl. Some parents want a brown-eyed child and they get a blue-eyed child. Some want a big, tall son and they get a short one. Some of them want a daughter of average height and they get a big, tall one. No parents hope for a handicapped child, but they get children who have speech and language problems. They have youngsters who have orthopedic problems, and so forth.

Number Three—probably the most important point or guideline that I can make for working with these parents is that time is needed for acceptance. This was true of Mary and Bill. But, once the parents are able to accept the handicap, this is a tremendous step forward. There are regressions. You will work with parents who, you think, really accept their child's problems, and you feel you have gone down the road a long way, and then in a month or two when you talk to them again they've slipped back.

Number four—I think we must help parents to realize that it is not the handicap that hinders the child's adjustment so much as how the parent himself feels about it. Doctor Benjamin Spock wrote a book, *On Being the Parent of a Handicapped Child.* After spending several months in an outpatient clinic, he reported that when he found a happy, well-adjusted child, he found serene parents. There have been some very interesting studies done recently in the area of compensatory education. In Southern California, researchers in some of the very poverty-stricken communities where many of the youngsters are doing poorly in school found that if the children are not motivated, they're not succeeding. Out of these very poverty-stricken homes, where the environmental factors are much the same, with the same type of housing, crowded conditions, and bilingual parents, every once in a while there emerges a shining light—some youngster who is really achieving. In several structure studies it has been discovered that if the mother has had some degree of education, even though she is living in this squallor and in these very poverty-stricken conditions, she is able to motivate the youngster to desire more learning. The more education the mothers can get, the greater the chances for school success for their children. We have to realize that in many cases we cannot change the environmental factors. The home is a difficult situation, and we can help with counseling, but sometimes we'd like to say, "If we could only take that youngster and put him in another home, all our problems would be solved." But, we don't dare wait until that happens, and it probably isn't going to happen anyway. We just have to set out to do what we can do and not be discouraged because we haven't solved all the problems.

We can help parents by getting them to appreciate the potentialities of their child. What are his assets? Now Bill was beginning to say their boy was going to have good hands. There were many things they were going to teach this boy to do with his hands, even though he was probably never going to walk. But, we have to be careful about overencouragement because unrealistic goals lead to trouble. Parents must realize that their children are fundamentally like all other children. They need food and rest and physical activity, and even when they are handicapped, they have the same personality needs that all of us have.

Also, handicapped youngsters like new experiences just the same as all children. Too often the handicapped child is left at home with a babysitter because it's difficult to take along a handicapped youngster. Sometimes, especially if he's in a wheel-chair or he isn't able to use the organized facilities in a public building, taking youngsters who are handicapped on a picnic is difficult. In fact, when I think of these youngsters trying to fulfill their personality needs, I'm reminded of a story about a three-year-old who was on an elevator for the first time. On the second floor a very large lady got on in front of them and the mother noticed that the lady jumped a couple of times and departed rather quickly at the next floor. After she had left, the mother turned to her little boy and asked, "Jimmy did you do something to that lady?" He replied, "Well Momma, she sitted on my face, so I bited her." I think this is what happens when handi-capped youngsters try to meet those personality needs. They get pushed back in the corner because of their problems, and as a result they bite back at mothers and fathers and brothers and sisters and fellow students.

Let's move on now to the parent conference. All of you are going to be involved in parent conferences at one time or another in your work. We usually expect the school principal to establish some boundaries for the parent conference, suggesting ways in which parents can help with the conference. If this is not done, the clinician cannot force this issue; however, the principal could indicate to the parents some of the information that could be helpful to the professional person holding the conference. For example, what is the relationship of the child to other children in the family? Does he fight with his brothers and sisters all of the time? Do they, when he gets home, pick on him so much that he retreats into a corner? What are his emotional reactions in the home to frustrating experiences? If he doesn't get to go along with his mother and dad everytime they do, what happens? What is his attitude toward school? What is the attitude towards speech? Sometimes you'll have a youngster with whom you think you're getting along well. He gives the impression that he likes to come to speech. But, he goes home and tells mother that he hates it and hates that woman he has to see for thirty minutes a day.

Let's consider the conference itself. We suggest that a speech/language clinician have some concrete material available. We suggest that you have samples of daily work dated and ready. What are some of the concrete materials that a speech therapist might have ready for parents? Are you going to want them to do some practicing of activities in the home? Perhaps you are going to be able to suggest a game, or at least you can show the mother some of the materials that you are using at school, why you're using them, and what you're trying to accomplish. If the parents feel that the session in speech therapy is the biggest waste of time that the youngster experiences at school, how much do you think is going to come out of that? The attitude is going to spill over on the youngster whether the parents say it in front of him or not. So, it's terribly important that you communicate with parents what you're doing and why you're doing it, and what you're getting accomplished.

We suggest making the initial greeting as relaxed as possible. Remember that many of the parents that you will be seeing have had some negative experiences with schools, and some of them may even be dropouts. The school environment may trigger memories of their miserable experience when they were "kicked out" of high school in their junior year and never did get that diploma. In other words, make parents feel that this is a comfortable, friendly situation.

Be sure that you discuss the whole child and not just limit the discussion to some articulatory problem. When you give the parent some suggestions, it helps to use the third person instead of the first person. Instead of saying, "This is the way I would do it," say "This is the way some people have done it"; you will find that you get a better response from parents if you try to put as much as possible in the third person instead of using the big "I." Be hesitant about giving advice. A parent will say to you, "You may feel that you're not progressing with the speech problem because the youngster isn't getting enough rest. I can't get Johnny to go to bed. What shall I do?" You can probably think of three good ways to get him to go to bed, but then you'll say, "Well, I'd do it this way," and the parents say, "I've already tried that." Where does that leave you? Pretty soon they have you in the corner. None of the ideas that you've given are any good. When the parents say, "I can't get Johnny to go to bed, what shall I do?", ask what they have done. Let them get their points out on the table and then, after you have looked at their points, you will probably be able to add one or two that they haven't tried, and they will be more willing to listen.

I would urge you in dealing with the negative and hostile feelings of parents not to argue with them. You don't have to indicate approval or disapproval, just listen. One way of dealing with this is to repeat back what they've said. Every once in a while a parent will say, "My child has had speech therapy now for seven years and it hasn't done a bit of good. He hasn't improved one bit." Then just say, "The child has been to speech therapy for seven years and hasn't made a bit of progress." They will be surprised when they hear this played back—"Well no, now he is making certain sounds better and he's talking more than he did." They just forgot about some of the progress that is being made or some of the things that have been done. Don't argue, but play it back to them. Out of a very negative situation you will bring a positive light, and then you can build from there.

You must control the conference; it has to be yours. You can't let the parent take over the conference and run down the road with it and never get anything accomplished. I think you have to be careful that you don't digress too much. They will want to talk about the neighbors' youngsters who are taking speech therapy. You have to say sometimes that we have a limited time so let's stay on Johnny's problems. You have to decide when there's time for a digression and when you should stay with the point. You'll get the very talkative mother. When that happens, give her a question that can be answered with *yes* or *no,* and then you can pick up the discussion right away. However, if you have a parent who just answers all your questions with *yes* and *no,* phrase a question so she cannot do that. Instead of saying, "Does Bobby like school?", where she can say "yes" or "no," "Does Bobby like speech?", ("yes" and "no") ask her how Bobby feels about his speech lessons. This will bring a parent out who is reluctant to talk. But, if you get one who is too talkative, phrase that question so there's only one answer, either "yes" or "no." Then you can come in and take over the conference. These are just simple little techniques, but they do work in controlling the conference.

Handling parent conferences is a very vital part of the job that you're going to face. People tell me out in the field that it is one area for which they feel they are not adequately prepared. Some of our teachers have found it helpful to keep notes on the parent conference, and they do this by jotting down the main points as they go along. I suggest that you say, "If it's all right with you, I'd like to keep some notes and I will give you a carbon copy so you can take it home. You may want to talk it over with your husband, and also this will give us a starting point for our next conference." If you start writing down a lot of material without explanation, you are going to ruin your conference. If the parents show any uncertainty about having a written record, don't push it at all. But, if they are willing, this makes a wonderful way to summarize the conference. The other parent who hasn't been there is informed, and it gives you a starting point at the next conference.

You ought to evaluate each of your conferences with parents. A few guides for evaluating a conference will be discussed here. What portion of the time was used by the therapist in talking? Did you talk about 90 percent of the time? If you did, that is probably too much. Were the topics covered pertinent and of direct value to the child's situation, or did you spend most of the time talking about the new Buick® the family bought? Your control over this is important. Did both the parent and teacher feel comfortable at the conclusion of the conference? I would urge you to avoid ending the conference on a negative note. You want that parent back. Sometimes a speech therapist will say, "Well, I really got to Johnny's father today and I bet he does something." You may be sure he's going to do something. That something he does is to never come back to see you again. So, end the conference on a friendly note; go until you are com-

municating in a friendly way. If you were to repeat the conference, what would you do differently? Just pause after your
conference and say, "Now, if I were to do this over, how could
I improve it?" When you finish and the parent has gone home,
say to yourself, "What did we accomplish?"

I wish you good luck in your work and good luck in dealing
with parents. It's challenging, and it's going to be of a tremendous
service, but also you need some techniques. You just can't go
in blind with the parents or you're going to find yourself terribly
frustrated. The best of luck to you.

CHAPTER 8

CLEFT PALATE

Robert Faggella, M.D. and Morris Val Jones, Ph.D.

A CLEFT LIP AND palate is a congenital deformity which is common to all races in all parts of the world. Egyptian mummies have been exhumed, showing this particular deformity. Medical literature through the ages has made reference to cleft lip/palate, both in description and in treatment. As with many other congenital anomalies, all types of supernatural fantasies, witchcraft, and demon possessions have been given as causative agents for the deformity. The first repair of a cleft lip as recorded in medical literature is attributed to an unknown Chinese surgeon at approximately A.D. 390. The common term for cleft lip throughout the centuries has been "hare lip," similar to the rabbit's natural cleft. The surgeons of the past all recognized the severe physical and psychological deformity that clefts fostered in the patient and the families. Very primitive techniques of closure were carried out, utilizing pins, needles, silk sutures, and even hot cautery.

In most communities today, the care of the child with cleft lip and palate is under the direction of a plastic surgeon. In some communities, this care may come under the direction of an oral surgeon or otorhinolaryngologist (ear, nose, and throat surgeon). The historical advancement of surgical techniques as well as understanding of embryology and muscular function has enhanced today's level of surgical precision. Such names as Lemesurier, Mirault, Brown-McDowell, Tennison, Skoog, and Millard are associated with classical types of repairs of cleft lips. Although there are many other names associated with surgical procedures for repair of labial clefts, all have contributed small variations to the work of these major men.

The history of palatal surgery began much later than labial surgery because of its dependence upon anaesthesia and sterilization. Wells (1971) has capsulized the beginnings as follows:

> The Frenchman Roux and the German von Graefe were the first in a group of surgeons who gave special attention to palatal repair during the nineteenth century. Others whose names would appear on any roster of well-known surgeons of the time included Johan Dieffenbach, Bernhard von Langenbeck, Philippus Gustavus Passavant in Germany; Alfred Velpeau and Philippe Blandin in France; Thomas Alcock and Joseph Lister in England; and Alexander Stevens, John Collins Warren and Jonathan Mason Warren in the United States. (P. 13)

Many of the surgical procedures developed by these "giants" are still the bases for modern surgical intervention.

Incidents

The incidence of cleft lip and cleft palate will vary from author to author and is given in terms of 1 in 500 to 1 in 1,000 live births. The classical statistics of 1 in 650 are those accumulated by Dr. Paul Fogh-Anderson, working in Copenhagen, Denmark. In this unique situation all cleft lips and palates in the country of Denmark and the State of Greenland are treated at one hospital; therefore, all statistics of live births can be accurately prepared, collected and tabulated. One surgical team performs the surgery. The data were published in 1962. Since then, there has been a very significant change in the social mores of birth. Abortion is prevalent; use of birth control methods is widespread; and, generally, birth rates after the skyrocketing periods of the late sixties are on a decline. More studies may show a change in this ratio. Statistics indicate that the incidence of cleft lip and the combination of cleft lip and palate is more prevalent in the male child, and the incidence of isolated cleft palate is more prevalent in the female.

Herbert Koepp-Baker stated the following facts in *Handbook of Speech Pathology and Audiology* (1971):

> Orofacial malformations appear more often among children of Japanese ancestry, and less commonly in American Negroes than among Caucasians. The incidence of these teratoses also appear to

vary in different parts of the world. A commonly published figure is one in 1,000 births, though some careful studies indicate that in some parts of the United States it may be as high as one in 600. About 25 percent of the malformations of the primary palate are bilateral. When they are unilateral about 30 percent involve the right side and 70 percent the left. It is generally asserted by clinicians that 85 percent of the bilateral clefts of the primary palate, and 70 percent of those that are unilateral, are associated with nonunions of the secondary palates. (P. 769)

Causative Factors

The overwhelming cause of cleft lip and palate appears to be hereditary factors. There are well-documented cases of familial cleft lip and palate. Some investigators attribute at least 60 percent of the problem to congenital and hereditary factors. There are many exogenous causes cited as causative agents for this malformation. In animal studies the entity has been brought about by the use of drugs, such as *Cortisone*®. It is difficult to transpose animal experimentation to human experience. Experimental data show that vitamin A deficiencies in animals will produce the same cleft problems. Radiation, also, will produce clefts. Thalidomide, a known teratogen, has produced this anomaly. The use of modern-day hallucinogens, such as LSD, has been cited but never definitely tagged as producing malformations such as cleft lip and palate. It is suspected that viral diseases, such as rubella, early in the pregnancy possibly would also account for orofacial anomalies. In many instances, several factors, both exogenous and indogenous, probably accumulate to produce the congenital malformation.

Muriel Morley (1970), the British speech pathologist, summarized the data of Fogh-Anderson as follows:

Fogh-Anderson investigated the geographical distribution of cleft lip and palate in Denmark but found an even distribution corresponding to the density of the population without any geographical variation between country and town. He also found no significant difference between the social classes, nor any relationship to birth rank when the first born and the last born were considered, either for hare lip and cleft palate, or for isolated cleft palate. However, he demonstrated a familial history of 30 percent of the families of 903 patients seen by him. (P. 19)

Embryology

The primordial germ layers of the embryo are the ectoderm, mesoderm, and entoderm. The ectoderm gives rise to the skin and its derivatives; the mesoderm, the connective tissues; and the entoderm, lining of the gastrointestinal tract. As the first few weeks of embryonic development take place, various folds, pouches, grooves, and migrations of tissue unfold. Most embryologists believe that cleft lip takes place some time before the tenth week of gestation and cleft palate by the twelfth week. The theoretical cause of the problem is the lack of penetration of the mesoderm with the subsequent breakdown or lack of fusion of the ectoderm, hence causing the cleft. Any exogenous factors, such as exposure to radiation, measles, drugs, etc., which affect this pregnant female after the twelfth or fourteenth week, therefore, have little chance of causing a cleft of lip or palate.

Classification of Clefts

Cleft lips and palates are classified according to their anatomical variation. A cleft lip may be complete or incomplete, depending on whether the cleft extends through all of the structures of the lip; that is, the red portion of the lip, the skin, muscle, and into the nose. The cleft can be unilateral or bilateral. Cleft of the palate is divided into the two anatomical parts of soft palate and hard palate, with the incisive foramen as the dividing point between the prepalate and the palate. The hard palate is that portion in the anterior or front of the palate with the bony roof, separating the oral and nasal cavity. The soft palate is the posterior musculature, which is the dynamic portion of the palate involved with speech. A cleft many involve only the soft palate or all of the roof of the mouth; it may be unilateral, meaning involving only one side of the vomer, or bilateral, involving the anterior portion between the two palatine shelves.

Treatment

The most significant aspect of treatment is the counseling given to the parent shortly after the birth of the malformed child. Ordinarily, the parent is in a state of shock from the recent encounter, disbelief of the fact that this could be his/her child. Due to the deformity and other aspects of fear and revulsion, the parents may have a subconscious rejection of the child.

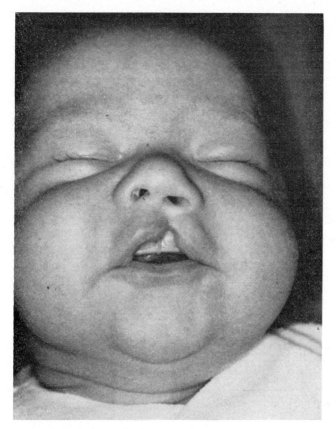

Figure 8-1.   Incomplete unilateral cleft lip, prior to surgery.

It is, therefore, very important to counsel the mother and father prior to the onset of a rehabilitation therapy program for the child. A careful explanation of possible causes is given; the proposed surgical intervention is outlined and prognosis is delineated in nonmedical terms. The discussion will also give reassurances to the parents that their problem is not unique and certainly not insurmountable.

Surgical Procedures

The initial treatment for closure of cleft lip will vary according to the medical personnel in charge. It generally depends upon the surgeon's own theory, feelings, experience, and training.

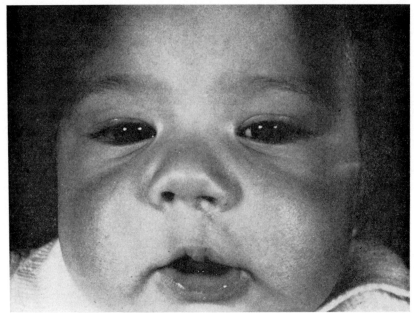

Figure 8-2.　Unilateral cleft lip, after primary surgery.

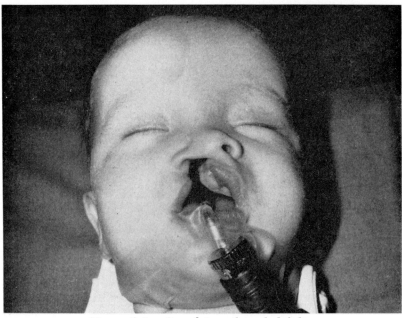

Figure 8-3.　Complete unilateral cleft lip.

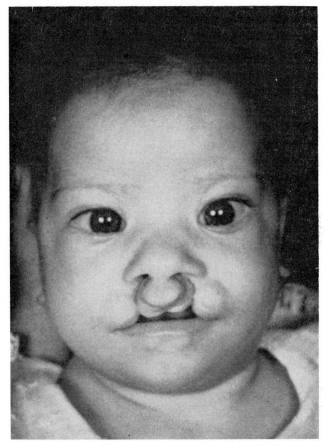

Figure 8-4.   Complete bilateral cleft lip.

The average closure time is around age three months. By that time the child weighs approximately 10 or more pounds; its physiological systems are well established and functioning adequately. Usually, the child can stand the rigors of surgery and general anesthesia without ill effects.

In most instances the surgery is carried out under a general anesthetic in a hospital; in some instances local anesthesia is utilized. The closure of a cleft palate will also vary with the training and experience of the plastic surgeon. Generally speaking, the palate is closed sometime between the ages of one and two. There is a theory, primarily prevalent in the Chicago area,

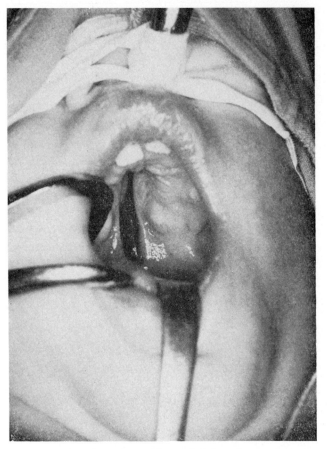

Figure 8-5.   Unilateral cleft palate.

that closure of the palate should not be carried out until age
three or four or longer. The theory for this late closure is less
possibility of interference with the normal growth that takes
place in the central area of the face. The primary surgical
procedures are structured so that, hopefully, secondary surgical
procedures will not be required. There is a possibility that, as
growth and development proceed, minor revisions of the lip may
be necessary between the ages of four and six.

   The main speech patterns from the malformed palate may
not become manifest until about the ages two or three. By then,
speech and language can be fully assessed. If velopharyngeal

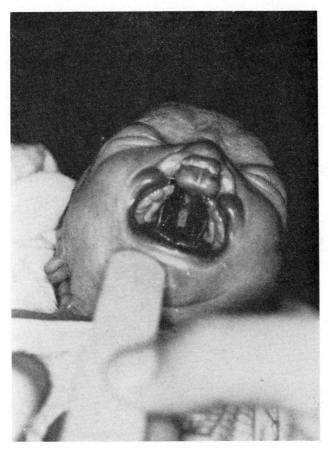

Figure 8-6. Complete bilateral cleft palate.

insufficiency is prevalent, it generally will necessitate a surgical procedure to close the aperture in the posterior pharynx. Velopharyngeal insufficiency is due to a lack of closure involving the soft palate, the lateral pharyngeal walls, and the posterior aspect of the pharynx. The tonsils and the adenoid mass are included. In the normal course of speech, as the air is brought forth over the vocal folds into the pharynx, the main thrust of the air should come forth through the mouth. With an opening in the velopharyngeal port, portions of the air will escape through the nasal cavity, thus giving the typical rhinolalia heard in severe cases.

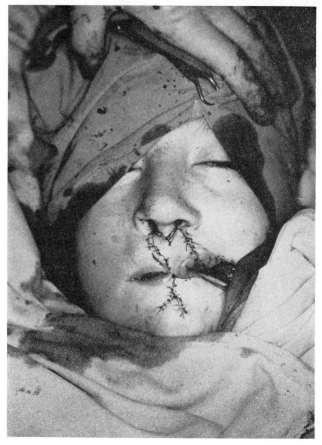

Figure 8-7. Abbé flap to transfer tissue from the lower to the upper lip.

Most plastic surgeons are anxious to have their cleft palate children under the guidance of speech pathologists at an early age. True enough, the very young child has a very short attention span, and working with this child is very difficult. But, as the child progresses in the school system, working with him to expand his vocabulary, improve his pronunciation, and control his musculature, the speech/language clinician can aid significantly in diminishing the velopharyngeal insufficiency problems.

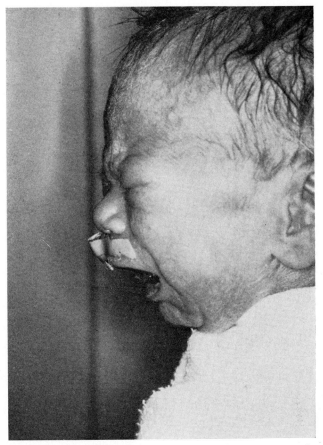

Figure 8-8. Pièrre Robin syndrome. A Logan bow protects the surgery of the upper lip.

*Velopharyngeal Insufficiency**

Velopharyngeal insufficiency (VPI) has been described by Bradley (1972) as the ". . . physiological condition in which the soft palate fails to reach the posterior wall of the pharynx and functionally separate the nasal from the oral cavity" (p. 56).

---

* The research for this section was done by Vivian Kaita, student in the Department of Speech Pathology and Audiology, California State University, Sacramento, California.

The inability of the soft palate to reach the pharyngeal wall may be due to insufficient tissue or to the deficient mobility of the existing musculature (Perkins, 1977).

In a longitudinal study of cleft palate children, Coccaro, Pruzansky, and Subtelny (1967) noted the nasopharyngeal growth of this group resulted in a nasopharynx which was "shorter in velar length and with greater dimension through which the soft palate must move to contact the posterior pharyngeal wall." This, they postulated, ". . . could explain the development of inadequate velopharyngeal closure for some cleft palate individuals as a consequence of growth" (p. 225).

Although cleft palate is the problem most commonly associated with velopharyngeal insufficiency, cleft palate is not necessarily a prerequisite. Many persons with VPI who do not have cleft palates enter speech clinics or approach cleft palate teams for treatment. Also, according to Williams and Woolhouse (1962, as cited by Bradley, 1972), 20 to 40 percent of the patients with repaired cleft palates still demonstrate VPI. Therefore, although the cleft no longer exists, VPI remains.

In attempts to determine the causes of velopharyngeal insufficiency, research and studies have resorted to describing conditions frequently associated with this insufficiency. Bradley (1972) categorized these conditions as being either congenital, acquired, or functional "associated causes." Although these have not been proven as causes of velopharyngeal insufficiency, determining which of these "causes" may be a contributor to the patient's condition is important in that it will determine which type of treatment and therapy must follow.

Reports submitted by parents of patients will often reveal histories of late acquisition of speech, regurgitation of foods and fluids through the nose, and frequent upper respiratory tract infections or frequent episodes of otitis media. These are indicative of congenital complications. One possibility is the presence of a submucous cleft, a condition in which the bones of the hard palate fail to unite but the mucous membrane over the cleft is intact. Concomitant with a submucous cleft is the displacement anteriorly of the velar aponeurosis, producing an increased distance between the velum and the posterior pharyngeal wall (Koepp-Baker, 1971).

The congenital condition of paresis of the soft palate muscles may also contribute to velopharyngeal inadequacy (VPI). This, in its mildest form, involves paralysis of the soft palate. In the more severe form it affects the tongue, lips, soft palate, and laryngeal and pharyngeal muscles. Hypernasality has been shown in case histories to be present from the onset of speech, as well as normal articulation errors associated with VPI (Worster-Drought, 1954 as cited by Bradley, 1972).

Another congenital condition which has been associated with VPI is that which Bradley titles *regional growth disturbances.* Some conditions included in this category are tongue impairment in maneuverability, unusual origin and insertion of the levator veli palatini muscles, and abnormal obtuse basicranial angle. All of these have been associated with hypernasal voice quality and, therefore, possibly a contributor to poor velopharyngeal function.

"Associated causes" which are acquired may include such disorders as pseudobulbar palsy, amyotrophic lateral sclerosis, diptheria, and myasthenia gravis. These are all types of neurological disorders or diseases which cause either paralysis or limited innervation of the muscles, thus reducing their mobility. Any neurological disorder may, therefore, cause VPI either during speech or during respiration.

Carcinoma of the palate or pharynx, as well as trauma to these structures, requiring removal of palatal or pharyngeal tissue, may also lead to palatopharyngeal insufficiency. If the missing parts can be replaced by prosthetic devices, speech can usually be restored to normal.

There are several viewpoints on the importance of the adenoids and the significance of their removal. Bradley (1972) cited Fletcher (1960) as proposing that the removal of the adenoids only unveils an already existing condition. She then refers to Roberts (1960), who indicated that adenoidectomies destroy the sphincterlike action of the pharyngeal musculature, creating a larger than normal pharynx and resulting in palatopharyngeal insufficiency without any other defects present (p. 58). Perkins (1977) took the following stand:

> Enlarged adenoids compensate for a soft palate that is too short or too immobile to reach a pharyngeal wall of normal depth; or, if

the velum is normal, they can compensate for an abnormally deep
pharyngeal wall. (P. 180)

Hypernasality has been known to be present in the absence
of any organic abnormality, although it is one of the main characteristics of velopharyngeal insufficiency. In a study by Williams,
Bzoch, and Agee (1958) as cited by Bradley (1972), it is
possible that what appears to be velopharyngeal insufficiency
may be inappropriate learning behaviors. Their study presented
deaf children who were able to obtain palatopharyngeal closure
on those sounds that do not require closure and were not obtaining closure on those sounds that do require it.

Two symptoms which seem to be present in all persons with
velopharyngeal insufficiency are distorted articulation and hypernasality. The reduction of intraoral pressure caused by insufficient
velopharyngeal closure prevents proper production of plosives,
and fricatives, particularly the voiceless consonants. Additional
characteristics which may accompany speech production are alae
pinching during the production of consonants, nasal emission
of air during sound production, and the presence of nonspeech
sounds. Attempts at producing sibilants may result in glottal
stops or pharyngeal fricatives. A variety of articulation errors
may be present if VPI is a by-product of neurological diseases.

An oral examination may provide some useful information for
recommendations for treatment and/or therapy. The presence
of a palatal or submucousal cleft may, up until this time, have
gone undetected. During examination, the extent of active movement of the velar and pharyngeal musculature may be observed.
However, it is becoming ever more popular to use radiography
and cinefluorography for a more accurate and objective assessment of velopharyngeal activity. Without these techniques,
judgment of the mobility of the pharyngeal mechanism is subject
to error, especially since one can observe these movements during
conversational speech (Skolnick, McCall, and Barnes, 1973).

Once palatopharyngeal insufficiency has been diagnosed, a
decision for or against treatment must be made. Treatment may
consist of speech therapy, surgery, prosthedontia, muscle training,
or any combination of these.

Speech therapy before physical modification of the oral

structures should place emphasis on speech and sound discrimination and articulation. The location and placement of the articulators should be stressed. If a good articulation pattern is developed before physical modification, less work will be necessary when the patient returns to therapy. As Perkins (1977) noted, neither surgery nor prosthetic repair can promise the disappearance of articulation errors. These treatments are for closure of the velopharyngeal port and will at best remove the voice quality problem of hypernasality. Even this, as Koepp-Baker (1971), Van Riper (1963), and Morris (1973) point out, is not totally obliterated. When discussing the possibilities of surgery or prosthedontia, the patient and the parents must be made aware that the possibility of therapy after surgery or prosthedontia exists. If the patient decides upon surgery after a period of speech therapy thinking his problems will disappear, he will be disappointed when he discovers he must return to therapy. The motivation of the patient is the key factor to successful therapy, and this type of situation should be avoided whenever possible.

Surgical treatment is applied in terms of the observed speech and the anatomical deficits of the patient. According to Koepp-Baker (1971), many surgeons attempt to combine the initial closure of the cleft with retropositioning of the palate or with pharyngeal implants to aid in velopharyngeal closure, thereby hoping to prevent secondary surgery (p. 788). One of the main purposes of secondary surgery is to improve speech. Therefore, if necessary, pharyngoplasty, pharyngeal implantations, and pharyngeal flap techniques may be performed at a later date.

There are those patients whose oral deformity is so extensive that surgical closure of the palate is not recommended. In these patients, surgery may render the velopharyngeal mechanism totally inadequate. Prosthedontia appears to be the only alternative.

One last bit of treatment to be mentioned here is that of muscle training. The purpose of this therapy is to strengthen the pharyngeal musculature through appropriate exercises. In most cases, increased velopharyngeal activity and achievement of velopharyngeal closure for speech can be seen after one month of training if therapy is pursued at home and if improvement is at all possible (Cole, 1971).

There are basically three techniques to muscle training. The first is the indirect method. It consists mainly of standard speech drills as well as yawning and swallowing exercises. The second technique is called the semidirect method. The goal is improvement of the velopharyngeal function without any direct physical contact with the musculature. Peterson (1973) questions the effectiveness of these first two techniques. She feels such tasks may not require velopharyngeal closure. Even if such tasks did strengthen the velopharyngeal musculature, this development of improved closure on nonspeech tasks may not generalize to speech.

The third technique is the direct method. The therapist employs some type of instrument to "touch, stroke, manipulate, or apply resistance to the palatal and pharyngeal muscles," the purpose of which is to bring to conscious awareness and to bring under voluntary control the motor acts which are essentially involuntary and reflexive in nature (Cole, 1972). The primary aim of muscle training is to incorporate into normal speaking the muscle activity necessary for velopharyngeal closure. If significant velopharyngeal closure or a significant increase in muscle activity has not occurred by the end of the third month of training, it is unlikely any significant changes will occur in subsequent training sessions. The patient may be referred to a surgeon or a prosthedontist. If he has not already seen one, he will be assessed for either surgery or initial fitting of an obturator. Or, if the patient had already had surgery and/or an obturator, follow-up examinations should be made to see if secondary surgery or obturator adjustments need to be made.

In most instances, if the velopharyngeal insufficiency problems persist after age eight, the surgeon must contemplate a surgical procedure. The testing for insufficiency is carried out by radiologists, utilizing a cinefluorographic technique. One can see and hear at the same time the sounds and the defect in the palate on a cinefilm. This gives the surgeon and others treating this child a better and more clear-cut idea of the problem existing in the posterior pharynx. There are a variety of surgical techniques available to overcome velopharyngeal incompetence. These techniques utilize the transfer of tissues, either from the palate, from the lateral pharyngeal walls, or from the posterior pharyngeal wall. In all of these instances, the purpose is to add length to the palate and bulk to the general velopharyngeal area in the hope of closing off the flow of air into the nasal cavity. Other methods utilized in selected cases include the use of bone grafting or the use of synthetic materials, such as silicone or Teflon®. These substances are inserted or injected in pockets developed through incisions in the posterior pharnyx. Again, the goal is to add bulk and block the passage of air into the nasal cavity. In some instances, prosthetic devices attached to the teeth are used. The general principle is the same: one of trying to add a blocking agent to the flow of air into the nasal cavity.

Speech and Language Characteristics

Cleft palate cases present a similarity of speech and language symptoms, collectively recognized as "cleft palate speech." Bzoch (1972) and his staff at the University of Florida assessed these deviations and tabulated the data. The following listing appears in the order of frequency of occurrence in 1,000 consecutive longitudinal case studies. Each aspect of abnormal speech can be reliably identified and rated or measured under specific and controlled test conditions. The categorical aspects of deviant speech are as follows:

1. Laryngeal and pharyngeal gross substitution errors of articulation for consonant sounds. (564)
2. Delayed speech and language development. (502)
3. Hypernasal resonance distortion of voice quality for vowel and syllabic sound elements. (431)
4. Distortion of consonant sounds due to audible nasal emission alone. (423)
5. Developmental dyslalia. (340)
6. Dysphonia characterized by aspirate voice. (313)
7. Lisping and other articulation distortions related directly to dental or occlusal abnormalities. (128)
8. Hyponasal resonance distortion of voice quality affecting vowels or nasal consonants, or both. (120)
9. Dysphonia characterized by a rough or uneven fundamental laryngeal vibration (hoarseness). (150 sic)

10. Articulation deviations related to loss of hearing acuity. (60)
11. Communication problems from visual distraction of the listener due to nasal and facial grimacing. (42) (P. 111)

Spriestersbach, Darley, and Rouse (1956), in an analysis of children with cleft lip and palates, found the consonants misarticulated in order of decreasing defectiveness were /z/, /th/, /s/, /ch/, /j/, /zh/, /th/, /sh/, and /t/. The five consonants giving the least difficulty were /m/, /n/, /h/, /y/, and /ng/.

McWilliams (1958), in a study of cleft palate adults, found the four sounds most freqeuntly misarticulated were /s/, /z/, /ch/ and /j/. They were essentially the same sounds frequently misarticulated by the children in the Spriestersbach study; /p/, /b/, and /m/ were among those sounds most infrequently in error.

The corroboration of these studies is an example of research findings that plosives and sibilants are likely to be defective in cleft palate speech; /s/ and /z/, along with /ch/ and /j/, present the most serious problems.

Studies indicate that the cleft palate population has least difficulty with the nasal consonants and greatest difficulty with the fricative consonants. Spriestersbach, Darley and Rouse (1956) made the following statement:

> . . . the data indicate that in general the nasal consonants are least often defective and the fricative consonants are most often effective with this sample of cleft palate children. Considering groups of sounds, the plosives seem to give more difficulty than the nasals but less difficulty than the fricatives with this sample of children. One reasonable implication of these results is that the cleft palate person does not have as much difficulty building up the momentary oral pressure required for the stop-plosives as he does maintaining oral pressure over a period of time such as would be required in the production of fricatives. (P. 442)

McWilliams (1958) found distortions to be the outstanding characteristic of adult cleft palate speech along with a high degree of consistency of misarticulation. She made the following statement in an article in the *Journal of Speech and Hearing Disorders*:

> We can readily see that the distortion of speech sounds is the outstanding characteristic of the articulation patterns of these adults with cleft palate. This differs from the findings of Spriestersbach,

Darley and Rouse to the effect that the articulation errors of cleft palate children were most likely to be errors of omission and least likely to be errors of distortion. However, the discrepancy between the findings of the two studies is compatible with Snow and Milisen's suggestion to the effect that the distorted speech sound represents a relatively higher level of development, which might be expected in adults, than do omissions or substitutions. (P. 72)

Morley (1962) characterized the substitutions of cleft palate speech in a discussion of glottal stops, pharyngeal fricatives, and tongue tip consonants:

The glottal stop is, therefore, usually substituted for any of all of the plosive consonants p, b, t, d, k, g, and may also be used for other consonant sounds. In some cases correct lip and tongue positions are used in conjunction with the glottal stop. (Chap. 5, P. 173)

The use of the glottal stop for the production of plosive consonants is usually accompanied by the substitution of some fricative sounds made in the pharynx or larynx for the normal fricatives /s/, /z/, /sh/, /th/, /th/, /ʒ/, and /f/ and /v/. These may be described as the "pharyngeal sounds." /s/ is the sound most frequently produced in this way. (Chap. 5, P. 173)

. . . The cleft palate child, on the other hand, uses the back of the tongue more readily than the tip and frequently substitutes /k/ or /g/ for /t/ and /d/. The consonants /k/ and /g/ may also be substituted for other anterior consonants, whilst fricative consonants, particularly /s/ are often made with the tongue approaching the /k/ position rather than the /t/ position. (Chap. 5, P. 176)

Spriestersbach, Darley, and Rouse (1956) found that the cleft palate children studied had significantly less difficulty articulating consonants as singles than in blends. They attributed this to "defective peripheral speech mechanisms" and hypothesized that the "rapid, precise placement of the articulators required in order to produce the several consonants in a blend overtaxes the ability of the speaker to compensate for his deficiencies" (p. 444).

Speech and Language Therapy

Morley (1970) has set a high goal for speech therapy:

The aim of any treatment for cleft palate is to produce normal speech, and by this is meant not merely intelligible speech, but speech which will defy any phonetician to discover the fact that the patient has ever had a cleft palate, and which is, in addition, natural and free from self-consciousness. (P. 213)

She discussed in detail the chief conditions which will influence the result of treatment:

1. The anatomical and physiological result of surgical treatment, including the development and mobility of the pharyngeal muscles
2. The intelligence of the patient
3. Acuity of hearing
4. The level and type of speech development at the time of operation
5. The degree of stabilization of the faulty neuromuscular patterns of speech and the patient's ability to inhibit these and incorporate normal articulation in fluent speech
6. The age when speech therapy begins
7. The environment and personality of the patient
8. Cooperation between the patient and therapist. (Pp. 213-227)

Wells (1971) has listed a series of subgoals in achieving as near normal speech as possible:

1. Motivation for modification of speech behavior, although it may preface other considerations, is a continuing goal
2. Development of awareness of the structures that will be used for new speech patterns
3. Achievement of adequate tonus and movement of the velo-pharyngeal and articulatory mechanisms
4. Control of the velopharyngeal sphincter
5. Proper direction of the stream of air, with or without voicing, through appropriate resonating, restricting, and impounding channels
6. Adequate production and use of the sound units in syllables, words, and sentences
7. Combination of velopharyngeal valving and articulatory movements in sequences of utterances
8. Ability to monitor performance and compare it with models presented
9. Retention of acquired skills if structures are modified by management or growth
10. Correction of speech skills with linguistic self-expression in a social environment—the automatization of speech. (P. 226)

Van Hattum (1974) has enumerated the basic principles to rehabilitation practices for cleft palate cases:

1. The success of speech therapy is determined by the structures.
2. The earlier the treatment, the better prognosis.

3. Parental counseling, guidance, and participation are important.
4. Language needs early and continuing attention.
5. The client must experience success in therapy and be convinced that he is capable of producing acceptable speech.
6. Exercises should not require strenuous activity that cannot be adapted to the rapid transition required for speech.
7. Auditory acuity and auditory discrimination must be as nearly normal as possible.
8. The single most important factor is velopharyngeal function.
9. The air stream must travel along an open and relatively unencumbered path.
10. Occasionally, the success of therapy is related to the client's ability to control his rate of speech.
11. The greatest improvement in communication will come from improved precision of articulation.
12. Tactile and visual stimulation are of more help than auditory stimulation in developing acceptable production of speech sounds.
13. Mental health is a desirable and necessary consideration in habilitation. (Pp. 325-330)

Numerous techniques have been developed by speech/language clinicians to rehabilitate the cleft palate individual. Most of these methods have been discussed in the chapters on "Articulation" (Chap. 2) and "Voice Problems" (Chap. 4). One continuing issue has been the use of blowing exercises as a part of the clinical intervention program. Two authors who suggest extreme caution are Wells (1971):

> The evidence suggests that blowing has little value in a speech training program for children with repaired or obturated clefts. If the velopharyngeal gap is not great, other methods of achieving closure may be more useful than blowing. If the gap is wide and the soft palate is inadequate in length of mobility, closure may not be possible for blowing; and attempts to succeed in blowing exercises may result only in further experiences in sending the stream of air through the nose as well as the mouth. (P. 234)

and McWilliams and Bradley (1965):

> The investigators suggest that, because speech demands velopharyngeal behavior that is physiologically different from that required for blowing, blowing exercises could be providing a kind of therapy that is diametrically opposed to the physiologic demands of some speakers. (P. 50)

In all cases speech therapy should be started as soon as possible so that a preventative program can be established with the parents in order to avoid faulty habits that would have to be eliminated later. Hahn (1972) has written extensively about how to set up home-centered therapy sessions.

Cleft Palate Guidance Group

It is important to realize that the care of a cleft lip and/or palate child is a multidisciplinary problem. The anatomical problem causes all sorts of other chain reactions which affect both the child and the family in many ways. There are distinct problems with hearing, teeth, social development, physical development, mental development, growth, speech, and general health. The cleft palate guidance group brings together all of the disciplines that would be working independently with this child and family. The child is presented before the group in a case presentation, generally preexamined by all the members of the group either before the meeting or at the individual offices. In this type of setting, the combined opinions then are collected and discussed. A more coordinated program involving the entire child can then be formulated and presented to the specific doctors, dentists, therapists and school authorities, state and local agencies, and all others concerned with the progress of the child. Cleft palate groups may be found in university settings, as well as in private hospital and other agency settings. They are existent in any community where there are significant numbers of cleft lip palate surgeries being performed. The direction that the specific group will take is dependent upon its members. It may be very dynamic; that is, seeking aid for the child, follow-up on the suggestions rendered by the various panelists, pushing the parents and the various agencies for progress. Or, it may be strictly a recommendation situation in which opinions are given, and the further disposition of these opinions will be dependent on the various agencies and people involved. In all cases, the cleft palate guidance group is a most important part of the rehabilitation of the child and family.

Wells (1971) emphasized the unique contribution of some members of the cleft palate team:

The surgeon—He uses "primary" or "secondary" procedures, depending on the point at which he sees the patient. Procedures used to close clefts in the hard and soft palates and to provide additional length often involve flaps of various kinds. The procedure that connects a strip from the posterior wall of the pharynx to the velum, the pharyngeal flap, was used and abandoned in the nineteenth century, then revived about 1924.

The orthodontist—If he takes part in the early orthopedic procedures to modify the alveolar arch and align the maxillary processes with the premaxilla, the orthodontist may be involved from the onset. Otherwise, orthodontic management of children with congenital clefts is relatively limited in the first six years of life.

The prosthodontist—Prosthetics involves the replacement of an absent part with an artificial one. Prosethetic management is the science and art of utilizing artificial materials to provide a separation of the oral cavity from the nasal cavity or to replace missing or extracted teeth.

The speech pathologist—He assesses the communicative abilities of the patient and provides remedial measures to improve speech and language. Additionally, he may serve effectively as a liaison agent between the team and the parents, assist the child to understand the procedures that will be carried out by surgeons and dentists, and interpret his terminology and procedures to other professional members of the team. (Pp. 147-174)

An outstanding Consultative Cleft Palate Panel has been developed at the Center for Craniofacial Anomalies, School of Dentistry, University of California, by its chairman, Egil P. Harvold. The panel meets once each month to evaluate from six to eight individuals with problems related to orofacial anomalies, most of which are cleft lip and palate. Many of the others have speech characteristics similar to those of the cleft palate individual. The following areas of specialty are represented on the panel (listed alphabetically):

Audiology	Pedodontics
Dentistry	Plastic surgery
Neurophysiology	Prosthodontics
Orthodontics	Radiology
Otolaryngology	Social services
Pediatrics	Speech pathology

Following individual specialty examinations, the panel members give their reports. After general discussion of each case, the panel makes recommendations for management to the referring medical personnel and to others, including the parents, who are connected with the patient. For older patients, such recommendations are discussed directly with the client. The panel members also consider the education of students, such as speech/language clinicians, a part of their responsibility, and they allow sponsored groups to view the proceedings of the total panel case presentations. At these meetings the students can see the patients as they are interviewed by the speech pathologist, view the cinefluorographic films, and listen to the discussion and the final recommendations.

REFERENCES

Bradley, Doris P.: Congenital and acquired palatopharyngeal insufficiency. In Bzoch, Kenneth R. (Ed.): *Communicative Disorders Related to Cleft Lip and Palate*. Boston, Little, Brown and Company, 1972.

Bzoch, Kenneth (Ed.): *Communicative Disorders Related to Cleft Lip and Palate*. Boston, Little, Brown and Company, 1972.

Coccaro, Peter J.; Pruzansky, Samuel, and Subtelny, J. Daniel: Nasopharyngeal growth. *Cleft Palate J*, 4:214-226, 1967.

Cole, Richard M.: Direct muscle training for the improvement of velopharyngeal function. In Bzoch, Kenneth R. (Ed.): *Communicative Disorders Related to Cleft Lip and Palate*. Boston, Little, Brown and Company, 1972.

Hahn, Elise: Directed home training programs for cleft palate infants. In Bzoch, Kenneth R. (Ed.): *Communicative Disorders Related to Cleft Lip and Palate*. Boston, Little, Brown and Company, 1972.

Koepp-Baker, Herbert: Orofacial clefts: Their forms and effects. In Travis, Lee E. (Ed.): *Handbook of Speech Pathology and Audiology*. New York, Meredith Corporation, 1971.

Koepp-Baker, Herbert: Treatment of orofacial clefts: Surgical, orthopedic, and prosthetic. In Travis, Lee E. (Ed.): *Handbook of Speech Pathology and Audiology*. New York, Meredith Corporation, 1971.

Massengill, Raymond, Jr. and Phillips, Phyllis P.: *Cleft Palate and Associated Speech Characteristics*. Lincoln, Cliffs Notes, Inc., 1975.

McWilliams, Betty Jane: Articulation problems in a group of cleft palate adults. *J Speech Hear Disord*, 1:68-74, 1958.

McWilliams, Betty Jane and Bradley, Doris P.: Rating of velopharyngeal closure during blowing and speech. *Cleft Palate J*, 2:46-55, 1965.

Morley, Muriel E.: *Cleft Palate and Speech*, 7th ed. Baltimore, Williams and Wilkins, 1970.

Morris, Hughlett L.: Velopharyngeal competence and primary cleft palate surgery, 1960-1971: A critical review. *Cleft Palate J, 10*:62-71, 1973.

Perkins, William H.: *Speech Pathology: An Applied Behavioral Science,* 2nd ed. St. Louis, The C. V. Mosby Company, 1977.

Peterson, Sally J.: Velopharyngeal function: Some important differences. *J Speech Hear Disord, 38*:(1), 89-97, 1973.

Powers, Gene K.: *Cleft Palate.* Indianapolis, The Bobbs-Merrill Company, Inc., 1973.

Ross, R. B. and Johnston, M. C.: *Cleft Lip and Palate.* Baltimore, The Williams and Wilkins Company, 1972.

Spriestersbach, D. C.; Darley, F. L., and Rouse, .: Articulation of a group of children with cleft lip and palates. *J Speech Hear Disord, 21*:436-445, 1956.

Spriestersbach, D. C.; Darley, F. L., and Rouse, V.: Articulation of a group *Communication.* New York, Academic Press, 1968.

Stark, Richard B. (Ed.): *Cleft Palate: A Multidisciplinary Approach.* New York, Harper and Row, 1968.

Van Hattum, R. J.: Communication therapy for problems associated with cleft palate. In Dickson, Stanley (Ed.): *Communication Disorders: Remedial Principles and Practices.* Glenview, Scott, Foresman and Company, 1974.

Van Riper, Charles: *Speech Correction Principles and Methods,* 4th ed. Englewood Cliffs, Prentice-Hall, Inc., 1963.

Wells, Charlotte, G.: *Cleft Palate and Its Associated Speech Disorders.* New York, McGraw-Hill, 1971.

Wicka, Donna K. and Falk, Mervyn L.: *Advice to Parents of a Cleft Palate Child.* Springfield, Charles C Thomas, Publishers, 1970.

CHAPTER 9

BRAIN DAMAGE AND/OR APHASIA

MORRIS VAL JONES, PH.D.

ALTHOUGH BRAIN DAMAGE in adults, particularly cerebral vascular accidents ("stroke"), has been a part of medical literature (Licht, 1975) since ancient times, the concept of brain damage in children has had a relatively short existence. Among the first professionals to specialize in writing about this childhood condition were Strauss (1951) and Doll (1953). Over the past forty years, the term *brain-damaged child* has been used to designate a certain pattern or set of patterns of behavioral disturbance.

According to Birch (1964), considerable confusion has resulted from the use of the term for two reasons:

1. evidence that children exhibiting the behavioral pattern described do in fact have damage to the brain is poor, and
2. many children with known and independently verified brain damage (i.e., nonbehavioral neurologic or anatomic evidence) do not exhibit the patterns of behavior presumably characteristic of "brain damage." (P. 4)

A listing of symptoms which are usually basic for motivating parents or educators to refer children for a neurological work-up includes the following:

Disordered behavior: the child is often described as overactive.
Short attention span: attention may best be described as capricious —now will-o'-the-wisp and again fixed with glue-like intensity upon socially irrelevant and educationally impertinent aspects of the environment.
Emotional liability: conduct is characterized by rapid shiftings of mood and affective expression.
Social incompetence: social failure may produce aggressive behavior, tears, withdrawal, or all of these in sequence or pattern.
Defective work habits: some tasks are pursued *ad nauseum* while others receive only intermittent and unevenly energized notice.

196

Impulsiveness and meddlesomeness: the child is apparently unable
to refrain from touching, moving, and handling objects. Lack
of inhibition may extend to all aspects of social functioning and
be reflected in unacceptable sexual displays, unprovoked aggres-
sion, and verbal outbursts.

Specific learning disorders: reading achievement is below age level;
there is difficulty in mastering arithmetic, general incapacity in
dealing with abstractions, and poor transfer of learning from
one context to another. (P. 10)

DEVELOPMENTAL APHASIA

Aphasia literally means "without speech," but when applied
to children the term has been construed in various ways. The
major controversy about the subject seems to stem from three
groups:

. . . those who insist that aphasia must be acquired after speech
has developed; those who think that a predilection of aphasia can
occur congenitally; and those who believe that aphasia in children
is caused by a developmental lag which may or may not be transitory. (Wood, 1963, P. 571)

Myklebust (1971) defined aphasia as follows:

Childhood aphasia refers to one or more significant deficits in
essential processes as they relate to facility in the use of auditory
language. Children having this disability demonstrate a discrepancy
between expected and actual achievement in one or more of the
following functions: auditory perception, auditory memory, integration, comprehension, expression. . . . they are assumed to derive
from dysfunctions in the brain, though the evidence for such
dysfunctioning may be mainly behavioral, rather than neurological,
in nature. (P. 1186)

Popular opinions of causation state that aphasia is the result
of a defect or damage to the central nervous system (Monsees,
1959), cerebral damage or failure of cerebral maturation
(Eisenson, 1966). Wood (1963) referred to aphasia as ". . . an
inability or limited ability of a child to receive or express spoken
symbols" (p. 571). Wood further states that the child's problem
is most often associated with central nervous system impairment.

Clinical histories have revealed that most aphasic children
do not present "hard-sign" evidence of central nervous system

pathology (Eisenson, 1972). Many more aphasic children, however, show evidence of "soft-signs" associated with minimal brain dysfunction. Common examples of "soft-signs" include mild tremors, poor physical coordination, and exaggerated deep tendon reflexes (Bortner, 1968).

According to criteria mandated by the California Education Code 894, 6801.1(a), and defined in California Administrative Code, Title 5, 3600(g), a minor is aphasic when all of the following statements apply to him:

1. He has a severe speech and language disability.
2. The dysfunction or impairment is evidenced by a written diagnosis or determination (as appropriate) as aphasia or probable aphasia by each of the following:
    A. A licensed physician and surgeon who has training and experience in working with children who have neurological defects;
    B. A credentialed or certified psychologist;
    C. A teacher (or specialist) credentialed in the area of the speech and hearing handicapped, or a member of the staff of a speech and hearing clinic or center who holds certification by the American Speech and Hearing Association.
3. The disability is diagnosed or determined (as appropriate) by each of the persons described in (2) to be other than a speech and language disability associated with deafness, mental retardation, or autism, and to be an expressive, receptive, or integrative character, or any combination of such characters.

Eisenson (1972) observed brain-damaged children:

The ability to categorize, which is unconsciously and spontaneously arrived at by normal children, is retarded or impaired in brain-damaged children. If the normal acquisition of language is affected, as it is with aphasic children, categorization or concept formation is also impeded. (P. 136)

Menyuk (1974) asserted that aphasic children differ from normal children in semantic development. They do not use major linguistic categories in the variety of contexts and syntactical structures as normal children do. Stark et al. (1968) made the following statement:

Because it is difficult for them to classify events with verbal labels, and organize the words they know in appropriate phrases and sentences, their productions tend to be inordinately short and reveal a variety of structural inadequacies. (P. 149)

Ingram (1974) conducted a study of the language of six children who had been placed in an aphasic class. They ranged in age from 10-0 years to 10-10 years, with a mean age of 10-3. Six published tests were administered according to the established protocol:

1. Assessment of Children's Language Comprehension (ACLC)
2. Boehm Test of Basic Concepts
3. Illinois Test of Psycholinguistics (ITPA)
4. Michigan Oral Language Productive Test
5. Peabody Picture Vocabulary Test (PPVT)
6. Photo Articulation Test (PAT)

Although the sample population was too small to permit generalizations about children in other aphasic classes, the following performance trends were characteristic of the group:

1. Responses to the ACLC and the Boehm indicated the subjects had difficulty in processing lexical sequences containing four or more items.
2. Responses to the Boehm indicated the subjects had difficulty with the concept of *time*.
3. Responses to the visual subtests of the ITPA suggest that vision may be the best modality to use to train aphasic children.
4. Responses to the Michigan indicated that the subjects had difficulty with double negatives, auxiliary verbs, irregular comparisons, and past tense markers.
5. Responses to the PPVT indicated that one-half of the group had inadequate receptive vocabulary. The mean difference between the subjects' mental age was 12.66 months below the mean chronological age.
6. Responses by the subjects of this study indicated few articulation problems. (Pp. 26-27)

Myklebust (1957) stated that most aphasic children show definite and distinct motor signs during observations and on motor tests.

A disturbance of motor coordination can be considered as characteristic of the aphasic child. This motor disturbance can be described as mildly diffuse incoordination, inferior grasp, and awkwardness rather than as obvious disabledness or cerebral palsy. (P. 516)

Darley (1964) concluded that aphasia was due to brain damage but not attributable to motor dysfunction. Developmentally, the aphasic child is usually slower in acquiring standing and walking milestones, later in developing manual laterality, awkward in performing gross movements, and deficient in fine motor coordination (Eisenson, 1966).

The Development of Facilities for Brain-Injured Children[*]

Before World War II, facilities for the diagnosis and education of brain-injured children were nonexistent. Beginning in 1946, professionals throughout the United States began to focus on the learning problems of these children. Although University professors, such as Grace Fernald at the University of California, Los Angeles, developed specialized clinics, a great deal of the early work was done by professionals in nonuniversity settings. Representative programs, which have influenced the course of the education of children with central nervous system dysfunction, are now discussed in some detail.

The Cove School

The Cove School (at Racine, Wisconsin and Evanston, Illinois) was organized in 1947 as a very small private, nonprofit school for "brain-injured" children by A. A. Strauss and Laura Lehtinen Rogan. Its objectives were several:

1. To provide education through new understanding and specialized methods for children with diagnosed mild brain damage unable to learn effectively or function behaviorally according to the expectation held out by their tested intelligence level.
2. To provide a working model of an educational laboratory which might serve as an example or inspiration for public school systems desirous of extending their special services to the same classification of children.
3. To provide opportunities for the training of teachers so that they might translate the learnings and experiences gathered at The Cove Schools into local programs adapted to the conditions and needs of their own communities.
4. To continue research and studies in the psychology and education of these children.

The early researches of Dr. Strauss and his collaborators on the psychological and behavioral consequences of early brain damage were done with mentally retarded children. It was

---

[*] This section is based, in part, on a previous publication by the author, *Special Education Programs*.

demonstrated in a succession of studies that children with exogenous mental retardation performed differently from endogenous mentally retarded children on tests of visual perceptual organization and concept formation. Children in the exogenous group were observed to be generally poor in the performance of skilled motor activities, and many of them exhibited speech and language deficiencies reminiscent of adult aphasia yet not quite the same. Difficulties in sustaining attention, erratic thinking, and restless or hyperactive behavior were commonly observed. The researches sought to revise the prevailing treatment concept based on the presumed homogeneity of mental deficiency by establishing a relationship between etiology and mental organization. In the groups studied it was shown that while the Stanford-Binet IQs used as measures of intelligence were the same, the children who were retarded mentally because of early brain damage and who came from normal families with presumably normal genetic patterns differed in important ways from those children who were retarded intellectually because of familial, presumably inherited, mental defectiveness. The distinction between exogenous and endogenous types of mental deficiency seemed to have greatest significance for the educable group with IQs ranging from about 50 to 80.

It was this group of needful children which The Cove Schools was designed to serve—those with learning and adjustment problems resulting from perceptual, attentional, memory, conceptual, language, organizational, and coordination deficits due to early minor brain damage, but with normal or close to normal tested intelligence levels. Since the schools were intended to serve as a demonstration or exemplary facility, the number of children enrolled was limited so that those enrolled might be studied in depth and worked with in small groups. At the present time the schools enroll twenty-four children in the residence unit and thirty-three in the day program. The central focus is on a rather homogeneous group to a large extent free of the complicating variables of disadvantaged socioeconomic circumstances and primary emotional problems. These are children of parents who want to provide opportunities but are frustrated by their lack of knowledge and the child's deficiencies.

The complicating emotional factors which are present are judged to be secondary. In a controlled environment with appropriate demands, many of the unacceptable reactive behavior patterns can be expected to change for the better as the primary problem improves. Although the major emphasis is on the group described above, room is always left for a few children who differ in a more extreme way, that is, who present severe deficits in language, perceptuo-motor development, behavior controls and emotional development, or who have additional complicating conditions of sensory losses or motor involvement. The latter are children who would normally not be considered the responsibility of the usual public school special education program in contrast to the main group who belong within the sphere of public instructional provisions. With a few exceptions, therefore, the group served is today composed of children between the ages of six and twelve years, with an established medical diagnosis of central nervous system damage or dysfunction, no primary emotional disturbances, tested ability levels in the normal range or on the borderline of the educable mentally retarded classification, and failure to progress in the available school situation.

In working with children who have learning disabilities, it is easy to focus so narrowly on the details of their disabilities that one loses sight of the character of the forest while studying the trees. For this reason the staff finds useful the broad test patterns as revealed by the Children's Wechsler and supplemented by other tests when indicated. In a very general way these test patterns seem to be associated with observable learning characteristics and academic prognosis. Despite the discrepancy in favor of the verbal score often seen in these children and the irregularities in development reflected on the subtests, these children usually respond well to special teaching. They utilize the information given by the teacher and respond with insight when relationships are pointed out. They are frequently quite resourceful in developing compensatory behaviors to accommodate to or minimize the deficits of which they become aware. Despite their erratic and confused approach to learning, they give the impression of being alert, normal, and capable of some introspection and analysis of their own difficulties. Although they may have conceptual confusions, they do not have significant difficulty with the process of conceptualization. Once having mastered the basic academic skills, they can apply them in a meaningful way but usually continue to need help in higher level integrative processes such as summarizing and organizing. They often continue to experience inefficiency in various aspects of mentation for an indefinite period of time, making what appear to be careless errors of omission, transposition, substitution, etc.

Children with a discrepancy in favor of the performance score usually present a picture of relatively well-organized behavior, competence in table and group games, and enjoyment of visuo-motor activities for recreation. Generally they demonstrate auditory discrimination and retention difficulties and almost always have severe reading and spelling problems. Insight into arithmetical relationships is usually good, but recall for automatic combinations is poor. They progress slowly in academic learning, especially in reading and spelling, put often do very well in art, crafts, and mechanical areas. Many of the children demonstrate various auditory discrimination and retention difficulties, their thinking is often descriptive rather than generalizing, their vocabularies small. They are successful in games and activities depending upon good visuo-motor organization and usually have good grapho-motor skill. As academic work becomes progressively more verbal-abstract in the upper grades they find it increasingly difficult but continue to perform well in practical courses.

The teacher needs to be able to meet the child on the level appropriate to his general intelligence and maturity, yet not be surprised by the many gaps in understanding, conceptual confusions, or missed steps in learning which soon become apparent. These relate to the areas of disability or inefficiency of the system. It is not unusual to find that a child can comprehend the concept of the equator as an abstraction, yet be unable to locate it correctly on maps with different angles of projection. It is possible for a child to be working at a fourth-grade level of reading and arithmetic and not know his own telephone number or the months of the year, or just be learning for certain the spelling of his last name. Children with impairment in their capacity for visual perceptual organization will reveal inadequacies in their perception of unitary form, pattern, size, figure against disturbing ground, the relationship of parts to a whole, the analysis of wholes, discrimination of small differences, simultaneous awareness of several features of a stimulus configuration, and the ability to deal with space coherently by filling it and sectioning it in an organized way.

Difficulties in auditory discrimination and organization are important problems which often require specific attenton. It is usual for children enrolled in our setting to have developed mastery of such fundamental auditory perceptual processes as identifying a sound with the object which produces it and being able to sense its localization and intensity. Many, however, have not developed very keen discrimination for some of the speech sounds or the awareness of stress as heard in syllable accenting. Other problems involving the verbal-automatic levels of speech and the auditory memory functions are seen in problems in patterning (sequencing) sounds in words and words in sentences. The former leads to mispronunciations such as "bisgetti," "aluninum," "memeber" and the latter to problems in establishing automatic patterns of word order in sentences. Group work in discrimination and auditory analysis is given to all children in preparation for the learning of phonics. Individual attention is provided for the child with more severe problems for whom the group work is insufficient. Here again specific task-related exercises such as rhyming and sound blending are planned in reading and spelling.

Awareness of how one's body moves and how to relate oneself to the space in which one lives is usually also disturbed in the child with nonmotor brain damage and contributes to the impression of clumsiness he often presents (his impulsiveness, his hypertonic grasp, and jerky or poorly modulated movements do also). Three types of activities relating to knowledge of the body and its movement are a part of our program. Body image activities are used to help the child become aware of the various parts of his body and their relationship to each other; this knowledge will eventuate in an internalized scheme of body awareness or body image. Group activities in the form of games, such as "Do as I Do," "Did You Ever See a Lassie?" and "Simon Says," are enjoyed by the children and permit a wide range of bodily movements.

A somewhat more complex level of body awareness, involving sequential patterning and recall, is required in moving according to a defined pattern. The latter requires the corollary innervation and inhibition of movements and their integration into a smooth whole. Jumping, hopping on one foot, gliding, galloping, walking on all fours, skipping, walking backwards, jumping jacks, circling, are all movement patterns which require that the limbs be innervated in a particular sequence. Mastery of these activities, just as the mastery of any new learning, requires attention, perception, memory, feedback awareness, and integration and so is a valid learning experience. These activities, furthermore, form the basis for a large repertoire of later game, dance, and gymnastic patterns and so have a highly functional goal.

Further handicapping problems which seriously reduce the efficiency of learning or output of the minimally brain-damaged child relate not so much to actual disabilities as to the manner in which the central nervous system performs its work. When a task involves difficult material or much information to be processed (solving arithmetic problems or reading), successful performance requires elimination (or inhibition) of all irrelevant input. The minimally brain-damaged child experiences difficulty with this process and is called distractible or inattentive. Irrelevant information interferes with the processing of the focal information, so that the task requires longer to complete or is inefficiently or automatically done. On the other hand, the minimally brain-damaged child often seems to overdo the need to admit only part of the information entering by the sense organs. It is as though much of the nervous system needs to be reserved for the task in order to insure its successful performance and all other aspects of the environment wherein they themselves feel uncertain or lacking. Once shown that learning is within their grasp, they often make heroic efforts at mastery. The cumulative effect of many experiences which have demonstrated to the child that his peers seem to know all the answers, or that they develop rapidly and easily many skills which he must struggle to master, is to leave him feeling uncertain, dis-

couraged, or left out. In a low-risk situation offering little threat
to his self-esteem with a teacher who can show him how to
master the learnings he has missed so often he develops a strong
thirst for achievement and is willing to invest much of his energy
in it. The prime importance of a high level of motivation for
the child's future school success is self-evident.

Another important consideration is the work environment.
A quiet, orderly, disciplined classroom is essential. For children
who find the sounds and movements of the classroom disturbing,
an individual study carrel is made by using a screen to block
out the distractions. An attitude of self-discipline and individual
responsibility is established as early as possible. Since the lessons
are planned so that the child will be successful, he can be held
responsible for their completion. For most children with minimal
brain damage, rehabilitative education is a long-term process.
Intensive short-term measures applied during the years critical
for the development of literacy skills, work habits, and expectations for one's self may provide the foundation for later educational efforts. The effectiveness of the latter will depend upon
the strength of the child's drive to achieve despite what are
sometimes long odds and the willingness of the regular school to
program intelligently and sensitively for one more category of
handicapped child.

Marianne Frostig Center of Education Therapy

The Marianne Frostig Center of Educational Therapy is a
nonprofit institution operated by the Foundation of Educational
Therapy for Children, opened in 1947 in Los Angeles.

The Frostig Center has three main functions— service, professional training, and research. Services involve educational,
psychiatric and psychological evaluation, and training and treatment of children with learning difficulties. Learning difficulties
may be due to brain dysfunction, environmentally caused emotional disturbance, or an apparent lag in development without
known cause. Usually both causation and symptomatology are
multiple, with emotional disturbances a frequent factor in the
total clinical picture. Moreover, a child's problems do not affect
him alone, but involve the entire family. Therefore, parents

often need psychotherapy; nearly always they need advice on how to help their handicapped youngster and support in carrying it out.

To meet these difficulties the Frostig Center has developed a multidisciplinary approach, which brings together in one place the services of psychiatrists, psychologists, social workers, and educational therapists. Each child is provided with a comprehensive evaluation and treatment program, which covers all developmental areas and takes into account the needs of the whole family. The remedial training programs are precisely geared to the individual child's test results.

The procedures for evaluation and general program planning at the Frostig Center are based upon developmental psychology. The staff of the center learns from the writings of those scientists who study development as well as from those who have themselves developed educational methods on the basis of the research findings of others. For instance, Piaget's research has many applications in the classroom, and at the center specific methods are used to help the child to achieve what Piaget terms *decentration*— the ability to relate the different parts of the visual perceptual field to each other. These methods apply to training in figure-ground perception and spatial relationships, but transcend perceptual abilities by helping the child to gain increased freedom from dependency on immediate stimuli (*see* publications of Piaget, J. and Lambercier, *Arch Psychol,* Geneve, from 1942-1956). Piaget's theory of the development of thought processes has been adapted to helping children develop their abilities to judge, classify, draw inferences, and so on.

Similarly, the theories of Russian scientists, especially Luria (1961), Luria and Yudovich (1959), and Vygotsky (1962), concerning the development of language have yielded suggestions for remedial techniques in the area of language and thought.

Other contributions to the center's philosophy and practice have come from neurophysiology. Neurological and neurophysiological research and theory have only lately become applicable to psychological understanding and educational practice. They impress on the educational therapist the importance of giving equal consideration to the promotion of sensory input, motor behavior, and body awareness. They elucidate the influence of both motivation and alertness on the function of the nervous system, on the significance of laterality, and generally give much significant information in regard to the functioning of the nervous system and its relation to behavior and the influence of brain anatomy and physiology on learning. Of equal importance are the examples of educational methods introduced by educators themselves, such as the already mentioned Montesorri, and Ann Sullivan, whose work with Helen Keller is especially instructive; or the pioneer work with brain-injured children of Strauss and Lehtinen (1947) and Strauss and Kephart (1955). At present in the U.S., Kirk (1962), Cruickshank (1977), Kephart (1966), and Myklebust (1975) are among the leaders.

Anna Freud's (1946) studies are also most important for education. She pointed out that what was called *delinquency*, as well as what is termed *neurosis*, is an expression of early unresolved conflicts rooted in the family structure. Many nonlearners become able to learn when they are helped to resolve these paralyzing conflicts. The resolution of these conflicts results in a modification of their outlook and behavior and their relative freedom from guilt and anxiety, permitting them to marshal the capacities for learning which had previously been denied or immobilized. Heinz Hartman (1951), by redefining the concept of the ego and emphasizing its importance as the mediator between the individual and external reality, served further to bridge the gap between psychoanalysis and education. By helping the child to achieve initial satisfaction in mastery, education promotes the wish to master even more, to attempt new tasks, and to enjoy the growth of skills and new achievements.

Applying the concepts of ego psychology to education and its practitioners, Sheldon Rappaport has postulated that the teacher should have positive personality factors which enable the educational process to take place in what he calls the "relationship structure." The teacher is instructed to provide the pupils with a sense of mastery, a desire for genuine achievement, and an ability to accept limitations and to master impulses which would bring them in conflict with their environment. The teacher should use warmth and love to help children face their difficulties.

Erikson's work, as well as Hartman's, is most important for the education of children with learning difficulties. Erikson (1950) showed how endangered the child feels who cannot master his developmental tasks. Everyday observation in the classroom confirms his view; progress is indeed often at a standstill because the child is paralyzed by all-pervasive anxiety which may rise to panic when he is confronted with a task which seems too difficult for mastery or with a relationship which seems threatening. He is afraid to perceive and understand the everyday world and to face himself. In the center's classrooms, therefore, a great effort is made not only to help the children master their learning tasks but also to help them understand the significance of their act of learning—to perceive and to enjoy their own progress. When they begin to feel more positive about themselves and the world around them, ego development takes place.

PSYCHIATRIC SERVICES. In charge of the psychiatric department are the medical director and the chief psychiatrist, both psychoanalysts. The medical director is responsible for the overall medical supervision of the center. He oversees the intake conference, formulates a diagnosis on the basis of the comprehensive evaluation, and approves and is responsible for the final treatment plan. He works together with the executive director in charting the future course of the center.

The chief psychiatrist is responsible for the day-to-day psychiatric treatment. He supervises all therapists, including educational therapists insofar as they are concerned with behavior disturbances in the classroom. The supervisory meetings of both the chief psychiatrist and the medical director constitute seminars for the fellows in educational therapy or psychology. The chief psychiatrist works closely with the executive director and the medical director in formulating clinical policy.

PSYCHOLOGICAL EVALUATION. Extensive psychological evaluation is available for children from three years of age to adolescence who present a wide variety of problems. The major reason for referral to the Frostig Center may be a learning difficulty, but sometimes the emotional or social problems are even more serious. As a rule, multiple disabilities are found, and it is necessary to pinpoint the child's strengths and weaknesses in all developmental areas. A wide battery of assessment measures are used, which are reinforced by observation. The child is evaluated by a team of clinicians working independently. While the parents are seen by the social worker, the same child is usually seen more than once by each clinician and altogether four to six times.

The psychological test battery explores motor skills, language development, perceptual functions, intellectual aspects of the personality (verbal and nonverbal), emotional and social aspects of personality functioning, and academic achievement. Four tests are regularly employed with children of the appropriate age level: the Frostig Developmental Test of Visual Perception (1964), the Wepman Test of Auditory Discrimination (1958), the Illinois Test of Psycholinguistic Abilities (1961), and the Wechsler Intelligence Scale for Children (1949), but others are added at the discretion of the director of psychological services or of the examining clinician. The findings obtained are integrated with the case history and with psychological, educational, and medical findings obtained from other sources.

One of the senior psychologists summarizes the findings gathered by his team, makes recommendations based on these findings, and submits his report to the director of psychological services for extensive review. At the weekly psychology staff conference some of these reports are discussed; all are reviewed by the director of the department. Final recommendations and dispositions are made by the psychiatric intake team headed by the medical director. The findings are interpreted to the parents, and recommendations are made by the social worker who did the intake interview, together with one of the psychologists who participated in the test evaluation. The parents thus have direct contact with one of the clinicians who studied their child.

EDUCATIONAL THERAPY. While in Vienna, Doctor Frostig's observations of postencephalic children indicated that such children might have perceptual disturbances, and she concluded that they, too, might be beneficially affected by training in sensory-motor functions and development of body image. Unfortunately, no standardized instruments were available to measure either a child's perceptual efficiency or the nature and degree of his improvement after training. The observations remained only "hunches" which could not be proved. Much later, in England and in America, psychologists interested in perception, such as Thurstone (1944), Wedell (1960), and Cruickshank (1957), found that the process of visual perception included several relatively independent abilities. The inception of the center in 1947 made possible a close study of children with learning difficulties, which seemed to confirm the conclusions of these psycholigists that a number of perceptual functions could indeed be differentiated. Five visual motor and visual perceptual abilities seemed of particular relevance to school performance: eye-hand coordination, figure-group perception, perception of form constancy, perception of position in space, and perception of spatial relationships.

To explore these abilities and to provide age norms, construction of a developmental test of visual perception was begun in 1958. Pilot studies were conducted throughout 1959 and 1960. Criteria used for the final selection of items in each subtest area were good age progression and low degree of contamination with other abilities. An attempt was made to differentiate tests of reproduction from those of recognition of visual stimuli.

Perception is the chief developmental task of the child at the age of beginning school entrance. Correlations found between teacher ratings of classroom adjustment and scores on the Frostig Test for 374 kindergarten children indicate that a child at this grade level who scores low on the test is highly likely to have difficulties with initial school adjustment. A lack of integrity of the nervous system is most clearly expressed in the main developmental task during any phase of development.

Not only are visual perceptual disabilities frequently reflected in disturbed behavior during the four- to seven-year age period, but a child's ability to learn to read is also affected by his visual perceptual development. The test enables the educational therapist to gauge the range of perceptual dysfunctions directly and to infer the existence of other dysfunctions if no perceptual disabilities are evident. Perceptual disturbances, especially visual ones, are so frequently the cause of learning difficulties, and probably of behavioral difficulties, that there is a temptation to believe that they are always the main or the only precondition for successful school progress. In the same way intellectual or emotional disturbances have been considered the essential cause. Usually, none of these factors occurs alone; the causation is nearly always multiple. All developmental abilities of a child have to be explored to find possible reasons for a learning deficit.

The program for each child is based on assessment data in each of six developmental areas (sensory-motor functions, perception, language, higher cognitive functions, emotional and social development) evidenced by children referred to the center. It is considered with what relationships, if any, exist among these deficits; how the deficits manifest themselves in school behavior and achievement; whether such deficits may be ameliorated and, if so, by what means. The various departments of the center contribute basic data: results of assessment at initial intake, including a developmental history; observations and progress reports by educational therapists; psychotherapy notes; the social worker's report on family attitudes and practices; public school reports; results of retesting, and so on. Many articles in professional journals, as well as textbooks written by staff members, explain in detail the methods employed at the Frostig Center. Among these is *Learning Problems in the Classroom* (1973) by Frostig and Maslow. In 1972 an experimental edition of the *Frostig Movement Skills Test Battery* by R. E. Orpet was published. Standardized on 744 Caucasian elementary school children from kindergarten through grade six, it consists of twelve subtests. The full battery requires approximately twenty or twenty-five minutes for administration to an individual child; however, a group of three or four children can be individually tested in about forty-five minutes. Time is saved in the group procedure by explaining and demonstrating each activity to the group and then by having each child perform individually. The subtests are administered in the order listed below:

Subtest	*Ability Assessed*
1. Bead stringing	Bilateral eye-hand coordination and dexterity

2.	Fist/edge/palm	Unilateral coordination involving motor sequencing
3.	Block transfer	Eye-hand and fine motor coordination involving crossing the midline of the body
4.	Bean bag throw	Visual-motor coordination involving aiming and accuracy
5.	Sitting/bending/reaching	Ability to flex spine, back muscles and hamstring ligaments
6.	Standing broad jump	Leg strength
7.	Shuttle run	Running speed and ability to make quick stops, changes of direction, and changes of body position
8.	Changing body position	Speed and agility in changing body position from a lying to a standing position
9.	Sit-ups	Abdominal muscle strength
10.	Walking board	Ability to maintain dynamic balance
11.	One foot balance:	
	a. eyes open	Static balance with eyes open
	b. eyes closed	Static balance with eyes closed
12.	Chair push-ups	Arm and shoulder girdle muscle strength (P. 2)

California State Diagnostic School for Neurologically Handicapped Children

In response to the requests of parents and a few medical and educational leaders that the state provide a specialized program for cerebral palsied children, the California State Legislature, on April 23, 1943, passed a resolution requiring the State Department of Education and the State Department of Public Health to investigate "the number of such children in the state who are in need of and can be benefited by special treatment and education . . . and to report to the Fifty-sixth Session of the Legislature the result of its investigation and make recommendations as to the treatment and education of such children, together with the facilities required for such purposes and the costs thereof." This report was provided, and the Fifty-sixth Session of the California State Legislature authorized the establishment of two state residential schools for cerebral palsied children in conjunction with the state cerebral palsy clinics. The California State Department of Education was designated as the agency responsible for the administration of the schools.

In 1946 the school for northern California was established in temporary quarters near Redwood City, and the one for southern California was established at the Convalescent Home of Children's Hospital in Los Angeles.

In 1953, the legislature authorized funds for the construction of facilities for the northern California school in San Francisco, at Lake Merced Boulevard and Winston Drive and adjacent to the San Francisco State College. In 1955, the northern California school was moved from Redwood City to these facilities. In March, 1964, the southern California school was moved into new facilities near the California State College at Los Angeles. A third school was established in Fresno in 1971.

In 1955, the next major step was taken to meet the needs of children with central nervous system disorders when the legislature, at the request of the State Department of Education, broadened the scope of the program to include "other similarly handicapped children." The two schools for cerebral palsied children were authorized by this legislation to extend their services to children with central nervous system disorders even though the children did not have motor handicaps. In the past few years the accepted student population has been composed of children with central nervous system dysfunction with only minimal or no motor involvement. In 1967 the name of the facilities was changed to Diagnostic School for Neurologically Handicapped Children. Most recently the Schools have been adding facilities for autistic childern.

OBJECTIVES. Because brain-injured children frequently have multiple handicapping conditions — sensory, emotional, intellectual, and motor in varying degrees and combinations—it is necessary to make a thorough differential diagnosis of all aspects of each child's ability to function in each of these areas before the programs of treatment and education he needs can be determined. The children must be worked with in small groups, and highly specialized and individualized teaching techniques must be employed. Therefore, the objectives of the schools are as follows:

1. To diagnose the degree and extent of each child's disorder
2. To determine the kind of educational programs best suited to

meet the needs of children with cerebral palsy and other similar handicaps

3. To determine the type of medical program that will enable each child with CNS dysfunction to progress to the extent his capability permits

4. To provide services for children with CNS dysfunction whose need for education and treatment programs cannot be met in the children's communities

5. To serve as a resource in the training of teachers, therapists, and other professional personnel

6. To serve as a demonstration laboratory for the in-service training of professional persons interested in special education

7. To provide counseling and education services for parents of children enrolled in the state schools for children with CNS dysfunction that will help to secure for each child the type of treatment and educational opportunities he needs.

REFERRAL FOR ENROLLMENT. Any individual between the ages of three and twenty-one who is a resident of California and who is suspected of having a central nervous system disorder (brain damage) may be referred to the schools for evaluation and enrollment by the following individuals, groups, and agencies:

1. The physician directing the medical program of the school or school district in which a child is enrolled

2. The consultant physicians of the State Crippled Services Cerebral Palsy Clinics that are conducted in various communities throughout the state

3. The county superintendent of schools of the county in which a child resides, the superintendent of schools or the director of special education of the district in which the child is enrolled, or the principal of the school in which the child is enrolled

4. The child's family physician who, as a result of his study, has found or suspects central nervous system damage and desires to have an intensive study made of the child

5. The State Neurological Diagnostic Clinics operated under the auspices of the State Department of Public Health and conducted in hospitals in different communities throughout the state

6. The staff of a state school.

DIAGNOSTIC EVALUATION. Each state school maintains a facility for a short-term diagnostic study of the child. Each child who is accepted for enrollment is initially diagnosed to determine the scope of his problem and to determine the period of enrollment.

The study, which usually lasts for one week, includes an evaluation of the child's immediate physical, intellectual, education, and emotional status. It is an integrated and coordinated study by a staff of educators, medical personnel, psychologists, and therapists. The medical evaluation is supervised by the school's medical director, and medical specialists are employed to examine the child whenever such services are found to be appropriate.

The cost of the medical examinations is borne by the state through the Crippled Children Services, the State Department of Public Health, or by appropriations to each school for medical services. Parents and guardians are expected to pay the costs of transportation for the child to and from the school, the cost of meals eaten at the school by siblings and adults other than the child's parents, and the child's personal expenses.

Under the school's program, a child may be enrolled on an inpatient or outpatient basis, depending upon the place of residence of the child or upon his family's financial circumstances. At least one parent or the guardian is expected to remain with the child during the initial evaluation period, a period ranging from two to five days.

Upon completion of the short-term diagnostic study, the child may be treated in one of the following ways:

1. Referred to a special education class in his home community
2. Referred to an appropriate agency for further service
3. Enrolled in the school's program as a residential or day student, depending upon his requirements. (Such an enrollment is based upon the necessity to work intensively with the child in order to determine the kind of program which will be of the greatest benefit to him.)

LONG-TERM RESIDENTIAL PROGRAM. The long-term enrollment program is designed to meet the educational-medical needs of each child. Special education programs are conducted by the state school's teaching staff at the nursery, elementary, and secondary school level. The medical program, under the supervision of a licensed physician, includes prescription of routine nursing care, medications, and regular consultations by medical and dental specialists. Special drugs are used when approved jointly by the medical director and by the child's family physician.

Group and individual physical, occupational, and speech therapy are scheduled according to the need of the child. Social casework and psychological counseling are available for parents and children when need for them is indicated. Board, room, laundry, and minor repairs to the child's clothing are provided by the school without cost to the parents. Children are generally enrolled for a period of from three to nine months for intensive study and determination of a meaningful program.

Each child's educational program is individually designed to help him in the areas where he has the most difficulty, as demonstrated by psychological and educational testing. The teacher's goal is to discover techniques and approaches to help the child make gains in the fundamental academic subjects. The program for the children enrolled is coordinated by educational and medical personnel who understand each other's viewpoints and who employ all known techniques in their effort to secure for each child a diagnosis and prognosis that may be used as a basis to determine the treatment program he must have if he is to have a life that is as productive as his abilities permit.

Language comprehension and expression (oral, written, or by gesture) are essential for living and learning. Speech therapists contribute to the overall program by evaluating the children's language skills and by giving the children intensive training in the skills which enhance self-expression. The audiometric center provides the special equipment the speech therapist uses to obtain a hearing evaluation of each child.

The staff psychologists serve an integrative function in the diagnostic and treatment program by providing a comprehensive appraisal of the child's intellectual and emotional capacities. The findings of the staff are interpreted to all school personnel who work with the child.

Attractive four-bed dormitory rooms provide bed space for the children in residence. "Roommates" chosen for compatibility of social maturity and interests become close friends in this environment. A staff of registered nurses and resident attendants provides personal care for the children day and night.

Recreation rooms and playgrounds are provided for evening and weekend recreation. The children are divided into compatible recreation groups and are encouraged to participate in suitable recreation activities under the supervision of an attendant staff. The aim of the recreation program is to provide each child with opportunity to learn appropriate leisure-time activities. Every effort is made by the staff to carry out activities that are appropriate to classroom work.

Educational and medical personnel from the child's home community, as well as representatives of authorized social agencies, are invited to join with the school staff in the conference that it holds for each child on the results of his evaluation study. In this conference the group has opportunity to share information and data about the child, to discuss findings by the staff of the school, and to study the resources of the child's home community as a means of developing a long-term plan for the child. If it is decided that the child's development can be significantly accelerated by a longer enrollment for the purposes of instruction, treatment, and training, then such an enrollment is suggested to the child's parents and to the officials of the school in the child's home community.

A conference of staff members of the State Diagnostic School and the parents or guardian of a child is held during the enrollment period if the members of the staff think that the conference will produce results that may be helpful in making the diagnosis of the child's needs and in determining the kind of program that is likely to be most beneficial. During the enrollment period and at the end of it, the parents or guardian of the child meet with members of the professional staff of the school to discuss recommendations which the members have made. Every effort is made to assist those responsible for the child to understand and accept the staff evaluation and the recommendations of the staff regarding the program that the child should have.

SPECIAL CLASSES. *Language Disabilities* (*Aphasia*). Children who have been diagnosed as language handicapped are enrolled in the class for language development. The language handicap is of a symbolic nature, i.e. aphasia (which may be receptive or expressive), alexia, agraphia, or acalculia, or some combination of these. The language retardation is not due to a hearing loss, to mental retardation, or to emotional problems, but to brain injury. Varying degrees of these conditions may be manifest in the disorder.

Children are enrolled for periods up to one year for language therapy. The primary emphasis is upon determining methods by which each child can learn language, and this emphasis results in special attention being given to the educational techniques required to help the child progress academically. The program is individualized, and attention is given to avoiding the undesirable effects which frequently accompany neurological impairment, such as distractibility, perseveration, and perceptual problems.

In general, the teacher uses methods which follow the pattern of normal language development. Those situations, persons, and objects most immediate to the child's daily experiences supply the materials utilized. Materials are selected or prepared on the basis of their relationship to the child's present level of language development. Attempts are made to work with the parents of each child and with the school personnel in the child's home community who will continue working with the child when he leaves the State School so that improvement in the child's language development while he is in the state school may be furthered by the school he attends.

Perceptual Disorders (Dyslexia). The class is for children of normal and above intelligence whose major problems are in the area of reading and who exhibit a degree of neurological involvement. Some neurologically impaired children are unable to achieve mastery of basic academic skills even though their measured intellectual capacities are within the educable range. The primary handicap of these children is inability to integrate visual stimuli into meaningful information. They may have normal visual acuity but be unable to interpret relationships of size or relative position, to coordinate eye movements with body movements, or to attend to a major visual stimulus while screening out extraneous stimuli. Sometimes they are also unable to retain visual symbols in their memory. Any of these inadequacies can interfere with their profiting from participation in preschool activities to the extent that they have the prerequisites needed to acquire skills such as reading. These inadequacies are also responsible for many social and behavioral disorders as the child attempts to respond to a world which he perceives in a confusing and disorganized manner.

These children do not necessarily have additional handicaps of orthopedic involvement, speech problems, visual impairment, lack of hearing acuity, or mental retardation, but they may exhibit the characteristics associated with such handicaps. The major emphasis in a training program for perceptually handicapped children is to help them develop visual perceptual skills. Specially prepared materials that require the use of all forms of sensual impressions—touch, muscle sense, hearing—are used for this purpose.

Readiness and Remedial Class. The readiness and remedial class is for children who have a variety of problems, such as are caused by immaturity or visual or auditory difficulties that have prevented the children from being successful in school. Children in the younger age group with such problems usually need an intensive reading readiness program and a considerable amount of individual instruction before they can participate successfully in regular school programs.

The older children who have major problems in the basic school subjects, such as reading, writing, arithmetic, and spelling, are given the individualized help each one requires. Their problems may be due to a variety of causes: visual or perceptual problems, or both; visual-motor coordination problems; visual or auditory discrimination difficulties, or both.

After the learning disability is differentially and definitely diagnosed in the Medical-Educational Diagnostic Clinic, a child may enter the remedial program, where he will be given the specific type of help that he needs. The teacher's primary aim in this program, as in the other programs, is to reduce the discrepancy between a child's ability and his achievement.

Institute for Childhood Aphasia

The Institute for Childhood Aphasia (ICA) was established by Jon Eisenson as a unit of the Division of Speech Pathology and Audiology, School of Medicine, Stanford University, in September, 1962. The institute was initially funded by a grant from the Scottish Rite Foundation of California and, for the first two years, was almost entirely supported by Scottish Rite funds. At this time a major portion of financial support continues to come from this source, but additional funds have come from several government agencies including the Office of Education, the Children's Bureau, the National Institute for Neurological Diseases and Blindness, and the Chronic and Sensory Diseases Branch of the United States Public Health Service. In September of 1965 a sizable grant from the United Cerebral Palsy Foundation enabled us to institute and expand a three-year research program to establish differential criteria for nonverbal children. In 1973 Jon Eisenson moved the ICA to the campus of California State University, San Francisco.

OBJECTIVES. The overall objectives of the ICA may be summarized as follows:

1. To establish criteria for behavioral and linguistic impairments in children with congenital or early acquired (before age two) brain damage. Such criteria, it is hoped, will permit differential diagnoses for nonverbal or severely linguistically retarded children who may be perceptually handicapped (developmentally aphasic) from those who are primarily mentally retarded, severely impaired in hearing, or emotionally (affectively) involved (primary autism or childhood schizophrenia).

2. To provide opportunity for language clinicians, speech therapists and other professional persons concerned with problems of language retardation to develop specific and differential techniques for developing language in brain-damaged, nonverbal children.

3. To provide a laboratory for experimentation with learning approaches which directly or indirectly may help to establish cognitive functioning in aphasic children.

4. To provide diagnostic evaluations and recommendations as to appropriate therapy and training for children referred to ICA but who cannot be enrolled for long-term treatment. Such diagnostic evaluations may, when indicated, include periods of from one to ten weeks of "diagnostic therapy."

5. To provide interested clinicians, graduate students, and other professional persons with opportunities on a trainee, intern, resident, or fellowship basis to obtain experience with aphasic and other nonverbal children in the development of diagnostic and therapeutic skills. Training of professional personnel is to be carried on through an apprenticeship relationship with one or more members of the ICA staff.

THE PEDIATRIC NEUROLOGIST (MEDICAL COORDINATOR). The pediatric neurologist makes his assessment of the child as would any pediatrician or neurologist who routinely and periodically examines a child for health status. He observes the child's reflexes and his sensory and motor abilities. In brief, he determines whether the child has the basic equipment for normal development and for learning what he is expected to learn in and out of school. The pediatric neurologist determines what specialized medical examinations are needed for the individual child and arranges for them.

More specifically, however, the pediatric neurologist wants to have directed questions from other professional persons who have contact with the child so that he can make directed and specialized observations during his own examination. Therefore, he wishes to be informed if a teacher or a clinician observes that a child has lapses of attention, or of memory, or suddenly loses contact with his environment. He wants to know about inconsistencies and liabilities of behavior, of hyperactivity or of hypoactivity, or of catastrophic reactions. He needs to be informed if any behavior has been observed by others that might constitute or resemble a seizure.

The neurologist makes direct observations about motor difficulties, gross and fine. He observes tongue and hand movements for possible dyspraxic involvements. He listens to the child's vocalizations and, if possible, views the activity of the vocal bands for indication of nerve weakness or paralysis. He also observes inconsistent behavior and sudden extinction of responses as well as the child's ability to attend and to concentrate. All of these observations are correlated with his neurological findings and their implications for the child as to his ability and potential for learning.

The neurologist, at staff conferences, explains the significance of EEG abnormalities and how these may relate to fluctuations in attention and to deviant behavior. Where indicated, he prescribes medication for control or modification of CNS dysfunctioning. He is also mindful that all concerned—the parents, the teachers, and the language clinicians—must be informed of expected changes when medications are administered. Such changes may include temporary depressions in alertness and in the child's affective responses as well as in periods of nausea and dizziness. On the other hand, improvement may also be expected along these lines.

THE STAFF PSYCHOLOGIST. The psychologist, through the use of direct and sophisticated observation, as well as through the use of selected standardized diagnostic instruments and test batteries, seeks to assess the child's abilities and liabilities, his assets and impairments, so that a picture of the child's mental, emotional and social functioning may be obtained. The psychologist is concerned not only with present functionings but with potential for future functioning. In a very basic sense, the psychologist is engaged in an "extended neurological." The evaluation of a child's perceptual functioning provides information to the neurologist which may reinforce or set aside suspicion about possible neurological involvement. Sometimes, the psychologist's observation provides clues of a more subtle nature than those readily picked up by the neurologist in a routine examination.

The information and insights obtained by the psychologist provide one basis not only for a differential diagnosis but for training and educational procedures which are consonant with such a diagnosis.

PSYCHIATRIC SOCIAL WORKER. The psychiatric social worker is responsible for the nonmedical aspects of the initial interview with the parents. Ordinarily, such an interview seeks to obtain relevant information stated as far as possible in the parents' own words about the way the parents view their child and, specifically, as to the nature of the child's problem which brought him to our institute. Information is obtained about the family background with emphasis on siblings and other relatives who may have had or who have similar or related language problems. Information about the child's social development is obtained through informal questioning, through the administration of formal inventories such as the Vineland Scale of Social Maturity, and the Doll Preschool Attainment Record.

The psychiatric social worker also obtains information about parental relationships to the child, to siblings, and to one another. In addition, the financial status of the family is determined with a view toward deciding whether any need exists for financial assistance for expenses involved in assessment and therapy. The psychiatric social worker is also available for consultation with the parents should need for more than financial support be required. The usual function of assisting in the placement of a child with an appropriate educational or training agency is also assumed by our psychiatric social worker; so also are the usual duties of consultation with members of the family and the staff relative to problems within the family that influence the child's behavior and may be related to his language difficulties.

THE LANGUAGE CLINICIAN. Each language clinician has dual teaching-training roles—the training of the child and, through an apprenticeship relationship, the training of the student clinician or intern. In accordance with the diagnosis or designation for each child determined during our institute staffing, the language clinician develops an individualized program of therapy. Records are kept of each child's progress in therapy.

Specifically, the language clinician is concerned with the training of the child, individually as well as in small groups, in the establishment of sensory-motor skills basic to language development and in the development of language skills per se. The language clinician is also directly responsible for the supervision of student interns. In addition, the language clinician consults with parents regarding techniques and skills that may be practiced and reinforced in the home environment. For those children who attend schools or other educational agencies, the language clinician consults with teachers and supervisors so that training programs may be maximally coordinated. Each language clinician also serves as a member of the diagnostic team and participates in all staffings.

From the data collected at the Institute for Childhood Aphasia, the staff members have published numerous articles in professional journals. Tyack and Gottesleben (1974) published their version of language sampling; the director, Jon Eisenson (1972), published a book, *Aphasia in Children*, which has become a guidepost in setting up programs for the language remediation of children with central nervous system dysfunction. In this book, in addition to extensive coverage of the speech and language characteristics of brain-injured children. Eisenson outlines programs for specific areas of deficiency, which include the following:

Speech-sound processing
The hyperactive child
Establishing representational behavior
Establishing and developing language in congenitally aphasic children
The child with expressive disturbance: Oral apraxia.

ADULT APHASIA

Since more than 80 percent of speech/language clinicians are employed in settings which provide services for children, only a minority of these professionals work with adults. Hospitals, private speech and hearing clinics, local branches of the Society for Crippled Children and Adults, Inc. (Easter Seal Society), and some University Speech and Hearing Centers have facilities for adult aphasics. However, the most comprehensive facilities for the remediation of adult aphasia are within the Veterans Administration Hospitals; the present writer was able to visit more than thirty of these hospitals on a sabbatical tour during the spring of 1976.

The ancient Egyptians reported head injuries with loss of speech between 3000 and 2500 B.C. and the term *apoplexy*, often resulting in aphasia, has been a part of medical literature for centuries. In 1861, Pièrre Paul Broca reported to the Anatomical Society that aphasia was the result of a lesion involving the left frontal convolution. In 1874, Carl Wernicke described the symptoms of sensory aphasia which followed lesions to the left temporal lobe of the cerebrum. Since the observations and writings of these two pioneers, numerous aphasiologists have added to the literature concerning the loss of speech and language as the members of sequelae of trauma or cerebral vascular accident (CVA). At the present time a national organization, Academy of Aphasiology, meets annually to discuss the latest developments in the field. Another group, composed primarily of employees of the Veterans Administration Hospitals, has an annual Clinical Aphasiology Conference. There are also workshops and clinical sessions in connection with the annual conference of the American Speech and Hearing Association.

Although aphasia may be caused by external blows to the head (trauma) or by penetrating wounds, such as those caused by bullets, the majority of adult aphasics are probably the victims of some form of cerebral vascular accidents. Such accidents, popularly known as "strokes," are more frequent with individuals over the age of fifty, but they have been known to occur with children. Jon Eisenson (1971) has discussed the causes of aphasia:

> The possible causes of cerebral damage with which aphasic disturbances are associated are many and varied. They include direct trauma by externally applied force, tumors, cerebral vascular lesions (embolisms, thromboses, aneurysms, hemorrhages), infectious diseases affecting brain tissue, and degenerative diseases invading the brain. (P. 1241)

Characteristics of Adult Aphasics

The most notable characteristic is the loss of ability to use language, either receptive or expressive or both. The degree of loss may vary from slight to total and the recovery of the patient may occur in a few days or take several months. In more severe cases, the patient may never regain his premorbid linguistic abilities. His loss may be restricted to oral language, or it may include losses in the areas of written language and quantative thinking (mathematics). In some cases the patient may be able to carry on a conversation but be deficient in reading (dyslexia) or in writing (dysgraphia). The patient's articulation is usually affected, but he may be able to articulate those words and phrases which he can recall. He often swears quite intelligibly and can issue complaints without difficulty.

Victims of strokes may have varying degrees of physical involvement, from monoplegia (one limb) to quadriplegia (four limbs); in many cases they are far more concerned about an inability to walk than to talk. Jon Eisenson has observed the personality traits of stroke victims:

> Generally, the effect is to aggravate those traits which are on the debit side of a personality. However, with the possible exception of concretism in some instances, we do not find new traits but rather manifestations in an intensified form of old traits. Unfortunately, with language and the ordinary instrumentalities of expres-

sion impaired, the degree of intensification of old traits may be so great as to appear new, in the sense that they cannot be ignored by persons having close and frequent contact with the aphasic. (P. 79)

Speech and Language Rehabilitation

Hopefully, the aphasic will be in a setting where he can have a complete program with the services of a team of experts. These include the orthopedist, the orthotist, the physical therapist, occupational therapist, the nursing staff, the clinical psychologist, and the speech pathologist. There should be frequent consultation (staffing) among these team members in planning the long range rehabilitation program for the patient.

There is no doubt that many aphasics improve significantly in language skills, but there is controversy whether such improvement is due to language therapy or merely to spontaneous recovery. Sarno, Silverman, and Sands (1970) reported the results of therapy with thirty-one stroke patients, all described as severe expressive-receptive aphasics. At the outset, these patients had essentially no speech and little understanding of speech; some were able to say a few words and understand some simple commands. They were assigned to one of three treatment groups: programmed instruction, nonprogrammed instruction, and no treatment. Patients who were treated received up to forty hours of therapy. Testing, at termination of treatment and one month later, to determine the degree to which a behavior learned during the treatment period had been retained, revealed no significant differences among the three groups. There was adverse criticism of this study among aphasiologists, and many suggested that the number of patients was insufficient, that their degree of aphasia was too severe, and that the treatment period was too brief. Presently, there is a cooperative study concerning the efficacy of speech therapy with aphasic patients being conducted at five Veterans Administration Hospitals; the results of this longitudinal study should shed some light upon the situation.

One of the problems in assessing the degree of aphasic involvement and the effectiveness of speech and language therapy is finding a measuring instrument which is both reliable and valid. Adkins (1974) conducted a study in which a comparison was made of the family members' assessment of the aphasic patient's communicative functioning level with assessments made by an aphasiologist using a standardized test. The spouse of each of thirteen subjects was interviewed, using the Functional Communication Profile as a questionnaire, concurrently with the testing of each patient using the Porch Index of Communicative Ability. This procedure was performed twice with a time lapse of one month between testing. Statistical analyses, using nonparametric statistical tests based on ranks, yielded the following results:

1. Comparison of performance of the Functional Communication Profile and the Porch Index of Communicative Ability showed a significant but weak relationship, indicating no more than a general group trend for related scores.
2. During the one month period between the first and second test, the patients made significant gains on both measures.
3. The amount of change that occurred on the Functional Communication Profile was not related to the amount of change on the Porch Index of Communicative ability.
4. Both tests proved to be highly reliable from the first to the second test.
5. Further study is needed in order to identify or devise a measuring instrument that combines the advantages of both tests: the objectivity of the PICA with assessment of communicative functioning in real-life situations. Such an instrument is needed to more precisely determine effects of speech and language therapy for aphasic patients. (P. 22)

Within the Veterans Administration Hospital system, especially in the western half of the United States, the Porch Index of Communicative Ability is highly regarded and its author, Bruce E. Porch, chief of Speech Pathology at the Veterans Administration Hospital in Albuquerque, New Mexico, has received accolades at the Clinical Aphasiology Conference. He continues to collect data concerning the test, as well as to develop a similar test for use with children. Two other tests, also developed at Veterans Administration Hospitals, are the Minnesota Test for Differential Diagnosis of Aphasias (1965) and The Boston Diagnostic Aphasia Test (1972).

In spite of the lack of objective evidence that language therapy for adult aphasics is effective, the general consensus is that such therapy has beneficial consequences. Martha Taylor Sarno (1975) has summarized as follows:

> Since so few studies have been carried out, much remains to be learned about the natural recovery process and the role of speech therapy. Despite the unsatisfactory state of our knowledge, there is one conclusion we can draw: as in other spheres of application, rehabilitation does not imply return to normal. The patient must be supported psychologically, he must be taught to adapt to his altered condition, he needs assistance toward recovery of self-esteem and a knowledge that something is being done to help him regain his power of communication. It is for these reasons that the aphasic patient must have speech therapy, whether or not the therapeutic process adds substantially to natural restitution. (P. 398)

Aphasiologists who specialize in speech and language rehabilitation of adult aphasics work in numerous settings, such as rehabilitation units in hospitals (a setting in which the present writer was employed on a part-time basis for four years between 1972 and 1976), in independent or university-related speech and hearing clinics, and in private practice. A number of professional friends of the author have retired from their university positions as speech pathologists to develop full-time case loads with adult aphasics. Approaches to speech and language therapy differ according to the training and experience of the clinicians; some, following the writings of Bruce E. Porch, tend toward structured sessions based on the data obtained from administrations of the Porch Index of Communicative Ability; others prefer a more informal, almost psychotherapeutic approach in which they stress the vocabulary and phrasiology needed in daily living. In any event, in contrast to the lack of linguistic background of the child with developmental aphasia, the adult aphasic has had a fully developed language system which has broken down, and the remnants can be utilized in rebuilding his communication system. Bilingual patients often revert to their original language, so initial therapy conducted in that language may be more effective. Unfortunately, not too many aphasiologists are polyglots, but sequential language, such as counting, days of the week, and months of the year, can provide a starting point. Often, family members can be utilized to supplement the original language materials in the home situation.

Although prognosis is a professional responsibility of the aphasiologist, such predictions are tentative at best and usually must be based on unmeasurable attributes of the patient which come through to the experienced clinician. Many factors will affect the course of speech and language therapy in addition to the expertise of the clinician; among these are the age and physical condition of the patient, the motivation of the patient toward oral and written communication, the level of aspiration of the patient in communicative skills, the degree and type of aphasic involvement, and the support (without dependency) of the family in carrying on the speech and language program outside the clinic setting. As Eisenson (1973) has written, "Essentially, most aphasic learning is actually a retrieval or reestablishing of functions" (p. 158). Thus, the patient, the professional staff, and the family members must work in a unified manner to accomplish as much as possible in each individual case. Spontaneous recovery is considered to be limited to the first few months following the initial trauma, but a well-planned speech and language therapy program can be productive for many months or years. In general, therapy is less effective after two years and often tops out by the third year.

REFERENCES

Adkins, Carol S.: *Comparison of Two Measures of Communication in Adult Aphasics.* Master's thesis, California State University, Sacramento, 1974.

Becker, Leonard V.: Auditory-articulatory dimensions of reading and reading disability. In Hartstein, Jack (Ed.): *Current Concepts in Dyslexia.* St. Louis, The C. V. Mosby Company, 1971.

Birch, Herbert G.: *Brain Damage in Children.* Baltimore, Williams and Wilkins Company, 1964.

Blair, Francis X.: Programming for auditorially disabled children. In Fass, Larry A. (Ed.): *Learning Disabilities: A Book of Readings.* Springfield, Charles C Thomas, Publisher, 1972.

Bortner, Morton (Ed.): *Evaluation and Education of Children with Brain Damage.* Springfield, Charles C Thomas, 1968.

Cruickshank, William M.; Bice, H. V., and Wallen, N. E.: *Perception and Cerebral Palsy.* Syracuse, Syracuse University Press, 1957.

Cruickshank, William (Ed.): *Cerebral Palsy: A Developmental Disability,* 3rd rev. ed. Syracuse, Syracuse University Press, 1976.

Cruickshank, William M. and Johnson, G. Orville (Eds.): *Education of Exceptional Children and Youth.* 3rd ed. Englewood Cliffs, Prentice-Hall, Inc., 1975.

Darley, Frederic L.: *Diagnosis and Appraisal of Communication Disorders.* Englewood Cliffs, Prentice-Hall, Inc., 1964.

Darley, Frederic L.; Aronson, Arnold E., and Brown, Joe R.: *Motor Speech Disorders.* Philadelphia, W. B. Saunders Company, 1975.

Doll, E. A.: Mental deficiency vs. neurophrenia. *Am J Ment Defic,* 57:477-480, 1953.

Eisenson, Jon: Perceptual disturbances in children with CNS dysfunction and implications for language development. *Br J Disord Commun,* 1:(I), 21-33, 1966.

————: *Aphasia in Children.* New York, Harper and Row, 1972.

————: *Adult Aphasia.* Englewood Cliffs, Prentice-Hall, Inc., 1973.

————: Aphasia in adults: Basic considerations. In Travis, Lee Edward (Ed.): *Handbook of Speech Pathology and Audiology.* New York, Appleton-Century-Crofts, 1971.

————: Therapeutic problems and approaches with aphasic adults. In Travis, Lee Edward (Ed.): *Handbook of Speech Pathology and Audiology.* New York, Appleton-Century-Crofts, 1971.

Erikson, Erik H.: *Childhood and Society.* New York, Norton, 1950.

Freud, Anna: *The Psycho-Analytical Treatment of Children.* London, Imago, 1946.

Frostig, Marianne; Lefever, D. W., and Whittlesey, J. R. B.: The Marianne Frostig Developmental Test of Visual Perception. *Percept Mot Skills,* 19:463-499, 1964.

Goodglass, H. and Kaplan, E.: *The Boston Diagnostic Aphasia Test.* Washington, Lea and Febiger, 1972.

Hartman, Heinz: Ego psychology and problem of adaptation. In Rapaport, David (Ed.): *Organization and Pathology of Thought.* New York, Columbia University Press, 1951.

Ingram, Suzanne: *An Analysis of the Language of Children Placed in an Aphasic Class.* Master's thesis, California State University, Sacramento, California, 1974.

Jenkins, James J.; Jimenez-Pabon, Edward; Shaw, Robert E., and Sefer, Joyce Williams: *Schuell's Aphasia in Adults.* 2nd ed. New York, Harper and Row, 1975.

Johnson, Doris J. and Myklebust, Helmer: *Learning Disabilities.* New York, Grune and Stratton, 1967.

Jones, Morris Val (Ed.): *Special Education Programs.* Springfield, Charles C Thomas, Publisher, 1968.

Kephart, Newell C.: *The Slow Learner in the Classroom.* Columbus, Charles
E. Merrill, 1960.

Kirk, Samuel A.: *Educating Exceptional Children.* Boston, Houghton
Mifflin Co., 1962.

Kirk, Samuel and McCarthy, James P.: *The Illinois Test of Psycholinguistic
Abilities.* Urbana, University of Illinois Press, 1961.

Licht, Sidney: *Stroke and Its Rehabilitation.* Baltimore, Waverly Press,
Inc., 1975.

Luria, A. R.: *The Role of Speech in the Regulation of Normal and Abnormal Behavior.* New York, Liveright, 1961.

Luria, A. R. and Yudovich, R. I.: *Speech and the Development of Mental
Processes in the Child.* London, Staples, 1959.

Marty, Mary Jane: *An Evaluation of the Perceptual-motor Skills of Children
Classified as Aphasic.* Master's thesis, California State University,
Sacramento, 1975.

Mecham, Merlin; Berko, Martin; Berko, Frances, and Palmer, Martin:
Communication Training in Childhood Brain Damage. Springfield,
Charles C Thomas, Publisher, 1966.

Menyuk, Paula: The bases of language acquisition: Some questions. *J
Autism Child Schizo,* 325-343, 1974.

Monsees, E. K.: Aphasia in children: Diagnosis and education. *Volta
Review,* 59:392-414, 1959.

Myklebust, Helmer: In Travis, Lee Edward (Ed.): *Handbook of Speech
Pathology.* New York, Appleton-Century-Crofts, 1957.

—————: Aphasia in children: Language development and language
pathology. In Travis, Lee Edward (Ed.): *Handbook of Speech
Pathology.* New York, Appleton-Century-Crofts, 1957.

—————: Aphasia in children: Diagnosis and training. In Travis, Lee
Edward (Ed.): *Handbook of Speech Pathology.* New York, Appleton-
Century-Crofts, 1957.

—————: Childhood aphasia: An evolving concept. In Travis, Lee Edward
(Ed.): *Handbook of Speech Pathology and Audiology.* New York,
Appleton-Century-Crofts, 1971.

—————: Childhood aphasia: Identification, diagnosis, remediation. In
Travis, Lee Edward (Ed.): *Handbook of Speech Pathology and
Audiology.* New York, Appleton-Century-Crofts, 1971.

—————: *Progress in Learning Disabilities, Volume III.* New York, Grune
and Stratton, 1975.

Orpet, R. E.: *Frostig Movement Skills Test Battery.* Palo Alto, Consulting
Psychologists Press, Inc., 1972.

Perkins, William H.: *Speech Pathology: An Applied Behavioral Science,*
2nd ed. St. Louis, The C. V. Mosby Company, 1977.

Porch, Bruce E.: *Porch Index of Communicative Ability: Administration,
Scoring, and Interpretation.* Palo Alto, Consulting Psychologists Press,
1971.

Rappaport, Sheldon: Personality factors teachers need for relationship structure. In Cruickshank, William M. (Ed.): *The Teacher of Brain-Injured Children*. Syracuse, Syracuse University Press, 1966.

Sarno, Martha T.: *The Functional Communication Profile: Manual of Directions*. New York Institute of Rehabilitation Medicine, New York University Medical Center, 1969.

Schuell, Hildreth: *Differential Diagnosis of Aphasia with the Minnesota Test*. Minneapolis, University of Minnesota Press, 1965.

Sarno, Martha Taylor: Disorders of communication in stroke. In Licht, Sidney (Ed.): *Stroke and Its Rehabilitation*. Baltimore, Waverly Press, Inc., 1975.

Sarno, Martha T.; Silverman, M., and Sands, E.: Speech therapy and language recovery in severe aphasia. *J Speech Hear Res, 13*:607-623, 1970.

Stark, Joel; Foster, C.; Giddan, J. J.; Gottesleben, R. H., and Wright, T. S.: Teaching the aphasic child. *J Except Child, 35*:149-154, 1968.

Strauss, A. A.: The education of the brain-injured child. *Am J Ment Defic, 56*:712-718, 1951.

Strauss, A. A. and Kephart, N. C.: *Pathology and Education of the Brain-Injured Child*, Volume 2. New York, Grune and Stratton, 1955.

Strauss, A. A. and Lehtinen, Laura: *Pathology and Education of the Brain-Injured Child*, Volume 1. New York, Grune and Stratton, 1947.

Thurstone, L. L.: A factorial study of perception. *Psychometric Monographs, No. 4*. Chicago, University of Chicago Press, 1944.

Tyack, D. and Gottesleben, R.: *Language Sampling, Analysis and Training*. Palo Alto, Consulting Psychologists Press, 1974.

Van Allen, Maurice W.: *Pictorial Manual of Neurologic Tests*. Chicago, Year Book Medical Publishers, 1969.

Vygotsky, L. S.: *Thought and Language*. New York, Wiley and Sons, 1962.

Wechsler, David: *Wechsler Intelligence Scale for Children*. New York, The Psychological Corporation, 1949.

Wedell, K.: The visual perception of cerebral palsied children. *J Child Psychol Psychiatry, 1*:215-228, 1960.

Wepman, Joseph: *Wepman Test of Auditory Discrimination*. Chicago, Language Research Associates, 1958.

Wood, Nancy E.: Decision making: Childhood aphasia. *ASHA, 5*:571-575, 1963.

CHAPTER 10

GENERAL LEARNING DISABILITY (MENTAL RETARDATION)

CATHERINE McCORMACK AND MILES RICHMOND

Definition, Degree, and Frequency

ALTHOUGH THE TERM *mental retardation* is the most universally used and accepted one, the various professional fields and workers dealing with individuals who have this condition have developed many classifications and labels which seemed to be the most appropriate descriptions at the time. Therefore, such terms evolved as *feeble-minded, moron, imbecile, mentally deficient, educable,* and *trainable.* The term currently in use is *general learning disability,* as opposed to *specific learning disability,* which is described in another chapter.

In addition to the diverse attempts at labeling children with general learning disability were the many attempts at defining this condition, since these children comprise a widely divergent, heterogeneous group. One definition formulated by the American Association on Mental Deficiency attempted to encompass all cases:

> Mental retardation refers to subaverage general intellectual function-
> ing which originated during the developmental period and is
> associated with impairment in adaptive behavior. (Heber, cited in
> Kirk, 1972, P. 163)

"Subaverage general intellectual functioning" refers here to one standard deviation below the general population mean on a standard intelligence test and "impairment in adaptive behavior" refers to deficiencies in maturation, learning, and social adjustment (Kirk, 1972).

Surveys which attempt to show the prevalence of children in the United States with general learning disability vary depending on the methods and criteria used. For example, if the examiner used an IQ score of 79 as the cut-off point, he would get a higher prevalence figure than if he used an IQ score of 69 as his cut-off point. Surveys conducted between 1953 and 1962 showed prevalence figures ranging from 15.2 to 50.2 per 1,000 children. However, the generally accepted rate is that 2 to 3 percent of school children are mentally retarded (Kirk, 1972).

The 3 percent of school children with general learning disability can be broken down as follows:

1. The "mildly retarded" (IQ from 50-70), 2.6 percent of the total population and 85 percent of the mentally retarded.
2. The "moderately and severely retarded" (IQ from 20-49), .3 percent of the total population and 11.5 percent of the mentally retarded.
3. The "profoundly retarded" (IQ below 20), .1 percent of the total population and 3.5 percent of the retarded. (Schlanger, 1973, P. 8)

Within these three classifications, speech and language difficulties occur in varying degrees:

Typically, less than half of the mildly mentally retarded have speech and language difficulties and these are not usually severe, 90 percent of the "moderately and severely retarded" and all of the "profoundly retarded" will have deviations in some or all areas of communication. (Schlanger, 1973, P. 8)

Etiology

The general agreement among the many different professional disciplines which deal with the retarded for the grouping of principal factors causing mental retardation is as follows:

1. Hereditary or familial traits resulting in general metabolic disturbances, or those affecting the central nervous system in a special way (genetic).
2. Embryonic or fetal disturbances reflecting the harmful influences acting upon the parents, especially the mother (constitutional).
3. Infections, toxic, traumatic, and nutritional difficulties during the birth period (environmental).
4. Infections, toxic, traumatic, and nutritional difficulties during the life after birth (environmental). (Nichtern, 1974, P. 116)

Down's Syndrome

Characteristics

Mongolism, trisomy 21, or Down's syndrome, as it is more frequently called at this time, "is the most common serious problem in development seen in a newborn. . . . It occurs more frequently than any other specific kind of mental deficiency or any single error in early development . . ." (Smith and Wilson, 1973). It is a perinatal condition caused by one of four types of chromosomal anomalies. The most common of the four types is nondisjunction trisomy 21, which is a faulty chromosomal separation during the formation of an ovum (and more rarely of a sperm). This results in an unequal distribution of chromosome 21 among the resulting cells (Donnell et al., 1975). This accounts for more than 90 percent of the Down's syndrome population (Wright et al., 1967). The results are a constellation of signs and characteristics which causes similar facial and bodily features among these children.

Articulation

It is generally accepted that retarded children have higher incidences of articulatory defects than are found in the general population, and several studies show that children with Down's syndrome have more articulation defects than other retardates. In a review of the literature, Zisk and Baler (1967) stated that they considered the descriptions of the articulation of these children to be fairly adequate. However, they wrote that little advancement has been made in understanding the cause of the speech problems in terms of the specific biological and social characteristics which "predispose" the mongoloid child to the development of given speech problems:

> . . . the lack of progress may be due partially to the adaption of naive positions, such as: "mongolism causes defective speech." Misconceptions of that kind obviously hinder the development of corrective techniques since they imply that the defect can be alleviated only by "curing" mongolism. (P. 229)

Several factors may be responsible for the poor articulation of these children. Some of their physical attributes directly affect the oral peripheral mechanism. A child may have some or all of the following: hypoplasia (incomplete development) of the maxilla; protrusion of the tongue; a thickened, fissured lower lip which may enlarge and hang down in later life; and mal-occlusion of the teeth (Magalini, 1971)—all of which may contribute to the high probability of speech defects. They also have palate abnormalities which result in a palate both high and low, called a "steeple" palate. In addition, newborns with Down's syndrome have generalized hypotonia or flabbiness of the muscles, which indicates cerebral immaturity. This means the development of the central nervous system of these children has been halted prematurely (Benda, 1969). As a result of the hypotonia, the speed and accuracy of production necessary for articulation usage may not be possible.

Language Development

In a review of the literature, Zisk and Baler (1967) concluded that the only agreement which existed between all observers is that these children are language delayed when compared to normal children. Morley (1972) wrote that language delay occurs frequently in mongoloid children with even the higher functioning mongoloid often exhibiting a severe language disorder. She also stated that, as a group, there is considerable variation with many remaining at the holophrastic (one word) level while others acquire enough language skills to communicate satisfactorily.

Zisk and Baler (1967) concluded further that the contribution to our knowledge about the language of children with Down's syndrome is difficult to assess. The literature agrees that they have delayed language, but the behaviors which were assessed were vaguely defined, and the studies lacked adequate controls. Specific factors relating to language development such as physiological and social variables have not yet been considered. Studies concerned with these specific variables may further support the statement that the mental retardation of Down's syndrome children is only partially responsible for the language delay.

Personality

Conflicts also exist in the literature on the personality characteristics of children with Down's syndrome. Several authors consider the personalities of this population remarkably similar and describe them as affectionate, pleasant, and docile (Lenneberg, 1967; West, Ansberry, and Carr, 1957; Magalini, 1971). However, Evans and Carter (1954) wrote, "They were often dirty, destructive, noisy, and obstinate, and sometimes also aggressive" (p. 960). Blessing (cited in Evans, 1974) found that mongoloid children exhibited the full range of emotional and social responses, as emphasized by Evans:

> This is worth emphasizing because in the past especially, this "contented cabbage" expectation may have contributed to the belief that mongol children were especially unresponsive to attempts at remediation. (P. 23)

Yet, if, as Lenneberg (1967) stated, these children are eager to please, this could make them more amenable to the therapy process.

Apparent differences of opinion exist in the area of personality traits, but conclusions are difficult, if not impossible, to arrive at since the judgments are so subjective.

Effectiveness of Therapy

The prevalent opinions about the utility and prognosis of speech and language therapy for children with Down's syndrome or children with mental retardation in general have undergone a gradual evolution since the 1950s. Prior to this period, education was restricted to children with an IQ above 50; therefore, most children with Down's syndrome were excluded. For example, West, Ansberry, and Carr (1957) stated, "The mongol is particularly unresponsive to speech rehabilitation, and it is practically useless to attempt such training" (p. 296). Reports such as this, based on clinical observation rather than controlled investigations, led to a paucity of research dealing specifically with the speech and language of the mongoloid child (Zisk and Baler, 1967).

However, as education in the 1950s began to encompass the trainable or severely mentally retarded with IQs below 50, training and management techniques for these children evolved. Today, in the 1970s, children with Down's syndrome receive education and therapy extensively. Nevertheless, the measurement and quantification of the effectiveness of speech and language therapy are difficult, and research has yielded little definitive information, as Kirk (1964) has observed:

> There have been few studies on the effects of therapy in speech correction or of educational programs on the development of speech and language. Only one study used randomized control groups, and few researchers have tested the reliability of their measuring instruments. Reports in many journals typically consist of a brief description of an educational program and a report that improvement was observed by the teachers or by others on a subjective basis. (P. 87)

In addition to the pragmatic factors Kirk (1964) mentioned, which impede conclusions about the effectiveness of therapy for children with Down's syndrome, are the abstract factors previously mentioned by Zisk and Baler (1967). That is, until the misconception that "mongolism causes defective speech" is abandoned, and corrective techniques and research deal with specific biological and social characteristics of the mongoloid child which "predispose" him to the development of given speech and language problems, the effectiveness of therapy will remain difficult to evaluate.

Intelligence

There is some disagreement as to the intelligence level of children with Down's syndrome, but there is a general overlapping of opinion that they fall primarily in the categories of moderately to severely retarded. Magalini (1971) cited the IQ range as being from the 20s to the 60s.

Types of Therapy

The type of therapy used with the Down's syndrome population and the retarded in general has changed from teaching primarily living skills (personal grooming, buttoning, etc.) to language skills. Although living skills are still considered important, the emphasis is on the ability to communicate.

Although there are innumerable approaches to language therapy with the retarded, four of the basic categories are described here. These categories are described broadly, since they are meant to give only the basic assumptions underlying the many theories and therapy approaches which branch from them.

Rote Learning. One of the currently most popular approaches with speech and language clinicians is the rote learning method. In this type of approach, one area of syntax and grammar is concentrated on at any one time. The area to be worked on is based on the normal progression of language development. For example, if a child has one word utterances, he is conditioned to imitate two word utterances (usually beginning with *noun + verb*) until the utterances are spontaneous; if a child uses sentences such as *Boy run*, he may be conditioned to incorporate *is + verb + ing* for *Boy is running*. Enlarging the vocabulary may or may not be incorporated. The goal of this type of therapy is that these utterances will emerge in the child's own language. As the child masters each linguistic milestone, another is introduced, expanding both length and complexity of the utterances.

The clinician may use a formalized program or establish her own informal program. The formalized program outlines constructions to be taught in a sequential, prescribed order. With the informal program, the clinician takes a language sample and, from this, determines what vocabulary concepts and constructions would be most appropriate for each child.

Prelinguistic Concepts. This type of therapy is most useful for children with very limited spontaneous verbal language. It consists of teaching children the requisite behaviors for speech and language, such as imitating, pointing, matching, same/ different, and sorting. Since it is not possible to teach all the feasible forms of constructions, and rote learning of sentences in an artificial situation may have little carryover to a child's spontaneous speech, particularly if he lacks the requisite skills, teaching the prelinguistic concepts serves to give the child the necessary tools to create and expand his own expressive language.

Play Therapy. In this type of therapy, selected constructions and vocabulary are incorporated into an activity. The activity may be making pudding or playing house, for example. The activities are also designed to provide motivation to communicate verbally. If the child is nonverbal, the clinician may start with simplified self-talk, such as "Wash cup . . . put cup here . . .

Where glass? Oh, here glass . . ." The child eventually begins to participate by doing his own self-talk and learns to comment on what he sees or does (Van Riper, 1972). The clinician avoids commands and yes-no questions which decrease a child's spontaneous language. The clinician also increases the complexity of her language as the child achieves mastery over a previous level.

NONSPEECH MODES. In addition to the verbal mode of language, which uses oral symbols, is the gestural mode of language, which communicates through manual signs, such as those used by the deaf. For some children the verbal code is too complex to comprehend and/or reproduce because of cognitive factors, such as auditory discrimination difficulties, or physical factors, such as difficulties in maintaining the speed and accuracy of the articulators, which is necessary for intelligible speech. The clinician may choose to use formal signs (established signs commonly used with the deaf) or informal signs (gestures that would be universally understood by most people or ones that are meaningful to the child and those in his home environment).

Simultaneous signing (signing and speaking) gives the child additional visual cues. It gives a "picture" of the word being said to increase the child's comprehension. The clinician may also use signing to give the nonverbal or unintelligible child a more effective means of expressing himself with those with whom he communicates most frequently. This necessitates that the clinician also involve one of those people, usually the mother, in enough training sessions so the child's signing is understood in the home situation.

In another nonspeech language training program described by Carrier (McReynolds, 1974), severely retarded children were taught to produce syntactically and semantically correct sentences by placing color-coded geometric shapes as symbols on a response board. The geometric shapes are symbols for morphemes and are color-coded to indicate grammatical class (noun, verb, article, plural marker, etc.). Once conditioning to the task has been accomplished, the child is shown a picture and is rewarded for producing only complete sentences describing the picture. The training does not attempt to follow the normal acquisition of language. According to the author, "the normal development process does not appear to be efficient logically, and indeed, some language-deficient children may fail to learn language because of the inefficiency of that process" (Carrier in McReynolds, 1974, p. 49).

As the child "writes" the sentence, the clinician speaks the words being represented. Through rote learning many children in the study imitated the words and allowed the clinician's model to fade out. Reports also showed that one child began speaking in other environments using some of the complex grammar taught in therapy.

CONCLUSION. The types of therapy described above are not necessarily mutually exclusive. In fact, it may prove to be beneficial in some cases to use an eclectic approach or tailor an approach to suit the needs of a client. The goal is to do whatever is most efficient for the client.

Methods of Language Training for the Adolescent Retarded at the Grant Special Education Center

Purpose of Montessori Materials

Language is the key to understanding about the world and being able to share that understanding in communications with others. In working with the retarded child, it is well recognized that language plays an important role in the conceptualization of the child's thought for the purpose of reasoning. In the course of development, after the sensory-motor period is over, the child conceptualizes and begins making concrete judgments about events and conclusions about future events. This seems to be the end of the mental development for many retarded children who never advance into the abstract reasoning stage requiring more advanced symbolization.

In order to develop into the concrete stage, the child must use some sort of symbolization to help describe and order his thoughts. This, even for the retarded, takes place in the form of receptive and expressive language. To facilitate this, the process must be well understood so that appropriate remediation can take place in the schools to establish this very important development for the child.

For this purpose, the sensory-motor materials designed by Doctor Maria Montessori have been beneficial to the students at the Education Center. These materials are designed to increase the individual discovery about certain sensory/motor advances, but they also increase language. The use of language in the Montessori education is always consistent and never changes by naming an object one name one time and another name another time. Specific names need to be used for initial understanding, especially for the retarded. The orderly and structured classroom provides an environment for order and structure for the elements of language.

Language Incorporation

Language is not a single entity and must be understood to be interrelated. Motor activities, social activities, and number conceptualizations are also part of language development, as well as language being a part of them.

Motor Skills Program

A well-designed physical education program has proven extremely effective, as both the mind and body are stimulated. It increases oxygen to the brain and would seem to be a positive factor physiologically.

The use of learning objects, verbs, and especially the more difficult names for things such as prepositions, are best taught in a motor skills class. As an example, when a child actually goes "under" the ladder or "over" the box, the child is "experiencing the language." At the Education Center, motor experience is a must, and through play and sometimes formal exercise the retarded child gets the full meaning of running, crawling, or such prepositions as *over, beneath,* or *behind.* A formalized program of circles, squares, and triangles cut out of plywood is used for shape discrimination and also for practical motor skills. Painting shapes on the playground concrete can be more useful than numbers for the retarded child to identify. When music is added to the motor skills, the rhythm seems only natural to the rhythm in the language, and the child responds to directions with more motivation and understanding.

Application of Language Skills

Normally, naming objects or describing objects or events in isolation holds little meaning for the retarded child and, only when the child makes actual use of objects do they give any meaning to the word. The methods used in motor skills are applicable in other areas, such as incorporating the names *pot* and *pan* while teaching cooking skills. The child has his or her hands on the pot and begins to call it by name. Then and only then do the names have meaning.

In addition, the skills taught in the classroom must be well thought out in sequential steps for the retarded child. Showing or demonstrating and inviting the child to copy is a basis for teaching. Very little language should be used for instructional purposes, and it should be concise and consistent. Labeling objects in the room is also helpful.

Stimulating Expressive Language

Often in trying to elicit expressive language, little opportunity is given for expanded responses. Questions should be asked requiring more than a "yes" or "no" answer. Many children must be given more than a reasonable length of time to respond. Patience on the part of the teacher is essential. Sometimes the question needs to be repeated. It may be difficult to ask questions since the children may comprehend statements more easily than formulating responses.

The use of body language can be an aid to comprehension. One of the teachers in the school also uses simultaneous signing successfully with her students. Simultaneous language is the method of using the manual signs of the hand that is used with the deaf and also verbalizing the words. It is not only a completely different process of reception, but gives another process of motor responses. When language can be expressed, either by voice or some other means, then needs are expressed or feelings are shared, and classroom behavior changes. The retarded seem to respond differently to manual signing than voice reception and even differently when it is simultaneous.

However, one still must have something to talk about or to share or to feel. Social activities in the school are essential for these purposes. Anticipation and recall of the events create as much language as the actual activity. The students bowl once a week, and many of the children ask each day, "Bowling today?" An activity such as bowling or roller skating opens up a whole world of motor skill experience with names for things and events. The child anticipates, relates experiences with others, and has something to "talk about" with others the following day. The staff at the school tries to have as many activities as possible for students to look forward to in the future to "talk about." Even the environment at the lunch table can be conducive for children to have an opportunity to "say something." Round tables with more eye contact for each class member are much more beneficial than the long, rectangular institutional tables. Teachers or aides eating with students can stimulate language. Ample time should always be given for language to take place at the lunch tables. The lunch time gives the child a place to share with others through language. At different times of the day certain free social situations should be scheduled for such a purpose. "Play" is extremely beneficial for the instructor to be involved in working on language, especially syntax. Play also seems to be spontaneous where incidental learning takes place.

The staff at the Education Center continues to talk to students even though some of the students use little expressive language. The staff should never fail to speak to these children. This may be one error the inexperienced teacher or clinician commits when working with retarded children. Again, consistent and repeated language must be used over and over.

Conclusion

The study of language of the retarded child and what can be accomplished in schools is not a mystery. The study of expected child development and the process of how to bridge the "retarded" or "slowing down" process must be understood. The retarded child requires more time and processes more slowly. Each sensory element is not isolated, and the sensory system must be totally integrated. Hearing, seeing, feeling, tasting and smelling must be experienced more intensely for integration for the retarded, and some areas may not be as effective as others. The activities in school which may be the formal lesson, play, or the planned social activities all play important roles in effective language development for the retarded.

Vocational Training

The students at the Education Center have their last exposure to full-time academic work during their first two or three years there. Once this is completed, vocational training is initiated. Although some simple, practical reading and math are continued, the vocational training of the students is the primary focus. This program involves approximately thirty students with two teachers, one aide, and a couple of volunteers. It is divided into six main areas of emphasis which also serve to maintain the school community at the Center.

Food Services

The students are responsible for the daily operation of the food services for the whole school. They offer seven different luncheon menus which means that over a one-year period the students will have experience with preparing lunch approximately 200 to 300 times. This experience gives the students the basis for entry level skills into food services jobs as well as teaching self-help skills. In addition to being responsible for planning and serving the meal, they must do the shopping, the cooking, the setting-up, and the cleaning.

Prior to this experience, the students learned in their classrooms the requisite skills such as measuring and the names of the items used in food preparation.

Marketing Skills

One of the major school projects each year is that of cracking and peeling walnuts. Approximately $1,000 a year is allocated to purchase whole, quality walnuts. The walnuts are cracked, shelled, and sold to the public. With this activity, students learn to begin and finish a job and all the necessary skills. The marketing of the walnuts involves many job skills and is, therefore, like the other job training activities, divided into job levels. For example, there are: (1) *crackers,* who are taught to crack the walnuts so they come out in fancy halves; (2) *sorters,* who separate the halves from the pieces; (3) *inspectors,* who make sure all the shell pieces are removed from the meats; (4) *weighers,* who weigh the walnuts for packing; (5) *packagers,* who put the walnuts in bags, and (6) *preparers,* who ready the bagged walnuts for distribution.

There are also opportunities for promotion to the more prestigious jobs and rotation to learn other skills. The money earned from the walnuts goes for activities that would otherwise not be possible, such as a camping trip or a trip to Marriott's Great America®, a large amusement park.

Laundry Services

The Center owns all its towel and physical education clothes. Therefore, students are responsible for the washing, drying, mending, ironing, and folding of all the linens. For this purpose, the Center also owns a washer, dryer, sewing machines, irons, and ironing boards.

Grounds Care

The students are responsible for landscaping and maintaining the grounds. This involves such activities as watering, mowing, weeding, and cleaning.

Wind Chimes Production

The sheltered workshop in Sacramento sponsored by Opportunities for the Handicapped, Inc. (OFHI) makes and sells ceramic wind chimes. Therefore, students at the Center are taught the necessary skills in the event they later choose to work there. Some of the skills learned are making the forms in clay, loading a kiln, firing the clay, glazing and stringing the forms.

Development of the Arts

The students express themselves in differing art forms. One of the students, who is also deaf, did a painting of Ronald McDonald®, submitted it in a contest, and won $200 from McDonald's restaurants.

Limitations

All the jobs and activities are broken down into sequences through task analysis. Every attempt is made to break them down into small enough sequences so that every student can master every task; however, there are always some things some of the students cannot do. In contrast, the major difficulty with most of the students at the Center is not that they cannot master the manual skills, but that they cannot master the language and social skills necessary for full, independent employment. For example, a student may be able to adequately clean sinks in a routine and fixed manner but may become confused if an employer says, "The last two sinks you cleaned are still dirty. Go back and clean them like you did the first ones." A changing of routine may also confuse him or her. In addition, the students at the Center, in general, lack social perception. For example, they may arrive at work ten minutes late, walk into the boss's office when he is on the phone or obviously busy with something else and ask to get off early that day. They do not "perceive" that it is a bad moment to approach the boss.

In an attempt to overcome this difficulty, the school personnel attempt to integrate the students with the community by activities mentioned earlier, such as camping trips and bowling. They also do all their traveling on public buses; school buses are not used. In addition, there are seminars and field trips, for example on using the bank and the post office.

Although the students themselves have personal, internal limitations placed on them by the fact that they are retarded, the Center attempts to eliminate as many external limitations as possible.

REFERENCES

Anderson, Robert M. and Greer, John G.: *Educating the Severely and Profoundly Retarded.* Baltimore, University Park Press, 1976.

Benda, Clemens E.: *Down's Syndrome.* New York, Grune & Stratton, 1964.

Carrier, Joseph K., Jr.: Application of functional analysis and a nonspeech response made to teaching language. In McReynolds, Leija V. (Ed.): *Developing Systematic Procedures for Training Children's Language, ASHA Monographs Number 18.* Washington, ASHA, 1974.

Donnell, George N.; Alfi, Omar S.; Rublee, Jo C., and Koch, Richard: Chromosomal abnormalities. In Koch, Richard and de la Cruz, Felix F. (Eds.): *Down's Syndrome (Mongolism): Research, Prevention and Management.* Mazel, Brunner, 1975.

Evans, David: Language development in mongols. *Special Education: Forward Trends,* 1:23-25, 1974.

Evans, Kathleen and Carter, C. D.: Care and disposal of mongolian defectives. *Lancet,* 2:960-963, 1954.

Kirk, Samuel A.: *Educating Exceptional Children.* Boston, Houghton Mifflin, 1972.

Kirk, Samuel A.: Research in education. In Stevens, Harvey A. and Heber, Rick (Eds.): *Mental Retardation; A Review of Research.* Chicago, University of Chicago Press, 1964.

Lenneberg, Eric H.: *Biological Foundations of Language.* New York, John Wiley & Sons, 1967.

Magalini, Sergio I.: *Dictionary of Medical Syndromes.* Philadelphia, J. B. Lippincott, 1971.

Morley, Muriel, E.: *The Development and Disorders of Speech in Childhood.* Edinburgh, Churchill Livingstone, 1972.

Nichtern, Sol: *Helping the Retarded Child.* New York, Grosset & Dunlap, 1974.

Schlanger, Bernard B.: *Mental Retardation.* Indianapolis, Bobbs-Merrill, 1973.

Smith, David W., and Wilson, Ann A.: *The Child with Down's Syndrome (Mongolism).* Philadelphia, W. B. Saunders, 1973.

Van Riper, Charles: *Speech Correction: Principles and Methods.* Englewood Cliffs, Prentice-Hall, 1972.

West, Robert; Ansberry, Merle, and Carr, Anna: *The Rehabilitation of Speech.* New York, Harper & Brothers, 1957.

Wright, Stanley W.; Day, Robert W.; Muller, Helga, and Weinhouse, Roger: The frequency of trisomy and translocations in Down's syndrome. *J Pediatr, 70*:420-424, 1967.

Zisk, Paulette K. and Bialer, Irv: Speech and language problems in mongolism. A review of the literature. *J Speech Hear Disord, 32*:228-241, 1967.

CHAPTER 11

CHILDHOOD AUTISM

Evelyn Bowling, M.A. and Morris Val Jones, Ph.D.

With a Case History by Robert Gerould, *Father of an Autistic Child*

Tʜᴇ ǫᴜᴇsᴛɪᴏɴ ᴏғ education and training for autistic children becomes increasingly critical as public schools open their doors to these enigmatic children. Solving the problem of finding efficient techniques for remediating the deficits these children have and searching out new methods to discourage their bizarre behavior patterns will now become the focus of many public school teachers, speech pathologists, and other educational specialists. However, since Kanner first described the autistic syndrome in 1943, a plethora of literature has accumulated, world-wide in scope, numbering more than a thousand books and articles. The task of identifying the literature is complicated because of the use of varied labels for the behavior Kanner called "early infantile autism." Such labels as childhood psychosis, symbiotic psychosis, atypical children, childhood schizophrenia, primary autism, and secondary autism are used throughout the literature according to each individual author's preference. Kanner's position was that infantile autism is a distinct clinical syndrome and that autistic children differ in many respects from all other instances of childhood schizophrenia.

Kanner (1972) summarized his early findings regarding this special population:

> In 1943, I reported eleven children whose withdrawal tendencies were noted as early as in the first year of life. I have suggested for the condition the term *early infantile autism*. More than 150 "autistic" children have been seen in our clinic since then, and many observations by others have been published. The common denominator in all these patients is a disability to relate themselves in the ordinary way to people and situations from the beginning of life.

250

Their parents referred to them as always having been "self-sufficient," "like in a shell," "happiest when left alone," "acting as if people weren't there," "giving the impression of silent wisdom." The case histories indicate invariably the presence from the start of extreme autistic aloneness which, whenever possible, shuts out anything that comes to the child from the outside. Almost every mother recalled her astonishment at the child's failure to assume the usual anticipatory posture preparatory to being picked up. (Pp. 699-700)

The cause or causes of infantile autism have been, and remain, a mystery. DeMyer (1975) has listed some of the etiological theories extant in the 1950s and 1960s.

Bettleheim (1959)	Parental rage and rejection.
DesLauriers (1962)	Theory within framework of psychoanalytic ego psychology. Inability to establish contact with reality.
Pavenstedt (1955)	*Folie a deux* between mother and child.
Rosenberger and Woolf (1964)	Children overwhelmed by affection from mentally ill parents.
Knight (1963)	Failure of establishment of oral primacy leads to shifting of cognitive development from exteroceptive to interoceptive ego.
Szurek (1956)	Both parents have disordered personalities. Child's reaction is a magnifier.
Clerk (1961)	Severe anxiety regarding management of aggressive impulses in mother. Communication problem in mother and child.
Ferster (1961)	Parents reinforce development of symptoms.
Bender (1955)	Disturbed area of CNS function (schiz.). Disturbance in maturational patterns using Gesell norms.
Colbert and Koegler (1958)	I° or II° dysfunctions of vestibular pathway, mental deficiency, and abnormal EEG.
Rimland (1960)	Conceptual impairment due to malfunction in reticular formation.
Fish (1960)	Problem in uneven timing of perceptual-motor level due to neurological factors.
Macmillan (1961)	Defect in states of cortical inhibition and excitation (Pavlov).
Pasamanick and Knobloch (1963)	Many cases have Chronic Brain Syndrome (CBS) and negative feelings of mother result from behavior of the child rather than cause it.

| Rees (1956) | Chemical imbalance exerting anesthesia-like effect on brain. |
| Schain and Yannet (1960) | Limbic system likely locus of dysfunction. (P. 395-396) |

The possibility of an organic basis for childhood autism has been explored. Rimland (1964) has accumulated numerous case studies in which vitamin deficiency played a role. In 1974, Rimland discussed possible hereditary factors as the source for the *overselection phenomena* recently delineated by research. He suggested that autistic children may inherit an excessive amount of the ability to concentrate through the genes of their parents. This ability may become so overly concentrated that he cannot decipher more than a single cue at a time. Since learning is largely a matter of pairing, the autistic child, perceiving one stimulus, would fail to make associations essential to learning. Simon (1975) discussed the possibility of an organic basis:

> There are, as yet, no neuropathological data on specific brain lesions in infantile autism. However, more and more children with autistic symptoms are now being described as displaying some signs of central nervous system dysfunction. (P. 473)

At the University of California Medical School, Irvine, research is being conducted to determine the relationship of nystagmus and childhood autism.

EVALUATION METHODS

Several methods of speech evaluation have been used to measure and describe the speech of autistic children. Usually these measurements have used spontaneous or elicited speech responses. Three scales of the Behavior Rating Instrument for Evaluating Autistic Children (BRIAC) included areas important to speech evaluation. The authors of BRIAC, Ruttenberg and Wolf (1967), outlined the Relationship, Communication, Vocalization and Speech Development subtests, which they used to compare three different populations of autistic children. Shapiro and Fish (1969) described a method to study language deviation in which speech was rated for developmental and functional levels in three twenty-minute language examinations over a six-month period. Davis (1967) described a clinical method of appraisal of language behavior of autistic children that was a language inventory designed to evaluate inner, receptive, and expressive language. Cunningham (1966) counted incidences of thinking aloud, answers, questions, complete sentences, incorrect omissions, incomplete sentences, and use of personal pronouns, as well as action accompanying speech. Wolff and Chess (1965) counted the total number of words, number of different words, and average length of utterances in their study of sixteen autistic children. Ward and Hoddinoth (1968) classified the verbal behavior in one autistic child from 540 three-minute samples spaced at five-week intervals over an eighteen-month treatment period. The authors suggested this method as a means of evaluating changes in verbal behavior.

Weiland and Legg (1964) used the first 750 words obtained in individual sessions to determine the frequency of various parts of speech. As a result of these studies and many others which used similar techniques, a comprehensive description of the characteristics of autistic speech and language is possible.

RESULTS OF EVALUATION STUDIES

The above investigators found that speech abnormalities were usually evidenced by a failure to develop speech, immediate and delayed echolalia, and also in impaired communicative behavior. The incidence of mutism ranged from a high of 61 percent in a sample of twenty-eight children (Fish, Shapiro, and Campbell, 1966) to a low of 28 percent in a sample of fourteen children (Wolff and Chess, 1965).

Immediate or delayed echolalia is the most common characteristic of the children who do speak (Rutter, 1965), and it is used both for communication and as repetitive or ritualistic behavior (Wing, 1966). The cause of the echolalic behavior is believed to be lack of comprehension, and the pitch level of echolalia is higher than that of other speech responses (Fay, 1969). The level of language development is higher in autistic children with fewer echolalic responses (Cunningham, 1966). However, echolalic children are more likely to develop use of spontaneous and more complex speech faster than children who were previously without speech (Lovaas, 1966).

The speech of autistic children has been described as overlapping into other diagnostic categories including aphasia, the brain damaged, the mentally retarded, and the nonpsychotic emotionally disturbed. The main characteristics reported by these investigators include lack of questions and informative statements, greater use of imperatives, few personal pronouns, limited verbal output, and frequent bizarre usage of words. Other descriptions include deviations in rhythm, pitch, and articulation with resultant atypical stress and inflection. The coordination of speaking with breathing is frequently lacking, which may account for some of the noticeable differences observed.

Studies showing the relation of speech development to other variables have also produced much helpful data. Nonspeaking children verbalize less in infancy (Ruttenberg and Wolf, 1967), are less alert and less responsive to sound in infancy, and manifest more autistic behaviors (Rimland, 1968). Self-mutilative behaviors and perceptual deficits are also more prevalent in nonspeaking children (Shodell and Reiter, 1968).

THEORIES AND EXPLANATIONS FOR AUTISTIC LANGUAGE DEFICITS

The evidence from research clearly indicates that the kind of speech development in autism relates to many other areas of functioning, and hence, many theories are expounded to explain the basic nature of the language deficit and to select the appropriate method for remediation. Demonstrating the assumption that a hierarchy of speech development moving from babbling to echolalia to words, phrases, and sentences must be followed to expand the speech of autistic children, Rubin, Bar, and Dwyer (1967) gave social reinforcement to the children's vocal responses and reported good results in increased vocalization in five of six children.

On the other hand, Wing (1966) states that the same programs for normals or subnormals are not necessary for autistic children and that the pattern of higher performance and lower verbal skills should form the basis for a treatment program. He concluded that teaching autistic children should be considered in terms of learning disabilities rather than emotional illness.

Emphasizing the fairly strong relation between autism and speech development, Rutter (1965) stated, "In so far as one may be due to the other, it is more usually the speech abnormality which is primary and the autism, secondary." However, Pronovost, Wakstein, and Wakstein (1966) suggest that perceptual problems are the most significant factors underlying impaired language development and should be the focal point of treatment. Numerous theories and treatments are based on the deficit in interpersonal relationships (Ruttenberg and Wolf, 1967).

Poor speech models have also been described as the cause of difficulties in language development in autistic children (Goldfarb, Goldfarb, and Scholl, 1966). This study has received criticism from other investigators because the mothers used in the study were not matched with their controls for age, education, IQ or social class, and because the researchers failed to report selection methods or mother-child correlations demonstrating a direct relation between mother-child speech patterns (Klein and Pollack, 1966).

Other explanations for the skewed speech development in autism include psychopathology (de Hirsch, 1967), retardation in ego development (Weiland and Legg, 1964), lack of empathy, and poor discrimination of social reinforcers (Cunningham, 1968).

METHODS OF TREATMENT

The methods of treatment for speech and language problems relate directly to the beliefs concerning causation of the problem of autism. A group of investigators who believe that the autistic child's lack of speech is related to his stress when withdrawing from hostile environments report that language improves as interpersonal relationships improve. According to Bettelheim (1955), autistic behavior is a defensive denial of the self against the threat of total destruction in a world perceived as hostile and rejecting. He believes the symptoms result from pathological characteristics within the parents, particularly the mother. The pathogenic understimulation or overstimulation prevents the child from effectively acting on his environment in a meaningful, growth-producing manner. Bettelheim's treatment environment does not involve parents and utilizes many permissive play therapy techniques which he feels promote autonomous personality growth.

Investigators who consider autistic speech to be another type of behavioral deficit have used primarily behavior modification techniques as the primary means of increasing speech production. Since 1964, more than twenty-five studies have used reinforcement therapy to expand the verbal responses of autistic children. One of the first studies involved increasing the frequency of a three-year-old autistic child's responses to one word vocal cues by using singing and rocking on the knee as reinforcements (Kerry, Myerson, Michael, 1965). Candy and visual color displays have also been used as reinforcers for vocalizations (Fineman, 1968). Actual speech was developed over an eighteen-month period in a four-year-old autistic boy in 1965 (Hewett, 1965). In another study, reading skills were developed in three autistic children (Hewett, 1966).

Lovaas has described the shaping of vocalization of two children through the technique of reinforcing successive approximations. After both subjects had developed imitative speech, Lovaas found that they imitated speech without rewards, thus indicating that imitation in itself had become rewarding. Later, the imitative vocabulary was used to develop more spontaneous speech (Lovaas, 1966, 1971). The behavior modification technique of rewarding successive approximations to the desired behavior was taught by Resley and Wolf (1966) to parents of an autistic child. The same investigators also developed spontaneous speech in four echolalic autistic children (CA 7-0 to 12-0) by using verbal prompts and fading (1967).

The comparison study by Ney (1967) attempted to determine which kind of therapy is effective for autistic children. Matched groups of psychotic children were divided into play therapy and operant-conditioning groups, and each received fifty forty-five-minute sessions directed toward developing speech. The group receiving behavior therapy showed more improvement in speech and in Vineland scores than the play-therapy group. In another instance (Martin et al., 1968), language development was carried out in a classroom situation, and seven out of ten psychotic children significantly improved. How many of these children were autistic was not specified.

The extent to which any of these techniques can develop spontaneous language is unclear, especially in the case of subjects who were mute. Reinforcement methods in an extensive training period to develop vocal responses in four mute psychotic children were reported by Hingtgen, Coulter, and Churchill (1967). A wide variation in results occurred with all subjects developing imitative speech, but the author comments that two were not able to make the initial auditory-visual and visual-vocal associations necessary for spontaneous speech. Other investigators have questioned whether mute psychotic children can ever develop more than rote speech (Weiss and Bern, 1967). Even if this is the case, most clinicians might regard rote speech as better than no speech. A recent publication by Lovaas (1976) describes in detail the use of behavior modification as the therapy approach of choice for the speech and language rehabilitation of psychotic children.

It is pertinent to note that the effectiveness in developing new responses stems from the emphasis on actively eliciting and rewarding specific behaviors rather than waiting for the child's hypothesized emotional disturbances to be resolved and for the new behaviors to spontaneously emerge. In addition, once considered normal except for severe emotional problems, autistic children have now been shown to have severe deficits in all other areas of development including behavioral, intellectual, perceptual, language, neurobiological, and social. Success in developing spontaneous or creative speech has been limited and appears to be directly related to the children's initial level of social and intellectual functioning. Clearly, more research into methods of developing speech and language in autistic children is needed to identify the approach which will achieve the highest level of language functioning possible. In addition, further specific observation is needed in the area of enumerating the basic communication tasks that autistic children at various levels can perform. This kind of precise data will enable the teacher to plan a curriculum designed to program an increase in verbal and nonverbal communication.

The Bowling Study

Bowling (1974) studied eight children who were enrolled in day classes at the Children's Center, a public school facility of Sacramento County in California. The children ranged in age from 5-0 years to 15-7 years with a mean age of 9-5 years (SD = 8.96 months). The children were placed in these special classes after a placement committee consisting of a psychologist, a school administrator, a teacher, a nurse, a speech pathologist, and a psychiatrist had reviewed and evaluated the available medical, developmental, psychometric and speech and language data concerning them and found them to be severely emotionally handicapped, functioning far below their potential, and not appropriate for a standard classroom placement. The children had all been described as autistic by psychiatrists who had evaluated their medical and behavioral records.

All of the children were living in their own homes. Two of the children's parents were divorced; in one instance, a step-father was part of the family constellation. In the second instance, the child had no contact with his father, and his mother remained single and was employed. These two children and one other in the sample had no siblings. The five remaining children in the sample had from one to four siblings at home. All of the parents cooperated in the activities and conferences that were planned as part of their child's participation in the Children's Center program.

Seven of the children were Caucasian and one was black. One child was from a bilingual background with his mother speaking Portuguese as well as English. Six of the children were from middle-class socioeconomic backgrounds and two were from families who required state economic aid.

THE TEST BATTERY. The test battery, Tasks for Evaluation of Communication in Autistic Children (TECAC), was developed by the author for use in this study. The fifteen TECAC categories were selected from the Verbal Language Development Scale (Mecham, 1963), the communication section of the Caine-

Levine Social Competency Scale (Caine, Levine, and Freman, 1963), the Parson's Language Sample (Schiefelbusch, 1963), the Communicative Evaluation Chart (Anderson, Miles, Mathey, 1963) and from the Communication Chart (Bangs, 1968). These categories were selected on the basis of the author's clinical experience with some fifty autistic children over a period of twelve years as a speech pathologist on the staff of two California State Hospitals and were considered by her to represent the body of information relevant to understanding the speech and language functioning of autistic children.

Tasks for the categories one through nine were devised by the author based on behavioral descriptions of the achievements in motor, adaptive skills, language, and personal-social skills of normal children from one to four years old. Tasks ten through fifteen were revised from similar tasks on the Parson's Language Sample. The areas covered ranged from the very basic behaviors of attending to objects and people to more complex receptive-expressive behaviors of following directions and repeating long sentences. A progression from easy to difficult tasks was not strictly adhered to in determining the order of presentation of the tasks. Since repeated task failure decreases interest and motivation, some relatively easy tasks were interspersed among the more difficult tasks to prevent this problem.

Tasks for Evaluation of Communication in Autistic Children explored the following aspects of interpersonal communication:

1. Attention to an object
2. Attention to a person
3. Responds to name
4. Imitates a movement demonstrated
5. Imitates a sound and movement
6. Imitates a rhythm
7. Imitation of a single word
8. Repeats a short sentence
9. Repeats a long sentence
10. Follows vocal and gestural directions
11. Follows vocal directions
12. Follows gestural directions
13. Indicates wants gesturally
14. Indicates wants vocally
15. Sings song

OBSERVED BEHAVIOR DURING TESTING. The incidental behavior of the children which occurred during the TECAC testing procedure was recorded on the test form under the category "Other behavior." It was this unique behavior which distinguished the performance of these children from that of retarded children on these tasks.

The sounds the children emitted during the test were a significant example of their unique behavior. Four of eight children made either constant or intermittent sounds including soft humming, loud moaning, tearful whining, or high pitched screeches. Occasional spontaneous jargon, mumbling, or whispering was also noted for four children.

Imitating a posture or action of the examiner occurred in the behavior of three children. The imitation of the examiner's movements took place before any test items requiring imitation were administered. For example, one child imitated the chewing movements of the examiner's mouth in eating the apple used in Task 1. Others moved their chairs closer to the table when the examiner did and crossed their legs when she inadvertently crossed hers. Two other children were imitative on a vocal level and repeated instructions or words the examiner used.

Other body movements during the TECAC administration furnished further descriptive data. Three children intermittently rocked during the session. Two others hit their own heads with their fists or banged their heads on the table when they became distressed. Two others grabbed at or hit at the examiner when she repeated a task that the child had rejected on the first presentation. Another mode of rejection of a task was covering their ears with their hands. Another child simply pulled his coat up over his head and sat very still. A third child rejected tasks by picking up the materials before him very quickly and placing them back on the shelf.

Three children used ritualistic movements involving their hands and trunks. Two other smelled, licked, twiddled, twirled, or manipulated in a bizarre manner small pieces of rubber, bits of plastic, or string they had brought with them. Even the two children who scored highest on the TECAC battery and received the highest level of BRIAC assignment made bizarre or inappropriate comments. The child who ranked third mumbled two alliterating names, "Lifeguard Louie," and "Doctor Donald," in various rhythmic phrases. The examiner knew of no concurrent factual or fictional referant for the phrases and could only surmise that the names represented strong protective figures to the child in this unfamiliar situation.

Six of the eight children did not remain seated at the table for more than a few minutes at a time. Some wandered, ran, hopped, or jumped about the room; others crawled under the table and across the floor and attempted to escape out the two doors. Two climbed on chairs to try to reach testing materials which were placed in brown bags high on shelves. This could be evidence for genuine curiosity or another part of the anxious behavior ascribed to autistic children when they note something unfamiliar in their environment.

Although two children hit at the examiner, other children tested her existence by stroking her arms or petting her hair as though she were their pet dog. One child attempted to explore her clothing. The suddenness of the behaviors without obvious specific stimulus was the quality that seemed to differentiate these behaviorisms from those observed in retarded children. In addition, inappropriate facial expressions, unusual posturing, and noises often accompanied the sudden tactual approaches to the examiner.

Two children demonstrated exaggerated eye blinking patterns during the first administration of the TECAC battery. Neither child retained these patterns during the second administration of the test. The eye blinking was the only observed behavior that did not reoccur on the second test. The reaction, therefore, probably was transitory and specific to this particular testing situation.

Unusual patterns of audible breathing, breath-catching sounds, and some breath holding were observed in three of the children. These patterns were of less intensity during the second TECAC administration and occurred only three times.

Difficulty in terminating some of the TECAC activities was a problem with seven of the eight children. Once the child began the task, such as pounding a peg, he seemed unable or unwilling to stop until the examiner removed the task items from the table. Three of the four children who had this difficulty showed no visible objection when the examiner removed the materials and interrupted their activity. The fourth child whined and tried to retrieve the object, but was soon distracted by the new material that the examiner placed on the table.

CONCLUSIONS. Findings of this study indicated that, within the limitations imposed by the sample, the measuring instrument, and the experimental design,

1. The TECAC is a reliable instrument for autistic children.
2. Autistic children perform best in following gestural directions (Task 12).
3. Autistic children perform least effectively in tasks that involve imitating a rhythm (Task 6), and in singing a song (Task 15).
4. Autistic children have great difficulty in tasks requiring speech on any level.
5. The behavior of autistic children during testing is atypical and difficult to manage.

CASE HISTORY

Numerous parent-written case histories of autistic children have been published (such as *Son-Rise* by Barry Neil Kaufman, New York: Harper and Row, 1976). The following account of Kevin Gerould was written for the authors by Kevin's father. It demonstrates, through being placed in the day-to-day reality of a parent, some of the psychological, physical, and social development of one autistic child. It also provides an example of the difficulties in diagnosis and in finding appropriate educational placement that are usually the hallmark of reports by parents of autistic children.

— — — — — — — — — — — — — — — — — —

Kevin seemed quite normal during the first few months of his life. His eyes were bright and shiny, and his reactions were very good. He did all of the normal baby things; he cried, he wet, he took his mother's milk enthusiastically, and he would lie on the floor, on his stomach, head up, and survey the world around him. My wife described him as a good baby. He made very few demands upon her outside of feeding and changing. Kevin was very quiet and seemed content to just lie there in his crib. As months went by, however, we became concerned. Unlike other babies, Kevin seemed indifferent to being held or played with. He didn't sit up by himself until he was a year old. Our first fear was that he was deaf, or blind, or both! Our own experiments and frequent visits to our family physican assured us that this was not the case. We knew what the problem wasn't, but obviously there was a problem.

Kevin didn't crawl or walk until he was three. He just didn't seem to be interested in going anywhere. He would sit for hours staring at the material on the couch, or rubbing his hand over the side of the refrigerator while staring into space. His indifference to being held gradually changed into active resistance. It may be that learning to walk (on his tiptoes) and to hop sideways resulted primarily from a desire to escape contact with other people. Our attempts to brush his hair or teeth were met with noncooperation, and he had to be tackled and held down to get pajamas on him.

Of course, this bizarre behavior drove us back to the family physician and, at the age of eighteen months, Kevin was diagnosed as mentally retarded. It didn't come as a surprise to my wife; mothers know these things, but it was a blow. Like most parents, we have dreams and hopes for all of our children. At first it seemed our dreams for Kevin had vanished. We have gradually learned that it's possible to have hopes for the future of a retarded child; they're just different hopes.

When Kevin was three, our family physician referred us to Alta California Regional Center for assistance in special education and training. Kevin's medical record was supplied to the physician at Alta, who examined him and, not surprisingly, also diagnosed him as mentally retarded, plus hyperactive and epileptic. At the doctor's suggestion, Kevin began attending classes at a developmental center for the multiple handicapped. By this time Kevin had begun other strange behaviors. He mouthed and licked almost everything. He constantly flipped his hands in front of his face and even when only slightly excited would begin jumping up and down. In an effort to control this, the doctors began prescribing various medicines. Phenobarbitol® made him so hyperactive he didn't sleep for forty-eight hours.

Other things they tried, such as Datril® and Veracillin®, sedated him, but made him drowsy and zombie-like, and he soon developed a tolerance to them.

At the development center, Kevin made limited progress. He learned to feed himself using silverware. He could be made to sit in a chair at a table, but he would not look at anything he was doing. It amazed me that he could catch a ball without even looking at it. The developmental center gave us our first opportunity to see Kevin in a group of retarded children, and it was obvious to us that he was different—he didn't "look retarded." Most of the other children gave indications of wanting some contact with others, but not Kevin. He was always alert and happy, but he always seemed to have his mind somewhere else. We were told that with luck and training Kevin might someday reach the level of a seven-year-old. We felt very helpless, for there was nothing we could do. It never occurred to us that the experts could be wrong.

When Kevin was six, we placed him in a small-group home about 75 miles away. The family he lived with had several normal children in addition to the seven retarded boys. He attended classes for the trainable mentally retarded at a school nearby. In our frequent visits we found the home to be full of love and affection, but with rigid rules and a strict schedule. With that many children around, it was really necessary to maintain a regular pattern and permit no changes. The woman who ran the home was opposed to the use of medicine to control the children, so she stopped giving Kevin his. When Kevin came home for vacations and holidays, we began noticing changes. He was calmer without the medicine. His vocabulary increased and he would randomly say things such as, "Kevin, you wet your pants." He fed himself well and would follow simple instructions such as, "Kevin, take your coat to your room," although sometimes he wouldn't get there or wouldn't come back.

Apparently Kevin's foster family had a strong religious conviction because we discovered that he would not begin a meal at home unless we said grace. Consequently we began saying grace at all of our meals and still do. Since returning to live with us and attending a local school, Kevin's attachment to grace before meals has spread to lunchtime at school. This in turn has caused his fellow students to take the practice home with them. Kevin may have started a new evangelical movement.

We were encouraged by Kevin's progress the year he was gone, but we wanted him back with us and enrolled him in a class for the trainable mentally retarded at the developmental center. For the next year Kevin made little or no progress. His bus ride to school lasted an hour and a half. By the time he arrived, all he could do was jump and flap. It normally took the teachers the entire first class period just to calm him down enough to get him to sit. TMR classes ran for twenty minutes, after which the students were moved to another classroom. The teachers felt this frequent change helped the students to concentrate when in class. For Kevin, however, it only increased his hyperactivity or drove him into fits of uncontrollable giggling. The teachers complained to us that they couldn't get him to look at them or at his studies. The only thing he learned how to do was remove his shoes, which he liked to flip in front of his eyes. During the course of the year he flipped several pairs out of the window of the bus. Kevin also developed a love for music, particularly Lawrence Welk and Elton John. He could also occupy himself for hours staring at a light or swinging on his swing in the back yard.

In the summer of 1976, when Kevin was eight years old, a psychologist from the school district, making a periodic visit to the developmental center, spotted Kevin; she too recognized that he was different. She attempted to test him, but he would only giggle or stare at the lights. That evening she called to tell us she thought Kevin was *autistic*.

Our reaction, even after we learned more about it, was one of relief. The label *mentally retarded* seemed such an all-inclusive term and one which did not appear to quite fit. Every book that we read describing the autistic child described Kevin. At least now we knew what was wrong! The psychologist told us about a program specifically for autistic children and invited us to observe the class. It was obvious from the beginning that this was the program for Kevin. There were three children in the class, with two speech therapists and two teacher's aides. The teachers are convinced that autism is a brain dysfunction affecting perception and are using behavior modification techniques to break through the autisms that are hindering the children's learning ability. It struck us that, perhaps unintentionally, the woman at the group home used similar techniques and got results.

We consider ourselves and Kevin lucky because he has been in that program for a year now. However, one of his teachers said that it was too bad he hadn't been placed in such a program when he was three or four instead of eight. That Kevin was improperly diagnosed and assigned to the wrong educational program for five years is unfortunately not unique. A misdiagnosis tends to influence subsequent diagnoses, resulting in the wrong placement and a lack of progress. Kevin was identified in a crowd by chance. One of the other children in his autistic class came from a class for aphasic children. A third child in the group was referred from place to place because it was obvious to his parents that he didn't fit in with each succeeding group. The Easter Seal Society eventually referred him to the autistic program. The fourth child is in the class because his mother has a friend who has heard of the program.

Since joining the class for the autistic, Kevin has progressed remarkably. His vocabulary has grown considerably and he can occasionally form a sentence. He has begun to use language appropriately, especially swearing, and can ask for most of the things he wants. Although he occasionally uses two word phrases, most of his expressive language consists of one word utterances. He is making progress at relating a three-dimensional object to the two-dimensional picture of that object. He can, for example, identify the pictures of his brothers and sisters. He takes the class attendance form to the school office each day and carries his own tray at lunch. Perhaps, more importantly, he is beginning to want to participate in activities with other children.

In the summer of 1977 we took all five of our children, Kevin's older two brothers and sister and a younger sister, in a car to New Mexico to visit their grandparents. Kevin enjoys riding and was no more problem on the trip than his "normal" brothers and sisters. We took along an ample supply of snacks for all the children and also brought a cassette tape recorder with a tape of Kevin's favorite music. Often we were able to get him to lie down and listen to music to pass the time. The first two days in New Mexico Kevin was quite upset with the changed environment and often requested verbally to go home by saying, "Ride in the car"? He wouldn't play with any of the toys his grandmother provided for him and became very attached to the tape recorder. We tried to give him some reassurance by letting him play in a bubble bath frequently, which he likes to do at home, and take him to McDonald's restaurant whose golden arches he can spot a mile away. By the third day he had adjusted fairly well and was eager to join his brothers in skipping races across the back yard. He became more manageable and seemed to get along well with the other people in the house, including an aunt he had never seen before. The return trip was uneventful, and Kevin seems to have dropped back into his old routine easily, although he occasionally asks for Grandma.

The trouble with autism is that there are as many treatment methodologies as there are books on the subject. This past year Kevin has been in a program that has worked for him. If it continues to work, there is no doubt in my mind he will surpass the seven-year-old level. How far will he go? Only God knows.

— — — — — — — — — — — — — — — — — — — —

Kevin's history dramatizes the challenge that awaits the speech specialist who tackles the job of teaching a class of autistic children. A summary of all the data from current research identifies fluctuations in response to sensory input, unevenness in all areas of development, disturbances in language with fixations on inappropriate levels, disorganized thinking, and motility disorders as the critical characteristics the autistic child brings to the learning situation. The speech specialist will be constantly challenged and frequently frustrated by these serious obstacles to progress. In reacting to the educational and social needs of autistic children, the therapist's role is an active, directive, comprehensive, and diversified one. As she relates on a personal level, she instructs, sustains, informs, corrects, protects, modifies, supports, limits, stimulates, reassures, intervenes, encourages, and physically guides the autistic child in his activities. The activities should provide purposed structure, and the therapist must be sensitive and alert to modify his approaches with each individual child. Some measure of success, no matter how small, needs to be built into every situation.

With a background in speech and language disorders, the speech specialist as the teacher of autistic children is particularly qualified to meet the demands of individual differences in receptive and expressive language. However, the current practice based on recent legislation allows the selection of teachers to include those with special education credentials, as well as those qualified in speech pathology. The differences in outcomes in speech and language growth should become the subject of future studies of autistic children since part of building a sound educational program is continuous evaluation of its effectiveness. At the same time, critical appraisal of the preparatory training specific to autism offered speech specialists and special education teachers should also be undertaken as part of an ongoing effort to identify the teaching that best ameliorates the handicaps of these children.

REFERENCES

Anderson, R. M.; Miles, M., and Matheny, P.: *Communication Evaluation Chart from Infancy to Five Years.* Cambridge, Educators Publishing Company, 1963.

Bangs, T. E.: *Language and Learning Disorders of the Pre-Academic Child.* New York, Meredith Corporation, 1968.

Bartak, Lawrence; Rutter, Michael, and Cox, Anthony: A comparative study of infantile autism and specific developmental receptive language disorder. *Br J Psychiatry, 126*:127-145, 1975.

Bettelheim, T. E.: Childhood Schizophrenia Symposium, 1955, #3 Schizophrenia as a reaction to extreme situations. *Am J Orthopsychiatry, 26*:507-518, 1956.

Bowling, Evelyn: *The Performance of Eight Autistic Children on Selected Communication Tasks.* Master's thesis, California State University, Sacramento, CA, 1974.

Cain, L. F.; Levine, S., and Freman, E.: *Cain-Levine Social Competency Scale.* Consulting Psychologists Press, 1963.

Cunningham, M. A.: A five-year study of the language of an autistic child. *J Child Psychol Psychiatry, 7*:143-154, 1966.

Cunningham, M. A.: A comparison of the language of psychotic and non-psychotic children who are mentally retarded. *J Child Psychol Psychiatry, 9*:229-244, 1968.

Davis, B. J.: A clinical method of appraisal of the language and learning behavior of young autistic children. *Journal of Communication Disorders, 1*:277-296, 1967.

DeMyer, Marian: Research in infant autism: A strategy and its results. *Biol Psychiatry, 10*:(4), 433-452, 1975.

Fay, W. H.: On the basis of autistic echolalia. *Journal of Communication Disorders, 2*:38-47, 1969.

Fineman, K. R.: Visual-color reinforcement in establishment of speech by an autistic child. *Percept Mot Skills, 26*:761-762, 1968.

Fish, B.; Shapiro, T., and Campbell, M.: Long-term prognosis and the response of schizophrenic children to drug therapy: A controlled study of trifluoperazine. *Am J Psychiatry, 124*:32-39, 1966.

deHirsch, Kathryn: Differential diagnosis between aphasic and schizophrenic language in children. *J Speech Hear Disord, 32*:(1), 3-10, 1967.

Goldfarb, W.; Goldfarb, N., and Scholl, H. H.: The speech of mothers of schizophrenic children. *Am J Psychiatry, 122*:1220-1227, 1966.

Hewett, F. M.: Teaching speech to an autistic child through operant conditioning. *Am J Orthopsychiatry, 35*:927-936, 1965.

Hewett, F. M.: The autistic child learns to read. *Slow Learning Child, 12*:107-121, 1966.

Hingtgen, J. N.; Coulter, S. K., and Churchill, D. W.: Intensive reinforcement of imitative behavior in mute autistic children. *Arch Gen Psychiatry, 17*:36-43, 1967.

Kanner, Leo: *Child Psychiatry*, 4th ed. Springfield, Charles C Thomas, Publisher, 1972.

Kerr, N.; Meyerson, L., and Michael, J.: A procedure for shaping vocalizations in a mute child. In Ullmann, L. P. and Krasner, L. (Eds.): *Case Studies in Behavior Modification*. New York, Holt, Rinehart and Winston, Inc., 1965.

Klein, D. L. and Pollack, M.: Schizophrenic children and maternal speech facility. *Am J Psychiatry, 123*:232, 1966.

Lovaas, O. Ivar: *The Autistic Child: Language Development Through Behavior Modification*. New York, Irvington Publishers, Inc., 1976.

Lovaas, O. Ivar: Considerations in the development of a behavioral treatment program for psychotic children. In Churchill, D. W.; Alpern, G. D., and DeMeyer, M. (Eds.): *Infantile Autism: Proceedings of the Indiana University Colloquium, 1968*. Springfield, Charles C Thomas, 1971.

Martin, G. L.; England, G.; Kaprowy, E.; Kilgour, K., and Pilek, V. (Eds.): Operant conditioning of kindergarten class behaviour in autistic children. *Behav Res Ther, 6*:281-294, 1968.

Mecham, M. J.: *Verbal Language Development Scale*. Minneapolis, American Guidance Service, 1963.

Ney, P.: Operant conditioning of schizophrenic children. *Can Psychiatr Assoc J, 12*:9-15, 1967.

Pronovost, W.; Wakstein, M. P., and Wakstein, D. J.: A longitudinal study of the speech behavior and language comprehension of fourteen children diagnosed atypical or autistic. *Except Child*, 33:19-26, 1966.

Rimland, Bernard: On the objective diagnosis of infantile autism. *Acta Paedopsychiatr*, 35:146-161, 1968.

Rimland, Bernard: *Infantile Autism*. New York, Appleton-Century-Crofts, 1964.

Risley, T. and Wolf, M.: Experimental manipulation of autistic behaviors and generalization into the home. In *Control of Human Behavior*. Glenview, Scott, Foresman and Company, 1966.

Rubin, H.; Bar, A., and Dwyer, J. H.: An experimental speech and language program for psychotic children. *J Speech Hear Disord*, 32:242-248, 1967.

Ruttenberg, B. A. and Wolf, E. G.: Evaluating the communication of the autistic child. *J Speech Hear Disord*, 32:314-324, 1967.

Rutter, M.: Classification and categorization in child psychiatry. *Journal of Child Psychology and Psychiatry*, 6:71-83, 1965.

Rutter, M.: Prognosis: Psychotic children in adolescence and early adult life. In Wing, J. K. (Ed.): *Early Childhood Autism: Clinical, Educational and Social Aspects*. London, Pergamon Press, Inc., 1966.

Schiefelbusch, R. L.: Language studies of mentally retarded children. *J Speech Hear Disord, Monograph Supplement*, No. 10, 1963.

Shapiro, T. and Fish, B. A.: A method to study language deviation as an aspect of ego organization in young schizophrenic children. *J Am Acad Child Psychiatry*, 8:36-56, 1969.

Shodell, M. J. and Reiter, H. H.: Self-mutilative behavior in verbal and nonverbal schizophrenic children. *Arch Gen Psychiatry*, 19:495-497, 1968.

Simon, Nicole: Echolalic speech in childhood autism: Consideration of possible underlying loci of brain damage. *Arch Gen Psychiatry*, 32:471-490, 1975.

Ward, T. F. and Hoddinott, B. A.: A study of childhood schizophrenia and early infantile autism. *Can Psychiatr Assoc J*, 1:377-382, 1965.

Weiland, I. H. and Legg, D. R.: Formal speech characteristics as a diagnostic aid in childhood psychosis. *Am J Orthopsychiatry*, 34:91-94, 1964.

Weiss, H. H. and Born, B.: Speech training or language acquisition? A distinction when speech training is taught by operant conditioning procedures. *Am J Orthopsychiatry*, 37:49-55, 1967.

Wing, Lorna: Counseling and the principles of management. In Wing, J. K. (Ed.): *Early Childhood Autism: Clinical, Educational and Social Aspects*. London, Pergamon Press, Inc., 1966.

Wolff, S. and Chess, S. A.: A behavioral study of schizophrenic children. *J Child Psychol Psychiatry*, 6:29-41, 1965.

CHAPTER 12

REMEDIATION FOR THE DYSLEXIC

JOAN M. SMITH, ED.D.

I'M NO GOOD. . . . I can't read. . . . I can't keep a job. My kid reads better than me." These were the desperate words of a man who came to the learning center for help in reading. Paul Wells could not recognize words except for a few survival words such as *Stop* when it was on a red sign and *Men* on a door. He could not assign sounds to any of the alphabet symbols and had little skill in blending sounds. He was experiencing acute frustration in earning a living and constantly changing jobs rather than explain his difficulty in reading. The factor which seemed to be causing the greatest impetus to his need to read at this time was his son. He had just started first grade. He was trying to learn to read and insistently asked his dad for help.

This man had one of the most severe reading disabilities that had been observed. His retention on a single visual symbol association was initially measurable only in seconds. After fourteen sessions he could extend his retention to two minutes. If an exercise in discrimination or identification of two symbols continued longer than two minutes, he would become totally confused. However, if the activity were changed for a short period and then the exercise resumed, retention was maintained.

As one observes the multiple skills necessary to retain words and comprehend meaning from graphic symbols, one begins to realize the complexity of the reading process. It appears that "learning" to read is not something everyone must experience. Probably a large number of the readers of this book cannot recall "learning" to read, and the majority of these individuals feel they "appeared with it" or "it just happened."

A great many individuals recall the experience of sitting in a reading circle trying desperately to pay attention to the oral reading of the child next to them. Visually they had already finished reading the page and were anxious to go on to the next page or were miles away with their own thoughts as the halting reading of their peers continued. For so many "automatic" readers there was and is little need for understanding the process of learning to read, but for between 30 and 50 percent of our school population "learning to read" is an ordeal. It is filled with failure, frustration, and fatigue. Depending upon the skill of the instructor in diagnosis, the training available, and other support factors, some of the pupils succeed and others continue to experience the three *F*s—failure, frustration, and fatigue.

LEARNING TO READ

Breaking the "learning to read" process into the individual skills is essential to understanding the complexity of a skill many take for granted. For the majority of our population these steps occur automatically or rapidly. Many steps are skipped and the skills occur "naturally" (with little effort). This does not happen for the dyslexic and/or the individual with a significant reading problem. For them one or more of the skills delineated under processing may not be functional. This creates at the minimum an inefficiency in processing or at the extreme renders the individual a nonreader or dyslexic.

A review of the individual skills necessary for effective processing can provide an understanding of the complexities in learning to read. The therapist, specialist, or teacher may then identify the area or areas of inefficiency or nonfunctioning and provide training intervention. The effective functioning of the processing skills is critical to remediation of reading difficulties. As the specialist provides remedial intervention the pupil will "plug in" or "bridge across" to functional skill areas to experience the gestalt of reading.

Each of the skill areas shall be described in detail with behavioral examples to assist the reader in identification of skill deficiencies. There are basic assumptions to the examples given. The first assumption is that the pupil has both vision and hearing abilities which make him capable of symbol awareness and sound awareness. Secondly, the pupil has the skill to attend to training for a one-minute period. While it is quite possible to train pupils with attention spans of less than one minute, it is likely that initial training for increasing attention span should be accomplished with more intriguing items than letter cards.

Throughout this discussion, *symbol* shall refer to a letter. Lowercase letters shall be used because of the frequency of use in reading and writing. The term *sound* shall refer to the letter sound, such as the sound *buh* for the symbol *b*. Alphabet-letter names are not useful in reading and rarely must be taught. Once the pupil is thoroughly familiar with the sound-symbol match, his learning should be sufficient to allow automatic retention of letter names as he experiences them in the classroom.

Learning to read requires the efficient functioning of our receptive channels, specifically vision and hearing. Adequate screening for interference with reading should begin with both hearing and vision testing. Generally both areas have been evaluated prior to the referral to the clinic or school specialist. The responsibility, however, lies with the specialist to review and evaluate the adequacy of the screening. Frequently in our public schools the vision screen consists of the pupil reading at a distance the E chart or Snellen chart. While this gives information for far-point vision, difficulties in near-point function may not become apparent. Scrutiny of the information will provide the specialist with information regarding its adequacy.

SENSORY CHANNELS FOR READING

The dyslexic or nonreader experiences an interruption in the processing and/or integration of input information. For reading purposes input is received through the two basic channels of vision and hearing. Inefficient usage of information received visually or auditorally contributes or causes reading difficulty. The information received through both of these channels is essential because it must be integrated so that meaning may be obtained from the word symbols.

In Figure 12-1 one can see the primary modes of receiving information, which lead into the processing center. The measurement of the input is obtained through the three channels of output illustrated in the figure.

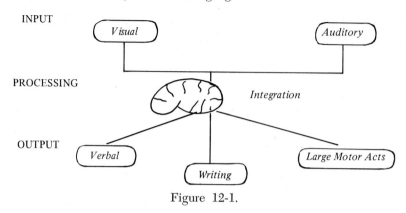

Figure 12-1.

The integration phase involves the actual processing of the symbolic and sound input. Each of the required levels is described in this chapter as a practical guide for identifying the dyslexic or nonreader's areas of inefficient processing. The actual process involves the use of both of the inner language channels: seen inner language and heard inner language. It is this internal language functioning which allows the processing to occur.

Seen inner language is the skill that most individuals develop allowing them to visualize an image. Visualization may include the imagination of a scene with which they have had some experience or one which is totally fantasy. Many individuals, especially those with reading disorders, are aware of their ability to visualize people, places, or objects but have never used their skill in visualizing symbolic information such as numbers, letters, or words. As an important part of the processing training there should be an attempt to determine if the pupil is using this internal language skill. He should be encouraged to do the suggested activities actively involving his visualization skill.

Most individuals readily will recognize that they have an active inner voice. The "voice in their head" talks to them and allows them to experience private thoughts. It is this inner voice which is referred to by the term *heard inner language*. The repetition of sounds, words, and sentences through our inner language moves us through the stages of experiencing sound retention, sound blending, closure on words, and finally experiencing meaning in reading.

The inner voice is necessary for active understanding in reading, and the identification of its existence is therefore important to the learner. Activities involving sound blending and auditory closure, when conducted on a subvocal level, may assist the pupil in developing improved reading performance.

The output channels described in Table 12-I are those most frequently required for school performance. During the early years, pupils are most likely requested to demonstrate their reading ability through oral reading or the verbal channel. As they move into third grade and above, most responses are required through the written modality. Workbooks, book reports, and completing the questions in the back of the chapter all require written output in order for the pupil to demonstrate that he read and understood the assignment. Through whichever of the channels the pupil is asked to respond, this is how his processing will be known.

TABLE 12-I

PROCESSING CHART FOR LEARNING TO READ

INPUT	PROCESSING				OUTPUT
	Level I ⟶	*Level II* ⟶	*Level III* ⟶	*Level IV*	Written
Vision	Visual				
	Symbol Constancy	*Symbol Discrimination*	*Symbol Seriation*	*Interpretation*	
				Integration	
					Verbal
Hearing	Auditory				
	Sound Recognition	*Sound Discrimination*	*Sound Sequencing*	*Language*	

PROCESSING LEVELS

Level I—Visual-Symbol Constancy

Letter symbols have basic properties through which they are identified. The retention of one symbol and the ability to recognize it in various positions, placements, and type sets is critical to achieving form constancy. The symbol *b* may appear quite different to the pupil dependent upon the angle from which it is viewed. The reader may experience this change by positioning this book to his right side and looking from this placement at the letter and then moving the book far to the left side.

$$\text{b} \qquad \text{b}$$

From the right-hand position the nonreader is likely to describe the symbol as a circle and a stick. From the left side it may appear more like a stick and a circle. The ability to recognize the constancy of form from various perspectives is the first step in being able to read. For the pupil to accomplish this level, activities in symbol identification should begin with the selection of one symbol. The symbol for *a* is usually a simple one and because of the frequency of use is economical to learn.

Placement of the symbol in many locations in the teaching room will afford the pupil multiple experiences in identification. As the pupil can identify the letter in isolation with accuracy, other shapes, numbers, and finally letter symbols may be included in the environment. At this level only the positive identification of the single symbol is required.

When the pupil can look at a page of letters and identify all of the *a*'s on the page, then the form constancy level is achieved for this symbol, and a second symbol may be introduced to achieve form constancy for another symbol. The specialist must also be aware that the pupil is moving into Level II. The pupil is required to discriminate between the two symbols and identify each of them; therefore, an awareness of likeness and difference is required.

Level I—Auditory-Sound Recognition

The ability to utilize letter sounds for the purposes of sound blending, auditory closure, and spelling begins with single sound recognition. The ability to identify a sound consistently and associate it with the appropriate symbol is a preliminary skill needed in beginning reading. A pupil cannot utilize phonics or word attack skills without adequate sound recognition.

In the same way that symbol retention may be difficult for the individual with perceptual problems, sound recognition is often especially confusing to the pupil with language disabilities or auditory memory deficiencies. Pupils who characteristically demonstrate poor listening skills may have a defect in sound recognition and retention. Careful observation and evaluation should be conducted so that there is early recognition of potential problems.

The training of sound recognition may begin with gross identification of words or object noises. The specialist may require the pupil to signal when he recognizes one noise, word, or sound. The signal should be associated with the sound and most efficiently would require tapping or pointing the letter symbol when the sound is heard.

The sound for the symbol being learned should be the first one selected. Both visual and auditory stimulation should occur together. This coupling of symbol and sound is the basic format for the entire learning-to-read behavior of recognizing words. The sound-to-symbol matching process is the basic skill for spelling, while the symbol-to-sound match is descriptive of reading. One recognizes a familiar sequence of letters and voices, internally or externally, the word being triggered by the visual combination.

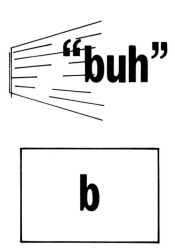

Level II—Auditory-Sound Discrimination

Sound recognition becomes complex when the pupil must differentiate between sounds with similar properties. As the pupil adds new sounds to his recognition level, certain ones will be difficult to assign to a symbol unless discrimination skills are developed. Sound combinations which may be confusing included the voiced-voiceless pairs such as v/f, z/s, b/p, d/t, g/k, or other related sounds such as m/n. The short vowel sounds are probably the most difficult for most learning readers. For this reason it is helpful to isolate and overteach the initial vowel sound introduced.

It is suggested that the vowels be presented for training using only the short sounds beginning with short /a/. The short /a/ has a high frequency of use in early linguistic readers and may be used in a large number of common three-letter words. With the nonreader the rapid beginning of reading is critical to combat the feeling of discouragement. The use of this one vowel sound coupled with the generally easier to learn consonants is usually learned quickly and encourages the pupil that he will read.

Vowel discrimination is a difficult skill for the nonreader because the vowel sounds are consistently distorted by their neighboring consonants. In addition to the variations of each vowel sound itself there are discrimination challenges for the learner between vowels with similar sounds. Short vowel sound such as /e/ and /i/, /o/ and /u/, and /a/ and /u/ or /o/ require sophisticated listenings. It is helpful to introduce the short vowels with the widest discrimination value first. Preferential order is /a/, /i/, /u/, /e/, /o/.

If one vowel is learned thoroughly before the next one is introduced, discrimination will be greatly aided. It will not be unusual with a nonreader or severely disabled reader to spend several months on the initial vowel sound before it has been thoroughly learned. Generally, the exercises from multiple books must be combined to provide enough rehearsal and review. Phonic books and reading programs rarely provide enough exercise depth for the nonreader. Programs are normally desig-nated to move at the pace of the average pupil. This even includes a number of programs marketed for remedial reading. The specialist can readily group the activities from multiple programs and provide the appropriate programming depth.

Level II—Visual-Symbol Discrimination

The combination of straight, curved, vertical, and the diagonal or horizontal line differentiates one letter from another. Many letters have components which appear so similar that they are difficult for the new reader to remember and differentiate. Some letters which exhibit these properties are m/n, h/n, w/m, t/j, q/g, b/d, b/p, and r/n. While there are many other combinations which have similar comparisons, it readily becomes apparent to the specialist which of these are confusing to the learner.

In initial phases of learning to read it is critical that the specialist present visual symbols which can be widely discriminated from one another. The presentation of both the *b* and *d* symbol in the same lesson would lead to certain confusion and probable continued difficulty for some time. For this reason it is most efficient to use one letter from the combination of each of the letters, practice these in isolation, and require discrimination from grossly different letters. The pupil's success in differentiating the differences and likenesses of letters will likely be related to the initial development of symbol constancy as reported previously.

Level III—Visual-Symbol Seriation

The recognition of symbols in a particular pattern is essential for reading success. The ability to recognize word configuration follows the ability to recognize individual symbols. While this seems quite apparent to the reader at this point, it is interesting to note that many specialists begin with word recognition rather than starting at the basic level of symbol recognition. The automatic ability to recall symbol constancy is crucial for success in long-term retention of words.

Programming for the pupil on Level III should begin with presentation of vowel-consonant or consonant-vowel sequences. Activities stressing the recognition of b/a and a/b as well as other vowel-consonant combinations will assist the individual in developing sound blending skills and the appropriate sequencing and seriation of symbols. When the pupil is comfortable with two-symbol combinations, the digit span may be increased to three symbols and more as the pupil is successful.

Level III—Auditory-Sound Sequencing

The purpose of sound sequencing in the reading development process is to allow for sound blending and auditory closure. The blending of sounds and the recognition experience of closure provide the pupil with the potential ability to read; however, the correct ordering of sounds is frequently difficult for the pupil. It is therefore important to begin with two sound sequences and only increase sequence capacity as the pupil experiences automatic closure on the digit capacity being rehearsed.

Activities which have proven successful include progression in the following manner:

b–a   ba
a–b   ab
ta
at
ba
rat
ch   a   p
chat

In each of the sequences, initially, the pupil works in isolation with the sounds until he can experience closure without sounding out a syllable. When recognition occurs and the individual experiences awareness of the sounds in combination, such as saying *ba* for *b* and *a*, then reading is beginning. It is the ability to experience syllable awareness and ultimately syllable closure that is most encouraging to the pupil.

It was at this level that the man, mentioned at the beginning of this chapter, realized he was going to be able to read. That awareness was incredibly exciting to both pupil and specialist. Mr. Wells was so excited that he had tears in his eyes as he said, "Just wait till I show my boy how to do this!"

Level IV—Language and Meaning

The integration of sounds and symbols is crucial for reading because without efficient functioning of this process we shall continue to experience reading problems. Once the decoding and encoding skills are working, reading for understanding can be achieved. In the majority of cases of dyslexia, and with most nonreaders, comprehension is not a severe problem. Most of these pupils find that once they can "get the words off the paper," pronounce the word, they can understand the meaning.

For pupils with asphasic disorders, vocabulary differences, cultural differences, non-English fluency, and even subtle language difficulties, the awareness of traditional English patterns is helpful. Activities to increase the awareness of common grammar transformations will assist the pupil in being able to predict what words will logically come next and evaluate the correctness of the reading of a sentence. For the pupil with language problems, programming is critical if the reading/decoding skill is to be useful.

An adequate vocabulary is equally crucial for reading effectiveness. In order for the pupil to experience auditory closure on a word, he will need an awareness of the word. The familiarity with the word being sound-blended will assist the pupil to experience closure. The pupil will need to experience a search of familiar words to identify the correct word. One pupil spent quite a while trying to figure out what a "ri . . . *ver*" could be. While "river" was in his vocabulary, he could not experience closure on it when he accented it in this manner. In other instances the pupil may not have the word in his vocabulary and, as a result, be unable to decide on the correct pronunciation because of a void in his internal vocabulary retention system.

OUTPUT CHANNELS

Pupils' reading skills are evaluated in basically two ways: verbal and written indications of understanding. In the early grades most reading evaluation conducted by the teacher utilizes the verbal response channel. Children are measured by how well they read aloud. In the later years they are evaluated by their effectiveness of written demonstration of what they have read.

Specialists should receive a caution at this point—some difficulties in reading are actually output channel deficiencies. Numerous pupils have difficulty expressing themselves in writing due to fine motor control and handwriting problems. Frequently these pupils are reported to have comprehension problems because they are unable to demonstrate their understanding of the information read.

SUMMARY

The isolation of reading levels is important for the understanding of the process for efficient reading. Pupils may experience stress at any of the levels or at many of the levels. The specialist who carefully evaluates the pupil's needs, programs at the success level, patiently allows automatic level processing to occur, and provides a reinforcing and encouraging learning environment will be successful as a reading facilitator. Even more important, the pupil will learn to read!

Mr. Wells can presently read at a mid-fifth-grade level. He has worked one hour weekly for two years to achieve this skill. Had he experienced sound-symbol training at an earlier age he might have been spared the frustration and defeat he suffered through school and as an adult.

When he was asked why he did not learn to read at school, he said with his toughest look, "Them teachers and me, we had an understanding . . . they didn't bug me and I didn't bug them." Mr. Wells is now a parent volunteer in a neighborhood tutoring program and proudly reports regularly the progress of his pupils . . . whom he is now teaching to read!

REFERENCES

Barsch, Ray H.: *Achieving Perceptual-Motor Efficiency.* Special Child Publications, 1967.
Cruickshank, William: *A Teaching Method for Brain-Injured and Hyperactive Children.* Syracuse University Press, 1961.

Ellingson, Careth: *The Shadow Children,* Topaz Publications, 1967.

Getman, G. N.: *How to Develop Your Child's Intelligence.* Dimensions Publishing Co., 1971.

Kephart, Newell C. and Roach, Eugene G.: *The Purdue Perceptual Motor Survey.* Columbus, Charles Merrill, Inc., 1966.

Money, John: *The Disabled Reader.* Baltimore, The Johns Hopkins Press, 1966.

Smith, Joan M.: *The Receptive-Expressive Observation.* San Rafael, Academic Therapy Publications, 1971.

Wagner, Rudolph: *Dyslexia and Your Child.* Scranton, Harper and Row, 1971.

CHAPTER 13

THE SEVERELY AND PROFOUNDLY DISABLED

Michael K. Grimes

INTRODUCTION

No other group of individuals in our society is more misunderstood and neglected than the group called "severely and profoundly disabled." For the most part, these children and adults are not in public school settings, but rather in state hospitals, convalescent and nursing homes, private hospitals or schools, and/or church-operated facilities.

They are often ignored because of the increased cost to care for them and the amount of time and personnel needed to provide even a minimal program. In the past five years many states have had to make fiscal cuts at the state hospital system, and this has meant that many of these children and adults were sent back to their local communities. They were initially absorbed by convalescent hospitals, church and private settings, and, more recently, the schools (Pub. L. No. 94-142 guarantees the full constitutional right of every school-age individual to a free education). The public sector has no other option but to plan and develop programs to meet the educational needs of these adults and children whose medical etiologies include the following:

Genetic-Based Diseases
A Down's syndrome (most common)—3 kinds
   1. Trisomy 21 (90% of all cases)
   2. Mosaic (8%)
   3. Other (2%)
B Homocystinuria (amino acids)
C Metachromatic leukodystrophy and sufatide metabolism (degenerative diseases of the nervous system)

284

D The following are due to infections: (prenatal)
1. Rubella or German measles
2. Mumps
3. Asiatic flu
4. Sytomegalic inclusion body disease
   a. virus infection in mother's salivary glands
   b. causes meningocephalitis
5. Herpes simplex and herpes zoster
6. Congenital syphilis
7. Various viral infections such as spirochetal, mycotic, and parasitic are common
8. Many toxics and poisons—X-rays—prenatal trauma—allergic reactions—birth complications

E Metabolic genetic errors
1. Tay-Sachs disease—most common in Jewish parents (60-70%)
2. Spielmyer-Vogt disease—enlargement of head
3. Kufs' disease
4. Gaucher's disease
5. Greenfield's disease

F Abnormalities of amino acid metabolism
1. Phenylketonuria (loss of pigment)

G Miscellaneous metabolic abnormalities
1. Wilson's disease

H Others include the following:
1. Tuberous sclerosis—skin lesions
2. Sturge-Weber
3. Ancephaly
4. Hydrocephalus
5. Microcephaly

I And many others

Along with these etiological factors are those associated with drug abuse, smoking, alcohol, and emotional trauma to mother during pregnancy. In most cases these children are not pleasant to look at, and in many states they are locked away until they die. It was not until the past decade that research has shown most of these individuals to be capable of acquiring more skills and achieving some academic success. As discussed earlier, recent federal legislation Pub. L. No. 94-142 has mandated many programs for these individuals, and the task now is for those of us in the speech and language field to develop, interpret, and, most importantly, help them to develop a communication system that is functional. All types of communication boards are currently being developed for the severely handicapped.

In many instances, this will be their first opportunity to become aware that an outside world exists. Developing a speech and language strategy for dealing with these exceptionalities musters all our training and insights. For the most part, we will be on our own with very few local resources. There are, however, a few therapists whose work does apply to this group.

Psycholinguistic Approaches to Language and Language Development — Therapists dealing in this realm include the following:

1. Kenneth F. Ruder of the University of Kansas, whose model is based on a generative transformational theory.
2. Lois Bloom of Columbia University, who deals with semantics and suggests from her data that it is possible for an observing adult to interpret the semantic intent of children's utterances from these data arrive at several treatments for language disorders associated with mental retardation, including the arrangement of words in sentences before attempts are made to teach morphological inflection, noun, verb, and adjective form.
3. Hass & Hass from Skimmer College, who assume that grammar should show how closely syntactic structure is bound to the basic features of communication. They are interested in the three faces of syntax: surface structure, semantic representations, and transformations.
4. Peter Rosenberger from Walter E. Fernald State School, who is concerned with the referential processes which underline human communication and the development of referential processes in children. In other words, how does a speaker select verbal repertoire in communicating with his listener?
5. William Bricher from George Peabody College who combines Psycholinguistic theory with a range of past research using the operant model.
6. Donald Baer, Douglass Guess, and Jeams Sherman from the University of Kansas, who deal with linguistic acquisition and the behavior functions of acquiring these skills.

Others include Jon Miller and David Yader, who believe that language programs for the retarded could be based on developmental language sequences that normal children follow; they have developed a syntax teaching program.

In the past five years there has been an increasing effort to integrate what have been isolated views in describing the human language system, its functions, and the process by which the human language system is acquired. This holistic and eclectic approach looks at and considers the semantic analysis of the child's language, the cognitive/constructive views of the child's language, and the socioconstructive views of language. (An in-depth discussion can be found in McLean's chapter on "Implications of Language Research" pages 295-317 in *Changing Perspectives in Special Education,* edited by Kneedler and Tarver— Merrill Publishing Company, 1977.)

What is basically happening is that a new humanistic-holistic approach is being developed that not only looks at past theories and views but also examines the newer trends in acquisition processes and treatment procedures. The new research becomes just as concerned with environment and social factors as with behavior, phonology, semantics, and morphological constructs. A few of the people involved in this new direction are Bloom, Bruner, Holliday, Luria, J. D. MacDonald, and Mahoney.

Some Assessment Ideas

Traditional assessment includes tools such as The Parsons Language Sample (Spradin 1963), The Houston Test of Language Development (Crabtree 1963), The Utah Test of Language Development (UTLD) (Mecham, Jex & Jones 1969), The Illinois Test of Psycholinguistic Abilities (Kirk et al. 1968), and The Zimmerman Preschool Language Test. These language tests may be appropriate. The problem is that, for many of these youngsters, a sit-down test is often impossible to administer. A speech and language specialist needs to have a sound basic knowledge of these tests plus the Peabody, McCarthy, Slingerland, Northwestern, and Carrow's Test of Comprehension and Linguistic Structure in order to develop a repertoire from which to base the language assessment. The specialist should also know how to interpret results from the Stanford-Binet, WISC, and Leiter. There is no one test that works or evaluates better than another, but the Speech and Language Specialist who has a working knowledge of these assessments can start to make some subjective evaluations as to where in the language hierarchy the evaluatee is. Observation and active participation in daily activities of the evaluatee are essential in a complete and thorough evaluation. If you as a Speech and Language Specialist are charged with the responsibility of providing an assessment, you must be willing to provide ample time for a diagnosis. The all-too-frequent one or two hour evaluation will not be adequate because it does not provide the Speech and Language Specialist the time to do a complete assessment. It must be ongoing. The assessment of a severely and profoundly handicapped person is one of the most challenging acts that will face a Speech and Language Specialist. It has been my observation that experience and exposure, not textbook strategies, are a Speech and Language Specialist's most useful tools in testing and evaluation.

After Assessment, What Next?

Providing a language remediation or a stimulus program entails the full cooperation of all support staff involved, i.e. parent, teacher, doctor, nurse, physical therapists, occupational therapist, psychologist, social worker, bus driver, and custodian. It is a total effort and one that should not be taken lightly. Basic language training must be consistent and should be taught in the same sequence that it is acquired by the normal child. Jon Miller and David Yoder's program on Semantic Development has been gaining increasing popularity. Studies by Woodward (1959, 1963), Sinclair (1969), Kahn (1975), and Wohlhueter and Sindberg (1975) cover a range of developmental achievements which demonstrate potential cognitive deficits of differences at particular stages of development compared to normal children. These studies support further exploration of cognitive behavior and its relationship to semantic aspects of language acquisition and to the development of language teaching programs for children with language deficits. Studies by Piaget, Morehead and Ingram (1973), Furth (1971), Cromer (1974), and Slobin (1972) all indicate that a direct focus on cognitive-linguistic behaviors of children with language problems will result in improved methodologies, clear decision-making procedures for individualized treatment program development, and an improved understanding of the important cognitive-language dimensions necessary for language growth. Commercial programs include the Peabody Language Development Kit, DISTAR, EDMARK, and SULLIVAN (BRL Programs). Some of the most proficient programs will be the ones that you as Speech and Language Specialist design for those individuals or groups you serve.

REFERENCES

Bartel, N. R.: The development of morphology in moderately retarded children. *Education and Training of the Mentally Retarded,* 5:164-168, 1970.

Bartel, N. R. and Hammill, Donald D.: *Teaching Children with Learning Behavior Problems.* Boston, Allyn and Bacon, Inc., 1975.

Bender, Michael and Velletutti, Peter J.: *Teaching the Moderately and Severely Handicapped* (3 volumes). Baltimore, University Park Press, 1976.

Bloom, L.: *Language Development: Form and Function in Emerging Grammars.* Cambridge, MIT Press, 1970.

Bloom, L.: *One Word at a Time: The Use of Single Word Utterances Before Syntax.* The Hague, Mouton, 1973.

Bowerman, M. F.: Discussion summary—development of concepts underlying language. In Schiefelbusch, R. and Lloyd, L. (Eds.): *Language Perspectives: Acquisition, Retardation and Intervention.* Baltimore, University Park Press, 1973.

Bruner, J. S.: From communication to language—a psychological perspective. *Cognition,* 3:255-287, 1974-1975.

Bruner, J. S.: The ontorgenesis of speech acts. *Journal of Child Language,* 2:1-19, 1975.

Chafe, E.: *Meaning and Structure of Language.* Chicago, University of Chicago Press, 1973.

Chomsky, C.: *The Acquisition of Syntax in Children from Five to Ten.* Cambridge, MIT Press, 1969.

Cromer, R.: Receptive language in the mentally retarded: Processes and diagnostic distinctions. In Schiefelbusch, R. and Lloyd, L. (Eds.): *Language Perspectives: Acquisition, Retardation and Intervention.* Baltimore, University Park Press, 1974.

Das, J.: Patterns of cognitive ability in non-retarded and retarded children. *Am J Ment Defic,* 6-12, 1972-1977.

Dunn, L. M. (Ed.): *Exceptional Children in the Schools—Special Education in Transition,* 2nd ed. New York, Holt, Rinehart and Winston, 1973.

Furth, H.: On language and knowing in Piaget's developmental theory. *Hum Dev,* 13:241-257, 1970.

Furth, H.: Linguistic deficiency and thinking: Research with deaf subjects, 1964-1969. *Psychol Bull, 71*:83, 1971.

Gay, B. and Ryan, B.: *A Language Program for the Non-Language Child.* Champaign, Research Press, 1973.

Guess, D. and Baer, D. M.: An analysis of individual differences in generalization between receptive and productive language in retarded children. *Journal of Applied Behavior Analysis, 6*:311-329, 1973.

Halliday, M.: Learning how to mean. In Lenneberg, E. and Lenneberg, E. (Eds.): *Foundations of Language Development: A Multidisciplinary Approach* (Vol. 1). New York, Academic Press, 1975.

Kahn, J. V.: Relationship of Piaget's sensori-motor period to language acquisition of profoundly retarded children. *Am J Ment Defic, 79*:(6), 640-643, 1975.

Luria, A.: Scientific perspectives and philosophical dead ends in modern linguistics. *Cognition, 3*:377-385, 1974-1975.

MacDonald, J. D.: Environmental language intervention. In Withsow, F. and Nygren, C. (Eds.): *Language, Materials and Curriculum Management for the Handicapped Learner.* Columbus, Charles E. Merrill, 1976.

Miller, J. and Yoder, D.: An onto genetic language teaching strategy for retarded children. In Schiefelbusch, E., and Lloyd, L. (Eds.): *Language Perspectives: Acquisition, Retardation and Intervention.* Baltimore, University Park Press, 1974.

Miller, J. and Yoder, D.: A syntax teaching program. In McLeon, J.; Yoder, D. and Schiefelbusch, R. (Eds.): *Language Intervention with the Retarded.* Baltimore, University Park Press, 1972.

Sinclair-de Zwart, H.: Language acquisition and cognitive development. In Moore, T. E. (Ed.): *Cognitive Development and the Acquisition of Language.* New York, Academic Press, 1973.

Slobin, D. I.: Cognitive prerequisites for the development of grammar. In Ferguson, C. A. and Slobin, D. I. (Eds.): *Studies of Child Language Development.* New York, Holt, Rinehart and Winston, 1973.

Woodward, M.: The behavior of idiots interpreted by Piaget theory of sensory-motor development. *Br J Educ Psychol, 29*:60-71, 1959.

Woodward, M.: The application of Piaget's theory to research in mental deficiency. In Ellis, N. (Ed.): *Handbook of Mental Deficiency.* New York, McGraw-Hill, 1963.

CHAPTER 14

ON BECOMING A SPEECH/LANGUAGE CLINICIAN

BARBARA HOADLEY AND SUSAN GOODRICH

T HE PRECEDING CHAPTERS have dealt primarily with the client and his/her problems with communication. We will now discuss the speech pathologist and/or audiologist and the requirements needed for the profession, both academic and personal, and the responsibilities thus entailed. As a speech pathologist and/or audiologist, your primary responsibilities will be the assessment and management of the client's speech, language, and/or hearing problems. In order to fulfill that responsibility, certain require-ments must be met and credentials obtained to guarantee eligi-bility in any work setting. The following four documents are generally recommended in any state with a master's level cre-dential and a licensure act:

1. A state credential in speech pathology and/or audiology
2. A state license in speech pathology and/or audiology
3. The American Speech and Hearing Association's certificate of clinical competence (ASHA CCC)
4. The Master of Arts degree (M.A.) in speech pathology and/or audiology or the equivalent.

The state credential is compulsory for working in the public schools, whereas the state license is required in order to work in any setting other than the public schools or federal agencies and institutions. The American Speech and Hearing Association (ASHA) issues the Certificate of Clinical Competence (CCC), which is the only nationally recognized measure of competence in the fields of speech pathology and audiology. A Master of Arts degree or equivalent training, in addition to a specified number of client contact hours and clinical competence, partially fulfills the criteria for these documents. The prospective professional must then be employed for a period equivalent to nine months of full-time employment and receive a passing grade on the appropriate National Testing Service Examination (NTSE) before receiving the license or the CCC in speech pathology and/or audiology.

In fulfillment of the academic requirements for these documents, certain courses are required as part of the student's training program. Through training and practical experience, the student develops a basic knowledge of the normal processes involved in human communication. By studying the deviations from the normal patterns, one can begin to diagnose and remediate both receptive and expressive communication problems. Though each training institution maintains its own particular requirements, most require a group of courses dealing with basic information imperative to a thorough understanding of knowledge in the field. The following is a general list of the topics or contents included in these courses. Courses in both speech pathology and audiology are usually grouped together at the undergraduate level but are separated sometime during the student's progression through the program. At this point prospective speech pathologists customarily continue to focus their concentration on diagnosis and methods of remediation for articulation, language, fluency, and voice problems, while prospective audiologists focus on the diagnosis and remediation of problems of the hearing impaired, with special emphasis on acoustics, assessment, and rehabilitative instrumentation and methods.

> *Phonetics*: A study of the physical production and acoustic characteristics of American speech sounds, their symbolization in phonetic and phonemic alphabets, and practice in broad transcription.
>
> *Anatomy and Physiology of the Speech Mechanism*: A study of the normal structures and functioning involved in respiration, phonation, resonance, and articulation.
>
> *Introduction to Speech and Hearing*: An overview of the speech pathologist's and/or audiologist's role, with a general explanation of the problems dealt with and the work settings in which the professional operates.
>
> *Articulation*: A study of both the normal and deviant development of articulation, including functional and physical etiologies, with theories and methods of assessment and remediation of articulation disorders.

Normal Language: A study of the normal development of language, including functional and physical etiologies.

Language Disorders: A study of the deviant development of language, including functional and physical etiologies, with theories and methods of assessment and remediation of language disorders.

Fluency: A study of both the normal and deviant development of fluency, including functional and physical etiologies, with theories and methods of assessment and remediation of fluency disorders.

Voice: A study of both the normal and deviant development of voice, including functional and physical etiologies, with theories and methods of assessment and remediation of voice disorders.

Note: The physical etiologies that may cause articulation, language, fluency, and voice problems include cleft palate, the cerebral palsied, mental retardation, and congenital deformities.

Introduction to Audiology: A study of anatomy and physiology of the ear, and the physics of sound as related to hearing measurement.

Audiometric Testing and Hearing Conservation: The administration and interpretation of individual and group hearing tests in both the public schools and the clinical setting; the development and administration of hearing conservation programs.

Aural Rehabilitation: A study of the theories and methods of rehabilitation for the hearing impaired.

Hearing Aids: A study of amplification systems and their use as rehabilitative devices.

Diagnosis and Management: A study of differential diagnosis, placement, and programming of those with speech, language, and hearing disorders.

Speech Science: A study of the physical aspects of the production and reception of speech signals, and methods and techniques of measurement employed in the speech and hearing sciences.

Research in Speech and Hearing: A study of research methods, statistical procedures, and the evaluation of data in speech pathology and audiology.

Research Writing: A study of format, style, and organization of materials for writing research and other reports in speech pathology and audiology, including the master's thesis.

Speech and Hearing Services: A study of the role of the professional in various work settings, the relationship of speech and hearing specialists to other professional personnel, and the purpose, organization, and administration of speech and hearing programs.

Counseling and Interviewing: The interviewing and counseling of parents of children and clients with speech, language, and hearing disorders.

Psychoacoustic Instrumentation in Audiology: A study of the fundamentals of electricity and electronic measurement; a description of measurement of the auditory processes and psychoacoustic experiments.

Clinical Audiology: A study of the methods, procedures, and instruments used in the measurement and diagnosis of auditory dysfunction.

Introduction to Clinical Methods: A study of the principles of modifying speech and language behavior; use of diagnostic tests, procedures, and clinical equipment.

Clinical Methods and Practicum—Articulation: A supervised clinical experience in the assessment and remediation of articulation disorders.

Clinical Methods and Practicum—Language: A supervised clinical experience in the assessment and remediation of language disorders.

Clinical Methods and Practicum—Fluency: A supervised clinical experience in the assessment and remediation of fluency disorders.

Clinical Methods and Practicum—Voice: A supervised clinical experience in the assessment and remediation of voice disorders.

Clinical Methods and Practicum—Diagnosis and Management: A supervised clinical experience in the differential diagnosis, placement, and programming of those with speech, language, and hearing disorders.

Clinical Methods and Practicum—Audiometric Testing: A supervised clinical experience in the measurement and diagnosis of auditory dysfunction.

Clinical Methods and Practicum—Aural Rehabilitation: A supervised clinical experience in the rehabilitation of the hearing impaired.

The primary purpose of the academic courses is to impart the theoretical concepts and practical knowledge of the field. In them, the student's competency can be demonstrated through traditional testing techniques, whereas clinical competence requires a more subjective judgment. The profession has established a minimum number of hours of supervised practicum experience necessary to assure that the student has attained competence.

Though each state establishes its own standards for credentials, the California State Credential in Language, Speech, and Hearing requires 300 hours of supervised practicum with children. If a speech pathologist also desires authorization to teach a class of aphasic children, an additional 100 hours of supervised practicum in an aphasic self-contained classroom are required for this authorization. The California state license requires 300 minor and adult hours, and each individual M.A. program also requires specified clinical experience. The CCC requires 300 hours of supervised contact with infants, children, and adults and regulates the following minimum number of hours in each respective area:

Speech Pathology			*Audiology*	
Articulation	30		Audiometric testing	215
Language	75		Aural rehabilitation	50
Fluency	25		Speech pathology not	
Voice	25		related to hearing	
Audiology	35		handicaps	35
Audiometric testing		15		
Aural rehabilitation		15		

In addition, 150 hours must be accrued at the graduate level, and 200 must be in the appropriate area of specialty, either speech pathology or audiology. Each speech pathology and/or audiology student must consult his/her own training institution to verify the number of hours required by the institution and state, as well as the age and type of clients needed. If the training institution is unaware of the requirements, the student may write directly to the State Department of Education or the ombudsman of the American Speech and Hearing Association to obtain the needed information.

We cannot emphasize enough that the above are minimum requirements, and it is highly recommended that the student plan to accrue more than these stated minimums. It is realistic to expect that most students will accumulate between 400 and 500 hours of supervised practicum within the time spent in the training program in order to fulfill all requirements. It is also important to note that the speech pathology and/or audiology student is solely responsible for the tallying and confirmation of supervised practicum hours accumulated. During one's course of study, both a vigilant recording by the student and verification of hours by an authorized supervisor are imperative to insure completion of the requirements for the desired documents.

Courses to Be Considered

Speech pathology and audiology are "people" professions, involving the interaction of human beings through communication, and incorporating the knowledge and experience of many varied professional areas in their implementation. Emerick and Hatten (1974) state that "the prospective speech clinician must acquire an impressive array of knowledge and skills if he is to perform his role effectively" (p. 23). Most training institutions' credentials, certificates, and licenses require elective courses in related areas such as linguistics, child and youth development, and exceptional children in order to provide a broad background of knowledge.

Speech pathology and audiology deal with all aspects of personal communication: speaking, listening, reading, and writing. Consequently, competency of the clinician is essential in these areas to insure accurate and adept communication skills which may be both taught and implemented proficiently. Any classes, particularly in the area of English, which promote the oral language skills of syntax, articulation, and diction, and the written skills of correct grammar, spelling, and punctuation should prove to be advantageous. Both as a student and as a professional in the field, the speech pathologist and/or audiologist must write reports, maintain files, and hold conferences and consultations, all of which require a competence in clear and concise expression. In addition to a proficiency in English, an accessory adroitness at typing would prove to be a valuable asset, considering the number of reports required of both students and professionals. With the advent of Public Law No. 94-142, and California's attempt to come into compliance with its Master Plan, professionals are held legally accountable for files and reports on each individual client. Though files are confidential, they are open to the client, the parents of the client, and all authorized professionals dealing with the client. In addition, individual program reports must be prepared and kept on permanent file; therefore, competency must be assured for cogent and efficient records. Accountability and consumer protection have become major considerations in all aspects of life. In our own profession, speech pathology and audiology, quality assurance of services rendered and peer review are currently being implemented in all work settings. This further indicates the need for competency in the preparation and maintenance of reports.

Public relations are an important adjunct to the responsibilities of the speech pathologist and/or audiologist in any work setting. The professions of speech pathology and audiology are not well known or understood by the general public, and it is therefore the responsibility of the professional to continually make visible the needs of the profession and the service it renders. In addition, the professions of speech pathology and audiology are dependent on the cooperation of other professionals and the community in general in order to function effectively. For these two reasons, if the professional is not able to communicate effectively, it is unlikely that s/he will be able to serve the client and his/her needs satisfactorily. One needs not only the skill to communicate the needs and justifications for such support to community service groups, school boards, and the like, but also to be able to promote cooperation among the professionals and personnel involved in providing services to clients. In order to be proficient at public relations, one needs both public speaking skills and an understanding and appreciation for the contributions to be made by others on behalf of our clients. A speech pathologist and/or audiologist may be very knowledgeable about his/her own profession, but if s/he is not capable of effectively communicating this knowledge to others, s/he cannot expect to gain the necessary support of parent groups, community service organizations, and/or school boards. The speech pathologist/audiologist must be appreciative of and capable of understanding the importance of the roles to be played by others in developing and implementing well-coordinated speech and hearing programs.

With the increased use of instrumentation and audiovisual equipment in the diagnosis and remediation of speech, language, and hearing disorders, a knowledge of the operation and maintenance of audiovisual equipment would be a valuable, time-saving tool. Though it is apparent why it is important to know how to operate equipment, it is equally important that one be able to perform basic repairs, as this can decrease the amount of time lost to the professional and his/her client in use of the equipment.

Any courses in the area of the behavioral sciences, such as psychology, counseling, and behavior modification, or in the basic sciences, such as biology, physics, and engineering, could prove to be directly or indirectly beneficial to working in speech pathology and/or audiology. Because ours is a profession dealing with communication, knowledge of normal processes of development and behavior will naturally complement diagnostic and therapeutic techniques.

The professions of speech pathology and audiology include people who perform research, provide clinical services, and administer programs. All of these segments of the professions require competent mathematical skills. The researcher needs these skills to apply formulas in the analysis of research data; the clinician, in reading research findings, and in the scoring and interpretation of assessment results; and the administrator, in developing program budgets and fund-raising activities.

A speech pathologist or audiologist is not a complete professional without basic skill and knowledge in these related areas.

Ethics

Before discussing the actual personal characteristics or traits the student needs to possess before becoming a speech pathologist and/or audiologist, we must first consider the code of ethics. The code of ethics of any profession establishes the rules and regulations by which the profession monitors itself and, therefore, guarantees to the public it serves that persons deemed qualified by the profession will give competent service. The following code of ethics is that of the American Speech and Hearing Association, and is presented here because ASHA is the nationally recognized organization of the professions of speech pathology and audiology.

Code of Ethics of the American Speech and
Hearing Association, 1976
(Last revised January 1, 1977)

Preamble

The preservation of the highest standards of integrity and ethical principles is vital to the successful discharge of the responsibilities of all Members. This Code of Ethics has been promulgated by the Association in an effort to highlight the fundamental rules considered essential to this basic purpose. The failure to specify any particular responsibility or practice in this Code of Ethics should not be construed as denial of the existence of other responsibilities or practices that are equally important. Any act that is in violation of the spirit and purpose of this Code of Ethics shall be unethical practice. It is the responsibility of each Member to advise the Ethical Practice Board of instances of violation of the principles incorporated in this Code.

Section A. The ethical responsibilities of the Member require that the welfare of the person he serves professionally be considered paramount.

1. The Member who engages in clinical work must possess appropriate qualifications. Measures of such qualifications are provided by the Association's program for certification of the clinical competence of Members.

(a) The Member must not provide services for which he has not been properly trained, i.e. had the necessary course work and supervised practicum.

(b) The Member who has not completed his professional preparation must not provide speech or hearing services except in a supervised clinical practicum situation as a part of his training. A person holding a full-time clinical position and taking part-time graduate work is not, for the purpose of this section, regarded as a student in training.

(c) The Member must not accept remuneration for providing services until he has completed the necessary course work and clinical practicum to meet certification requirements. The Member who is uncertified must not engage in private practice.

2. The Member must follow acceptable patterns of professional conduct in his relations with the persons he serves.

(a) He must not guarantee the results of any speech or hearing consultative or therapeutic procedure. A guarantee of any sort, expressed or implied, oral or written, is contrary to professional ethics. A reasonable statement of prognosis may be made, but successful results are dependent on many uncontrollable factors, hence, any warranty is deceptive and unethical.

(b) He must not diagnose or treat individual speech or hearing disorders by correspondence. This does not preclude follow-up by correspondence of individuals previously seen, nor does it preclude providing the persons served professionally with general information of an educational nature.

(c) He must not reveal to authorized persons any confidential information obtained from the individual he serves professionally without his permission.

(d) He must not exploit persons he serves professionally: (1) by accepting them for treatment where benefit cannot reasonably be expected to accrue; (2) by continuing treatment unnecessarily; (3) by charging exhorbitant fees.

3. The Member must use every resource available, including referral to other specialists as needed, to effect as great improvement as possible in the persons he serves.

4. The Member must take every precaution to avoid injury to the persons he serves professionally.

Section B. The duties owed by the Member to other professional workers are many.

1. He should seek the freest professional discussion of all theoretical and practical issues but avoid personal invective directed toward professional colleagues or members of allied professions.

2. He should establish harmonious relations with members of other professions. He should endeavor to inform others concerning the services that can be rendered by members of the speech and hearing profession and in turn should seek information from members of related professions. He should strive to increase knowledge within the field of speech and hearing.

3. He must not accept fees, gifts, or other forms of gratuity for serving as a sponsor of applicants for clinical certification by the American Speech and Hearing Association.

Section C. The ASHA Member has other special responsibilities.

1. He must guard against conflicts of professional interest.

(a) He must not accept compensation in any form from a manufacturer or a dealer in prosthetic or other devices for recommending any particular product.

(b) Public statements and announcements of services should serve to provide accurate and adequate information to the public about the professional and the services rendered by its practitioners. All Members must observe this principle as an affirmative ethical obligation under all conditions of professional practice. The Member should announce services in a manner consonant with highest professional standards in the community. The announcement may include identification by name, appropriate professional title and qualifications, services offered, fees, location, hours, and telephone number.

(c) He must not engage in commercial activities that conflict with his responsibilities to the persons he serves professionally or to his colleagues. He must not permit his professional titles or accomplishments to be used in the sale or promotion of any product related to his professional field. He must not perform clinical services or promotional activity for any profit-making organization that is engaged in the retail sales of equipment, publications, or other materials. He may be employed by a manufacturer or publisher, provided that his duties are consultative, scientific, or educational in nature.

2. He should help in the education of the public regarding speech and hearing problems and other matters lying within his professional competence.

3. He should seek to provide and expand services to persons with speech and hearing handicaps, and to assist in establishing high professional standards for such programs.

4. He must not discriminate on the basis of race, religion, sex, or age in his professional relationships with his colleagues or clients. (ASHA, January 1977, P. 41)

Having read the Code of Ethics, you are now aware that the client and your responsibilities to him/her have first priority. If recompense for services provided becomes of primary concern, then you may very well find yourself in conflict with the preceding Code of Ethics. The professions of speech pathology and audiology recognize the free enterprise system and are not politically advocating socialistic conditions, yet the person coming into these professions must be one who is rewarded by giving of himself and serving others. Service professions, by their very nature, require a diligent dedication and moral responsibility that determine the effectiveness of one's entire professional career. Now it would seem appropriate to examine the personal traits or characteristics of the person desiring to become a member of the professions of speech pathology and/or audiology.

Personal Characteristics

Throughout this chapter we have attempted to describe the program of training a person goes through in order to become a speech pathologist and/or audiologist. We will now address ourselves to the professional himself and what he personally must bring to the profession.

Some speech pathologists and/or audiologists appear organized, working within structured environments and with specifically developed methodology, whereas others appear to act on intuition and the reality of the situation at hand. Both ends of the spectrum can be accommodated within the profession as long as they share the common denominator of bringing to the client an appropriate combination of expertise in understanding, acceptance, determination, and dedication to do their work.

Persons in the field of speech pathology and/or audiology are not made up of one particular configuration of traits, and are thus not easily stereotyped into specific standard patterns of behavior.

We have stated that the primary purpose of the professions of speech pathology and audiology is to serve clients. What we have not dealt with is what this service entails. The service that is to be provided to the client involves change: a change of behavior that will allow the person to more effectively communicate with others in his environment and, therefore, allow him both to benefit from and to perform better in that environment. The ethics of the profession will hold you responsible for making the appropriate changes, but inherent in that is the fact that you will change the life of another human being. This fact is not peculiar to our profession but is shared with teaching, medicine, psychology, and social work, to name but a few. The point to be stressed is that, as a professional, you must be willing to take the responsibility of changing another person's behavior and to accept the concept that it is within your right to do so.

Another responsibility related to the services offered by our profession is to maintain the rights of the client. The client or responsible person has the right to accept or reject services. In order to make a reasonable judgment, the client or responsible person must be informed of the need for the service and what the service will offer in benefits to the client.

Public Law No. 94-142, passed by the United States Congress in 1975, states that service (change) can only be provided after the individual, or parent and/or guardian of the individual, has given *informed* consent. Certainly, the provider of the service would then share the responsibility for change with the client, which would include communicating to the client/parent the intended change, so that s/he indeed can give informed consent. The clinician must then realize for himself what constitutes *informed* consent. Is establishing a basic acquaintance with the service to be provided sufficient, or is a more thorough understanding of the processes involved necessary before the recipients of the service can be said to be *informed*? If so, how is the understanding to be measured and confirmed? The clinician must decide at what point the client/parent is truly informed of the service (change) to be provided. In addition, the professional must be responsible for developing the program to be followed in bringing about the change in behavior, and for insuring that the change is appropriate so that it benefits the client in interacting with his environment.

What kind of person possesses the traits that would allow him/her to operate within this framework? Several researchers have attempted to outline the personal characteristics which an individual wishing to pursue the profession should possess. They have listed objectivity, awareness, sensitivity, insight, patience, perception, responsibility, dedication, understandng, empathy, creativity, resourcefulness, enthusiasm, caring, loyalty, punctuality, virtue, open-mindedness, conscientiousness, sensibility, and many others. Certainly we have no argument with any of the mentioned traits, as each will be necessary at one time or another during one's career. The problem is in defining what these terms mean and measuring their existence in any human being. Rather than deal with these traits that we find undefinable and unmeasurable, we have chosen a different approach. Because acceptance of the responsibility to change a person's behavior is paramount to the rehabilitative process, this should and can be considered by the student prior to entering the profession. The other personality traits and/or characteristics will have to be considered by the student as s/he proceeds through supervised practicum with clients. As the student interacts with the client, a need for specific traits will be apparent, and the student will then have to determine if s/he possesses the appropriate traits or can develop them as a part of his/her learning. Identification and measurement of these traits cannot be accomplished apart from the process in which they occur. Subsequently, we may then judge from that process what qualities will be necessary for the person to possess. Only from understanding the whole of the professional's responsibility, rather than the parts or personal traits, can one truly evaluate whether or not s/he is suited to become a member of the professions of speech pathology and/or audiology.

Hopefully, the above-presented material has caused you to ask yourself the following questions: Do I want the responsibility of changing someone else's behavior? If so, am I willing to accept the charge of that responsibility through four years of scholastic study? Is this what I want? Will this profession be fulfilling and challenging enough to sustain a life's career? Am I willing to make the necessary commitment of time and effort to achieve the knowledge and competency necessary to fulfill the responsibilities of the profession's Code of Ethics? Am I also aware and willing to accept that this commitment is never-ending and will continue as long as I remain in the profession?

If, after reading through the credential, licensing, certification, and degree requirements, the courses and practicum indigenous to them, the Code of Ethics, and our own attempt at discussing personal traits and/or characteristics of the prospective professional, you still find yourself desirous of entering the professions of speech pathology and/or audiology, then we would like to welcome you to a most fulfilling and stimulating field of professional study and to a career in a very important area of health and education.

REFERENCES

ASHA, Volume 19, Number 1, January 1977, p. 41.

Emerick, Lon L. and Hatten, John T.: *Diagnosis and Evaluation in Speech Pathology*. Englewood Cliffs, Prentice-Hall, Inc., 1974.

CHAPTER 15

SUPERVISED PRACTICUM WITH EMPHASIS ON PUBLIC SCHOOL PRACTICUM

PAULINE STONE, M.A.

IN ORDER TO WORK as a Language, Speech, and Hearing Specialist in public schools, a specific credential is required. States differ somewhat in the credential's title and requirements. For example, in California, credentials are authorized by the California Commission on Teacher Preparation and Licensing. Currently, in California there are two kinds of credentials which enable one to serve as a Language, Speech, and Hearing Specialist in public schools. One is the Specialist in Special Education— Communications Handicapped. This credential requires a preliminary teaching document (credential) and a special education credential with advanced specialization in Communication Handicapped. This specialization is usually tracked into one of three areas—deaf education, language and speech, or deaf-blind.

The other credential, and the one we shall discuss in this chapter, is entitled The Clinical Rehabilitative Services Credential —Language, Speech, and Hearing. The minimum client contact clock hours of supervised clinical practice with minors, as well as the various competencies and training, are specified by law. Training institutions must submit to the Commission on Teacher Preparation and Licensing a detailed description of their program's conformance to state requirements and must receive that Commission's approval before they are authorized to grant this credential to students successfully completing their programs.

In California, the student who successfully completes an approved training institution's program qualifies for the basic credential listed above, and school districts may employ such, credentialed persons as itinerate Language, Speech, and Hearing Specialists. Such specialists identify, assess, and remediate pupils

305

with speech and language disorders in the public schools. They typically schedule these pupils for individual or small-group sessions of thirty to forty minutes and may see them once, twice, or more times per week, according to district policy or as staff time allows.

There is another public school setting in which the Language, Speech, and Hearing Specialist may work. This is the self-contained classroom for the severely language handicapped. These are pupils who have been identified as having normal intelligence, but whose receptive and/or expressive language is so disordered that they are unable to learn in a regular class-room. An older term for this condition is *childhood aphasia,* and that term is still frequently used. In any case, these pupils are differentiated from pupils whose language disorders are primarily due to hearing loss or mental retardation, since all these groups have different educational needs.

It has been found that these oral language handicapped children can best be served in a small, self-contained classroom where language remediation is intensive and all curriculum is modified and specially designed to meet the individual language deficit of each child. These programs are relatively new in public schools. In California it has been the Language, Speech, and Hearing Specialists who not only serve on the identification and assessment team in identifying these pupils' language problems, but also it is specialists with this training who are in charge of these classes. This has been appropriate, since a thorough under-standing of each child's individual language deficit is essential for intensive remediation. However, recent California regulations require that, in order for the Clinical Rehabilitative Services Credential to qualify persons to serve in this classroom setting, a special authorization is necessary. This special authorization requires that many specific additional competencies be demon-strated. Each training institution was asked to submit its method of insuring that their students meet these requirements. In our training institution we encourage all our credential candidates to earn the special authorization as well as the fundamental Clinical Rehabilitative Services Credential. This allows our graduates to be employed in either of the two public school settings.

Certain course work in educational curriculum and methods as well as the additional competencies and a specific requirement of a minimum of 100 supervised clock hours in a classroom for the severely language handicapped was therefore added. The competencies to be met in this added practicum are highly specific, and the student must not only clock the additional minimum 100 hours, but must demonstrate the ability to successfully conduct such a classroom. Also, it is specified by state regulation that the additional 100 hours for the specific authorization are indeed additional to the basic 300 hours minimum required for the Clinical Rehabilitative Services Credential in Language, Speech, and Hearing. Thus, the minimum supervised client contact hours with minors required for a California Clinical Rehabilitative Credential — Language, Speech, and Hearing with special class authorization is 400.

It is evident that public school practicum is a requirement specific to a state public school credential. In other words, for students not wishing to earn a public school credential, it is quite possible to earn a master's degree in Speech Pathology and to qualify to take examinations for the American Speech and Hearing Association Certificate of Clinical Competence in Speech Pathology and for state license as a Speech Pathologist. Successful passing of examinations and the completion of ASHA Clinical Fellowship year* and Required Professional Experience year* for state license would then qualify the speech pathologist to work in non-public school settings such as hospitals, rehabilitation centers, etc.

Since, however, in most parts of this country the largest number of speech pathologists are employed by public schools, most students prefer to qualify themselves so that they are eligible for all three documents. Indeed, the majority of training institutions have scheduled their programs of course work and clinical practice in such a way that successful graduates at the M.A. level can be trained and prepared to qualify for professional work in a variety of settings.

It must be kept in mind that, in order to meet client contact

---

* These require one year of employment under the supervision of persons holding these documents.

hours as required by the three basic documents, many more than the minimum hours are usually required. This is because, while the credential requires a minimum of 300 client contact hours plus the 100 hours for special endorsement, all with minors, the ASHA Certification of Clinical Competence and the State License require minimum hours with a variety of specific disorders, some of which must be with adult clients.

Many training institutions have found advantages to giving students a direct experience of exposure to the work of a speech pathologist before they get too deeply committed to the several years of detailed preparation. In our training institution we accomplish this by requiring each student with a speech pathology and audiology major to satisfactorily complete an assignment of a minimum of thirty-five client clock hours working as a task-trained student aide under the direct supervision of a Language, Speech, and Hearing Specialist in the public school. These hours do not count toward clinical hours required, but they are prerequisite to admittance to clinical practice and methods courses. This experience acquaints the student with clinical work in this field. It also acquaints him with the public school setting and working with children. It serves one more function. The current California credential requires that a certain knowledge of regulations, required record keeping, and other aspects of this profession's function in the public school setting be accomplished at the undergraduate level. We place this experience in the second semester of the student's junior year and attach to it certain competencies and assignments that guarantee the student's understandings of these matters according to the state's requirements for credential. We used the term *task-trained* in describing this early exposure the student is given in direct work with children who have speech and language disorders. Indeed, the student in his second semester in the program does not possess any of the professional expertise necessary to function as a speech and language clinician (or as a Language, Speech, and Hearing Specialist, as the speech pathologist is called in the public school setting). Thus, *task-trained* refers to a training technique which professional speech pathologists can utilize in enlisting the services of any untrained aide—

paid or volunteer — while maintaining complete professional direction of the client. It is a technique we consider quite important, one we include in the competencies which the graduate students must meet in their public school practicum.

In our training program, once the students have successfully completed this experience as well as all prescribed course work in their junior year, i.e. their first two semesters in the department, they are ready to enroll in the next sequence of course work and to enter the University Clinic for the first clinical methods and practicum work. They will have their first experience as clinicians. They will be carefully guided and supervised by a staff member who has the Certificate of Clinical Competency issued by the American Speech and Hearing Association as well as California State Licensure. They will have had the academic course work dealing with the disorders before they will be assessing and remediating these disorders, and they will take specific concurrent clinical methods course work given by the faculty member who supervises their clinical work.

Our clinical training and experience begins with a semester of assessing and remediating clients whose primary disorder is articulation and/or language of a functional nature. Great emphasis is placed on behavior management, assessment, and the writing and following of appropriate goals and objectives in a logical, sound, sequential order. As in all the clinical courses, the student is carefully observed, supervised, critiqued, and guided in connection with his work with clients. The student meets with the supervisor in regularly scheduled individual conferences and also attends the concomitant methods course in which principles and techniques are discussed. Students are instructed in the techniques of parent interviews, case summaries, and professional reporting, and they have actual, supervised experience in all these phases of clinical practice.

The next semester of clinical experience centers on in-depth diagnostic assessment and remediation, as well as more detailed case summaries of clients presenting severe and often complex speech and language disorders. Most of these clients are multihandicapped, and the understanding of interrelationships of several deficits is emphasized. Client and parent conferencing, as well as working with other professionals, is experienced in further depth.

Three more clinical courses follow: one devoted to clients whose primary disorder is stuttering; one devoted to clients with voice disorders; and one which deals with hearing testing and aural rehabilitation. In all clinical courses the students' clinical sessions are carefully supervised and critiqued. Individual instruction in the principles and techniques applicable to remediation is given immediately after the session and in individual conferences. In our training institution, in addition to the listed clinical courses, we require of persons who are preparing to qualify for the M.A. degree, ASHA certification, and state license specific hours of supervised practicum working with adult aphasics and with laryngectomized clients receiving therapy in esophageal speech.

In all these clinical courses the student participates in his own individual evaluation process both during and at the end of each semester. Gaining competence in the self-evaluation as part of the professional role is fostered throughout the training.

The careful logging of total client-contact clock hours according to type of problem is precisely recorded and initialed by the supervisor each semester. A separate individual log of clock hours in observation of ASHA certified clinicians working with clients is similarly recorded each semester. These records will be of extreme importance to the students later when they apply for credential, ASHA certificate of clinical competence, and state license.

We have given a brief overview of the supervised clinical training given our students primarily within the University clinic or in affiliated sites as required and sequenced in our training institution. These supervised clinical hours working with the various disorders are designed to help students meet requirements of the American Speech and Hearing Association and California State License as Speech Pathologist. We have come to feel it is important for students to have had all the required course work, as well as training and supervised clinical practice in assessing and remediating all types of speech and language disorders, *before* enrolling in public school practicum. What we have just outlined describes the clinical work prerequisites to public school practicum, which we shall now discuss.

Earlier in this chapter we mentioned recent credential regulations in California requiring each training institution to follow state guidelines and submit in detail to the State Board of Education the way in which competencies required are met. These same state regulations require the training institution to establish regular meetings with their Community Advisory Board. This board, made up of representatives of the various professional settings, gives ongoing input to us regarding all aspects of training provided. This has proved to be very valuable as we refine the goals, objectives, and competencies to be achieved by those students who complete our program.

An additional and very important source of input and guidance to us is the Master Clinical Group. These public school specialists meet with us both in scheduled meetings and informally throughout the year. They are the ones who work directly with our students in school practicum. They are paramount in advising us and submitting recommendations regarding the various competencies and procedures basic to the school practicum.

What is a Master Clinician? This term, as well as the role and responsibilities it entails, was chosen some years ago in California when the State Board of Education conducted an intensive, ongoing study on the subject of school practicum, with participants from public schools, training institutions, and student groups. The work of this group, which met in San Dimas, California, was invaluable in producing uniform guidelines for school practicum for the state of California. The guidelines defined Master Clinician as that public school Language, Speech, and Hearing Specialist who, in addition to accepting the defined responsibilities involved in "taking a student," also possessed ASHA Certificate of Clinical Competence in Speech Pathology, had a minimum of three years experience in a clinical itinerate school assignment, and had previous experience in the particular school district. The role and responsibilities of the training institutions and of the students were also set forth in the guidelines, and these guidelines were the product of concensus by all groups involved. Since the issuance of the "San Dimas Guidelines," the role of the Language, Speech, and Hearing Specialist in public schools has changed. The training institutions have refined student competencies to meet these changes, but always within the framework of close cooperation with the public school personnel, following the principles set forth in those original guidelines.

Because these San Dimas Guidelines preceded school practicum in self-contained classrooms for the severely language handicapped, and since such practicum hours do not apply to ASHA Certification and licensure, these criteria do not apply to Master Clinicians supervising students in that setting. However, this author feels much credit is due these Master Clinicians who guide students through the competencies needed to conduct programs in self-contained classrooms. The program is new and multifaceted. The Language, Speech, and Hearing Specailists who work with us in this connection have contributed immeasurably to working out this aspect of school practicum and continue to contribute to the facilitating of this experience. The added academic course work in curriculum and methods, which is a state requirement in addition to the minimum 100 practicum hours, appears adequate to give the students the necessary background for practicum experience in a self-contained classroom.

How do training institutions arrange and conduct school practicum courses? This varies somewhat from institution to institution, but in all cases the basic responsibility for this function lies with the training institution. In our opinion, wherever this responsibility has been met conscientiously, the school districts, the supervisors of public school programs, and the individual Master Clinicians have been magnanimous and enthusiastic in their cooperation.

At California State University, Sacramento, the Speech Pathology and Audiology Department feels its responsibility in this connection is to work very closely with the various school districts and Master Clinicians involved, to be responsible for all student assignments, to coordinate student supervision on a shared basis, and to be responsive to Master Clinicians' recommendations and implement them whenever possible. Thus, when and how the student schedules this experience is the result of this response and of the University and the public school personnel working together.

Based on public school recommendations, our students enroll in public school practicum *after* completing all clinical training and course work in the department. Thus, they come to this experience well qualified to work with all language, speech, and hearing problems. This allows them to concentrate on the many competencies germane to the public school setting and apply and refine their clinical skills within this new setting.

As we worked through the many competencies required of the student to qualify for assignment in self-contained classrooms for the severely language handicapped, the specialists recommended that this practicum needed to be scheduled on a concentrated, five-day-per-week basis in order to give daily continuity. The itinerate Master Clinicians concurred that such scheduling would lead to a more realistic experience in itinerate work as well. Thus, we evolved our final semester for graduate students applying for state credential as comprising a twelve-unit, full-time public school practicum. It currently entails six units for ten full-time weeks of itinerate practicum; three units earned in five full-time weeks of practicum in the self-contained classroom for the severely language handicapped, and three units of seminar—three hours weekly. Needless to say, the student is restricted from taking any other units of work—academic or clinical—during this semester. To achieve all competencies in this semester is indeed a full-time job.

What is meant by competencies in connection with public school practicum? These competencies as accepted by our state Commission of Teacher Preparation and Licensing refer to the objectives and experiences, along with their criteria and conditions, that make up the overall goal of competency in all aspects of conducting a language, speech, and hearing program in public schools. There are some thirty competencies (objectives) in the course for itinerate specialist setting and some sixteen for self-contained classroom setting. These objectives are further described in the course assignments, and the competencies they describe are demonstrated both as we observe the students actually conducting programs in the school setting and by the oral and written reporting the students bring to regular seminar meetings. The competencies the student is required to achieve resemble the duties described in a detailed job description for positions in both settings. Thus, the student who successfully achieves all of these competencies is prepared for a position as Language, Speech, and Hearing Specialist in both settings in which such specialists are employed in California Public Schools.

Some examples of the objectives leading to competencies will be discussed here. In the case of itinerate practicum they include such things as identifying pupils having communication handicaps by means of conducting screening programs and responding to teacher referrals, after preparing teachers for making such referrals. Contacting and interviewing parents and incorporating parent participation in remediation is an important competency. Conducting and reporting diagnostic assessments of identified pupils; selecting and reporting the goals, objectives, methods, and materials required for each pupil; establishing and scheduling a workable case load; and conducting the daily group and individual remediation sessions as scheduled are all vital competencies to be achieved. Such responsibilities as participating as a professional team member in placement staffings; the programming, task training, and supervision of communication aides; and maintaining all records required by state school law and district regulations are further examples.

Examples of specific competencies achieved in the orally handicapped classroom include such things as designing and implementing individual remediation educational plans in the various learning areas adapted to meet the language deficits of each individual student. Designing and conducting daily classroom schedules, including allocation of tasks performed by paraprofessionals, maintaining classroom management, and active participation in parent group and individual meetings are other important competencies.

What about supervision? How is this conducted and by whom? It is evident that, although the university has the ultimate responsibility, supervision is shared between the Master Clinician and the University Supervisor of School Practicum. The technique for this shared supervising responsibility used in our training institution is as follows. The Master Clinician is first, the daily, on-site supervisor who demonstrates while the student observes and soon thereafter is the observer and the guide of the student's performance, giving daily feedback to the student concerning his/her work. The University Supervisor makes a minimum of ten on-site observational visits to the students as they perform throughout the semester. The University Supervisor attempts to observe a minimum of three sessions of learning subject areas in the case of self-contained classroom practicum on each visit. Written feedback is furnished the student at the time of these visits, and conferencing with both Master Clinician and student is part of the process. In each of the two practicum settings during the semester, two three-way evaluation conferences are scheduled—once at the midpoint and once toward the end of both the itinerate and the self-contained classroom experience. The student, Master Clinician, and University Supervisor schedule meetings together for the purpose of these evaluations.

A few years ago, the Master Clinicians Group in our area recommended that the University adopt a uniform evaluation instrument for their use with our students, and we devoted some time to examining various forms that had been developed throughout the country. We finally accepted the Clinical Appraisal Form (The W-PCC) developed at the University of Wisconsin as our instrument of choice. We submitted it to the Master Clinicians Group for their experimental use, adapted it slightly, and received their approval for continued use. This has proved very useful for evaluating the student's proficiencies in the itinerate practicum. It covers all areas and skills involved and, on a ten-point scale, allows for appraising the student's independence of performance. Each student and Master Clinician is provided with a copy of this format at the beginning of the semester. They are asked to rate the performances independently so that the students rate themselves before coming to the evaluation meeting, which is conducted by the Master Clinician with the University Supervisor present. The Master Clinician interprets and explains his/her ratings and discusses with the student any discrepancies between the two ratings. (Students often tend to rate themselves somewhat lower than the Master Clinician.)

Both parties are asked to color code the midperiod and final ratings so that differences can be seen between these two ratings. This method has proved to be very helpful to students and extremely informative to the University Supervisor. Often the first evaluation meeting helps clarify not only those skills which will be emphasized over the second half of the assignment but also those experiences which must be furnished by the Master Clinician before the student completes all objectives.

In the case of the self-contained classroom experience, different skills and areas of expertise needed to be evaluated. We met with the Master Clinicians involved with that program, elicited their suggestions, and worked out a fairly brief evaluation form, which they accepted. Again, the same format of student self-rating and Master Clinician rating, as well as the midpoint and final three-way conferences with the University Supervisor, is utilized. Both these evaluation instruments are viewed as dynamic rather than static. Whenever changes, additions, or deletions are suggested, they are carefully considered and incorporated according to the desires of everyone concerned.

When the student first enters the practicum assignment, we find it helpful to promote immediate communication regarding the Master Clinician's expectations and philosophy. We request students to ask their Master Clinicians to list these factors in the order of the individual Master Clinician's feelings of priority. The students then record these and submit and discuss them in an early seminar meeting. This helps the student understand early in the experience what is expected in the particular situation, and the discussion helps him/her understand how these expectations differ slightly with each Master Clinician.

Whenever possible, we like to request students to list their own strengths and weaknesses as they perceive them and to discuss these about midpoint in the experience. Then, toward the end of each experience, we look at these together again and discuss any changes the students may feel have taken place. We find this can best be done in individual conference, but, in any case, the major purpose is to encourage students to evaluate their own competencies in a realistic and constructive way as they progress through experiences. Our objective is to promote objectivity and overcome any defensiveness regarding one's professional skills. Our hope is that, by reinforcing candid, objective self-appraisal and encouraging realistic goals for future growth, we are instrumental in fostering that quality as an important aspect of any professional role.

Another area in which we find scheduling individual conferences very useful is in the assignment of students' evaluations of their own audio tapes of group sessions. We schedule two such audio group session playbacks and self-critiques during the itinerate practicum and one during the self-contained classroom practicum. The students are given specific criteria by which to evaluate themselves—such things as numbers of pupil verbal responses versus clinician verbalizations; the appropriateness, accuracy, and specificity of clinician's verbal reinforcements, etc. In individual conferences with the University Supervisor the student is asked to replay and analyze the sessions. The focus on specific, preaudited and analyzed aspects gives structure to the conference, and the many other aspects that invariably come to both parties' attention prove useful as discussion points. The student hopefully will find this technique to be useful later.

In our experience we have found many advantages to the concept of a competency-based program—especially for professional work in a specific setting. By applying task analysis to these professional assignments, it is possible to list, teach, and allow the students gradually to demonstrate competencies in each aspect of the job. The skills required in school practicums are many and varied. The level of independent functioning required is high. However, by assigning these various skills as specific course objectives, naming the experiences in which they are to be met and the criteria and conditions under which they are demonstrated—and all of these are constantly reviewed and modified according to input from the public school personnel—we feel our students have the satisfaction of knowing they are well prepared.

Our seminar meetings serve many valuable functions. Aside from the clarification of objectives and the shared presentations of selected readings, many other aspects of sharing information are of value. Our students are assigned in different schools, different school districts, and certainly to different Master Clinicians. When each student presents methods and materials and procedures learned in his particular setting, all members of the group benefit. They learn new techniques and develop an appreciation for situations other than their own. This is especially valuable in learning differences of approach with students of different grade levels. There is much sharing, and an *esprit de corps* develops which we hope serves as a model for good staff relations in the professional experiences to come.

Our assignment involving students' attendance at professional meetings and workshops is also based on the "model for future behavior" concept. Since ongoing education is a vital part of the life of every professional person, we attempt to inculcate this notion by assigning these experiences during the practicum.

Each spring we invite a panel of Program Directors from the various districts in our area to address our students. Approximately twelve such persons attend and give individual descriptions of their programs and discuss their methods of interviewing for positions.

We introduce the students to the services of our University Placement Bureau and guide them in starting their professional placement files. We help them through the intricacies of applying for credential, American Speech and Hearing Association Certificate of Clinical Competence in Speech Pathology, and state license in Speech Pathology.

All the students' written assignments are carefully assembled in individual folders, which are returned at semester's end. These are planned in such a way as to serve as references concerning various procedures to be used in their professional positions later.

Thus, we conceive of our practicum semester in public schools as a period which helps students shift their self-images from that of university students to professional participants. We hope it serves as a bridge between these two important phases of professional life.

CHAPTER 16

THE END OF THE QUIET REVOLUTION: THE EDUCATION OF ALL HANDICAPPED CHILDREN ACT OF 1975*

ALAN ABESON AND JEFFREY ZETTEL

O<small>N THE OPENING DAY</small> of school in September 1978, a quiet revolution[1] will end. The end will not come silently, easily, or dispassionately. The officers and soldiers who led and fought the revolution will not fade away for they recognize that the passing of this revolution may merely be signalling the beginning of the next. Accompanying this end, however, will be celebration —celebration for children who are handicapped and who, since the beginning of public education in the United States, have been the victims of discrimination that often prevented them from receiving an education. On that day in 1978, it will be a violation of federal law for any public education agency to deny to a handicapped child in need of a special education an appropriate program. As stated by the National Advisory Committee on the Education of the Handicapped (1976), "In law and as national policy, education is today recognized as the handicapped person's right" (p. 143).

The beginning of the end of the final phase of the revolution to achieve public policy affirming the right to an education for every child with a handicap was on November 29, 1975, when President Gerald Ford signed into law Public Law (P.L.) 94-142, the Education for All Handicapped Children Act of 1975,

---

* Reprinted from *Exceptional Children*, October, 1977, by Alan Abeson and Jeffrey Zettel by permission of the Council for Exceptional Children. The Council for Exceptional Children retains literary property rights on copyrighted articles.

[1] In one of the early articles written about the litigation and education of the handicapped, the movement was titled "The Quiet Revolution" (Dimond, 1973).

which becomes fully effective in September 1978. This law, which concluded the policy revolution begun in 1970, was built heavily on the policy victories that were won since that time in the nation's courts and state legislatures. Additionally, the Act is based upon principles of sound educational practice that, although applicable to all children including the handicapped, were often pioneered and articulated by special educators.

Since the enactment of P.L. 94-142, it has been a central theme of discussion for virtually every element of the education community in the United States. The discussions have centered around strengths and perceived weaknesses of the Act and the implications for professionals and for parents. The settings of these discussions have extended from the Congress, the United States Office of Education, state legislatures, and state departments of education to local school boards and local education agencies.

Too frequently, however, the topic not discussed is implementation. It is implementation that begins for some children in October 1977 but that must be extended to all school age youngsters in September 1978. Too frequently as well, discussions of P.L. 94-142 have been based on misinformation or misinterpretation. Too often during these debates, the history is forgotten, administration reigns supreme, and the danger of this law becoming a comprehensive set of empty promises looms large. As will be discussed more fully later, the thrusts that lie ahead, while not revolutionary in the establishment of policy, may be in establishing appropriate practice.

In large measure, the burden for overseeing the effective implementation of this Act rests at least in part with special educators, many of whom are the veterans of the battles just concluded. Teachers, administrators, psychologists, therapists, and parents, for example, are all members of the implementation community. So too are all other members of the education community who may not be aware nor think of themselves as having responsibilities for children who have handicaps. One effect of the Act will be to bring about a closer alignment of all educators—a goal that is desirable so all children can receive an appropriate education. It is in the spirit of signalling the end of the quiet revolution, moving forward with implementation, and relating the recent history to the major policies contained in the Education for All Handicapped Children Act of 1975 that this article has been written.

PUBLIC POLICY AND THE EDUCATION OF CHILDREN

Educational public policy is established at the federal, state, intermediate, and local governmental levels by boards, legislatures, courts, and administrative bodies that often have responsibilities both within and outside educational settings. The purpose of these policies is to provide the basis for the total operation of the American education system. These policies, when totally considered, serve as the elasticity that permits variations between the federal, state, intermediate, and local education agencies yet maintains some commonality of purpose, procedure, and function.

P.L. 94-142, as a statute passed by the U.S. Congress, represents one expression of public policy regarding the education of children who have handicaps. Similar policy is represented by statutes that are passed by state legislatures. Other expressions of public policy can be found in rules and regulations, guidelines, and bylaws that are developed at both the state and federal levels to provide instruction and guidance to state and local education agencies, respectively, in their carrying out of each agency's statutes.

Occasionally, the intent, form, or substance of statutory or regulatory policies are challenged either substantively or for purposes of clarification. These issues are often dealt with in rulings by attorneys general who are most active at the state governmental level. A second and more well known setting for resolve is the nation's judicial system where case law is created. It was in a federal district court in Philadelphia in 1971 where the Pennsylvania Association for Retarded Children, now known as the Pennsylvania Association for Retarded Citizens, in a lawsuit against the Commonwealth of Pennsylvania, first raised the cornerstone of the quiet revolution—the right of every mentally retarded child of school age to receive a public education.

The significance of public policy in relation to the education of children requires emphasis. In reality, virtually every decision made in a public school setting is controlled by policy. For example, policy leads to definition of those children who are eligible to participate in programs; it defines the services to be provided; it leads to specification of the nature and quantity of personnel to be made available for the delivery of services to eligible children; and finally, it provides for the availability of resources such as dollars, space, and time to allow the above responsibilities to be implemented. Public policy also serves to provide for the stability, consistency, and continuity of program operations over time and throughout individual agencies. During the quiet revolution, the placement practices used in individual school buildings within local school districts were often described in court as arbitrary and capricious because their standards and procedures differed drastically from building to building. In part, such conditions occurred because little or no districtwide policies were available and in force to guide the behavior of the individual building teachers and administrators. Clearly, the presence of policy that is modern, written, and familiar to the entire educational community is in the best interests of all those employed or served by the public schools.

A RECENT HISTORY OF THE INADEQUACY OF EDUCATING CHILDREN WHO HAVE HANDICAPS

With minor exceptions, mankind's attitudes toward its handicapped population can be characterized by overwhelming prejudice. [The handicapped are systematically isolated from] the mainstream of society. From ancient to modern times, the physically, mentally or emotionally disabled have been alternatively viewed by the majority as dangers to be destroyed, as nuisances to be driven out, or as burdens to be confined. . . . (T)reatment resulting from a tradition of isolation has been invariably unequal and has operated to prejudice the interests of the handicapped as a minority group. (*Lori Case v. State of California*, 1973, p. 2a)

The manifestations of these attitudes occurred in schools in a variety of ways including the exclusion of children who have handicaps, incorrect or inappropriate classification, labeling or placement, and the provision of inappropriate education programs, as well as arbitrary and capricious educational decision making. While this listing is not exhaustive, it is lllustrative of the major practices in use prior to the initiation of the quiet revolution. To a large degree, the Congress designed P.L. 94-142 to respond at least in part to these illegal and inappropriate practices.

Exclusion, Postponement, and the Right to An Education

The Congress of the United States in the statement of findings and purposes that are a part of P.L. 94-142 (1975), indicated that "one million of the handicapped children in the United States are excluded entirely from the public school system and will not go through the educational process, with their peers" (Sec. 3, b, 4). Related is an analysis of 1970 census data done by the Children's Defense Fund (1974) who concluded that "out of school children share a common characteristic of differentness by virtue of race, income, physical, mental or emotional 'handicap' and age" (p. 4).

While this factual picture could lead to conclusions of condemnation against the educators who perpetuated this injustice, it must be acknowledged that in many jurisdictions, existing policy permitted—even sanctioned—the exclusion of children with handicaps from public school attendance. State compulsory school attendance statutes, for example, frequently permitted such steps when a local superintendent of schools, with or without notice to the state, determined (in an unspecified manner) that a child could not profit from an education or had learned all that he or she was capable of learning. If a child with a handicap was in need of transportation to get to a program or a program was needed but not readily available, then denial of service was considered in some jurisdictions to be legitimate.

Beginning in 1970 and continuing today, the legality of denying a public education to child with a handicap by exclusion, postponement, or by any other means has been successfully challenged in both state and federal judicial systems. The rationale for such litigation has been primarily derived from the equal protection clause of the Fourteenth Amendment of the United States Constitution, which guarantees equal protection of the law to all the people. In other words, where a state has undertaken to provide a benefit to the people, such as public education, these benefits must be provided to all of the people unless the state can demonstrate a compelling reason for doing otherwise. The language most often used to express this concept in education was the 1954 *Brown v. Board of Education* Supreme Court decision that proclaimed:

> In these days it is doubtful that any child may reasonably be expected to succeed in life if he is denied the opportunity for an education. Such as opportunity, where the state has undertaken to provide it, is a right which must be made available to all on equal terms. (74S. Ct. 686, 98L. Ed. 873)

Two of the most heralded and precedent-setting right to education lawsuits occurred in the early 1970s in Pennsylvania and the District of Columbia. It was in fact these cases that initiated the quiet revolution. In January 1971, the Pennsylvania Association for Retarded Children (PARC) brought a class action suit against the Commonwealth of Pennsylvania in Federal District Court for the alleged failure of the state to provide all of its school age children who were retarded with access to a free public education. The court supervised agreement which resolved that phase of the suit decreed the state could not apply any policy that would postpone, terminate, or deny children who were mentally retarded access to a publicly supported education. Further, it stated that all retarded children in the State of Pennsylvania between the ages of six and twenty-one were to be provided with a publicly supported education by September 1972 (*Pennsylvania Association for Retarded Children v. Commonwealth of Pennsylvania,* Consent Agreement, 1972).

Following the *PARC* decision, a second, similar federal decree was achieved in 1972. In *Mills v. Board of Education of the District of Columbia* (1972), the parents and guardians of seven District of Columbia children brought a class action suit on behalf of all out-of-school, handicapped children. The outcome of the *Mills* decision was a court order providing that all school age children, regardless of the severity of their handicap, were entitled to an appropriate free public education.

In both the *PARC* and *Mills* cases, allegations were made regarding the manner in which identification, evaluation and placement activities, and decisions were rendered regarding the education of children who have handicaps. Consequently, both the *PARC* consent agreement and the *Mills* decree required specific due process procedures to be established. Also litigated in these cases was the issue of where children with handicaps should be placed in relation to nonhandicapped children for receipt of their education. Both of these policy areas will be examined later in this article.

Following the precedents established by these two cases, the right to education principle became further solidified through the passage of a number of state statutes and regulations, thus adding to the impetus and policy breadth of the revolution. By 1972 it was reported that nearly 70 percent of the states had adopted mandatory legislation requiring the education of all children who have handicaps as defined in each state's policies (Abeson, 1972; p. 63). By 1975 all but two state legislatures had adopted some form of mandatory law calling for the education of at least the majority of its handicapped children (U.S. Congress, Senate, 1975). Today all but one state has enacted such legislation. Further, the Educational Amendments of 1974, P.L. 93-380, required that, in order for states to participate in the financial assistance available under the Act, they were to establish a goal of providing full educational opportunities to all children with handicaps.

Incorrect or Inappropriate Classification or Labeling

A major component of the quiet revolution, the labeling and classification dilemma also became the subject of litigation. It must be recognized, however, that Dunn in 1968 published a historic article that described the issue and brought it to the attention of the field. For purposes of litigation, however, substantial evidence was gathered which supported the claim that schools too often assigned labels, subjected children to individual psychological assessments, and altered their educational status without the appropriate supporting data and often without parental knowledge.

The classification of children with handicaps by categorical labels was shown to produce major problems (Abeson, Bolick, and Hass, 1975, p. 5). Among the adverse effects of inappropriate labeling are:
• Labeled children are often victimized by stigma associated

with the label. This may be manifested by isolation from usual school opportunities and taunting and rejection by both children and school personnel. In the latter instance, it may be overt or unconscious.

- Assigning labels to children often suggests to those working with them that the children's behavior should conform to stereotyped behavioral expectations associated with the labels. This often contributes to a self-fulfilling prophecy to conform with the stereotyped behavior associated with the label and ultimately does so. When a child is labeled and placement is made on the basis of that label, there is often no opportunity to escape from either the label or the placement.

- Children who are labeled and placed in educational programs on the basis of that label may often not need special education programs. This is obviously true for children who are incorrectly labeled, but it also applies to children with certain handicaps, often of a physical nature. The fact that a child is physically handicapped does not mean that a special education is required.

Other researchers questioned the alleged preponderance of minority group children found in special education classes. Studies conducted by the California State Department of Education, for example, discovered that while Spanish surnamed children comprised only 13 percent of their total school population, they accounted for more than 26 percent of the students in their classes for the educable mentally retarded (Weintraub, 1972, p. 4). Mercer (1970), examining the process of special educational placement in Riverside, California, found three times more Mexican Americans and two and a half times more black Americans in those programs than would be expected from their percentage in the general population.

In January 1970, *Diana v. State Board of Education* was filed in the District Court of Northern California. The suit, brought on behalf of nine Mexican American students ages eight through thirteen, alleged that the students had beeen improperly placed in classes for the mentally retarded on the basis of inaccurate tests. Coming from homes where Spanish was the predominant or only spoken language, the plaintiffs argued they had been placed in classes for the educable mentally retarded on the results of an IQ score obtained from either a Stanford-Binet or Wechsler intelligence test. When the nine were retested in Spanish, however, seven scored higher than the IQ cutoff for placement in classes for the educable mentally retarded.

On the basis of this data, the plaintiffs argued that the tests relied primarily on a verbal aptitude in English and ignored their learning abilities in Spanish and that the tests were standardized on white, native-born Americans and related in subject matter solely to the dominant white, middle-class culture (Ross, DeYoung, and Cohen, 1971, p. 7).

A similar landmark decision regarding the testing and classification of students was filed in late 1971 on behalf of six black elementary students attending the San Francisco Unified School District. The plaintiffs in *Larry P. v. Riles* (1972) alleged they had been inappropriately classified as educable mentally retarded on the basis of a testing procedure that failed to recognize their unfamiliarity with the white middle-class culture and that ignored learning experiences they might have had in their homes.

In resolving these suits, various agreements were established requiring the use of the following types of practices:

- Children were to be tested in their primary language. Interpreters were to be used when a bilingual examiner was not available.
- Mexican American, black American, and Chinese American children already in classes for the mentally retarded were to be retested and evaluated.
- The state was to undertake immediate efforts to develop and standardize an appropriate IQ test.

As with right to education, these cases and the growing literature led to the concept of nondiscriminatory evaluation. This concept was also added to state law in many states, particularly in the form of requiring school districts to consider multiple data and sources for consideration by teams of professionals prior to making classification and placement decisions. In addition, mandates appeared requiring that parents of children suspected of being handicapped be provided with notice and the opportunity to approve or reject evaluation of their child. These principles were also articulated in P.L. 93-380. Specifically required of the states was that they were to adopt procedures to insure that

testing materials and procedures used for classification and placement of handicapped children were to be selected and administered so as not to be racially or culturally discriminatory.

Provision of Inappropriate Education Programs

While the quiet revolution at times seemed to be focusing
on major rights issues, attention was also focused upon more than
simple access to the public schools. The evidence that emerged
in the process of documenting the effects of classification and
their resulting placements seemed to suggest that many assignments were made as a function of administrative convenience
rather than an awareness of the individual needs of children.
Consequently, the goal of access was modified and expanded
to include the concept of access to appropriate programs.

This concern was reflected in the judicial orders that emerged
from both the right to education and classification litigation.
Similarly, the emerging statutes qualifying the nature of the
education to be provided to children with handicaps was abun-
dant with the words "suitable" and "appropriate" and the phrases
"specialized instruction," "appropriate to the child's capacity,"
and "designed to develop the maximum potential of every handicapped person."

These qualifiers were further translated principally in state
statute and regulation into requirements for the development of
some type of individually designed and delivered program. A
notable example comes from Illinois, which adopted a regulation
(State of Illinois, 1974, p. 6) requiring that educational plans
be developed that include specific objectives to be attained by
each child.

Such directives were clearly related to the use of multiple
professionals in the evaluation process. Without such a procedure and goal, much of the valuable individual information
acquired about each child was lost and never considered in
relation to the unique needs of individual children. Further, it
became apparent as the revolution progressed that the spectre
of accountability was also going to be applied to the education
of handicapped children.

A major aspect of the suitability or appropriateness measure
of a handicapped child's program, which was further addressed

in the litigation, was where children with handicaps should be placed for educational purposes in relation to their nonhandicapped contemporaries. The conceptual basis for considering this issue came largely from Reynolds (1962) who portrayed the existence of a continuum of placements for children with handicaps ranging from the least restrictive, i.e. being placed in a regular classroom setting with considerable opportunity to interact with nonhandicapped children, to the most restrictive setting, i.e. a special school or a nonpublic school placement, such as a private institution, that would provide little if any contact with nonhandicapped individuals. It is well recognized, however, that the implementation of this continuum was never intended nor should be interpreted to mean that all handicapped children should be placed in regular classrooms. What is intended is that individual children, possessing individual needs, will be placed on the basis of these needs in the least restrictive setting.

As of 1974 only six states were required by law and eleven by regulation to adhere to the principle of least restrictive placement (Bolick, 1974). However, by October 1975, the National Education Association reported that twenty-two or half of their state affiliates reported having statutory or regulatory language requiring that children with handicaps were to be placed in regular classes at least some of the time.

Perhaps one of the clearest and most comprehensive statutory definitions of least restrictive environment as it applies to children with handicaps can be found in the following 1972 Tennessee state statute, which was essentially echoed in P.L. 94-142:

> To the maximum extent practicable, handicapped children shall be educated along with children who do not have handicaps and shall attend regular classes. . . . Special classes, separate schooling or other removal of handicapped children from the regular educational environment, shall occur only when, and to the extent that the nature or severity of the handicap is such that education in regular classes, even with the use of supplementary aids and services, cannot be accomplished satisfactorily (Tennessee Code Annotated, Sec. 23, Chap. 839, 1972).

Inappropriate Educational Decision Making

As has been briefly mentioned, the quiet revolution also was concerned with the manner in which education decisions were being made about children with handicaps in the public schools. The litigation revealed students were frequently misplaced and misclassified not only as a result of inappropriate evaluation instruments and procedures, but also because of inappropriate decision making occurring often in local schools. Traditionally, school administrators were able to decide whether a child with behavioral problems, a child restricted to a wheelchair, or a child who was especially difficult to teach could come to school and, if so, where that child was to be placed. Often these decisions were made unilaterally, without data, without legal basis, and without parental involvement or notice.

When these practices were brought to the attention of the court in Pennsylvania, the court ruled first, prior to consideration of the right to education question, that such practices must cease. To remedy the situation, the court first established the right of all children who are mentally retarded to the protection of procedural due process (in accordance with the 5th and 14th Amendments). This was contained in the 1972 *PARC* consent agreement which decreed that no child who is mentally retarded or thought to be mentally retarded can be assigned initially or reassigned to either a regular or special educational status or excluded from a public education without a prior recorded hearing before a special hearing officer.

Second, the court approved as part of the agreement a twenty-three-step process to meet the due process mandate. Some of the requirements included:

- Providing written notice to parents or guardians of the proposed action.
- Provision in that notice of the specific reasons for the proposed action and the legal authority upon which such actions can occur.
- Provision of information about the parents' or guardians' right to contest the proposed action at a full hearing before the state secretary of education or his designate.
- Provision of information about the purpose and procedures of the hearing, including parents' or guardians' right to counsel, cross examination, presentation of independent evidence, and a written transcript of the hearing.

- Indication that the burden of proof regarding the placement recommendation lies with the school district.
- Right to obtain an independent evaluation of the child, at public expense if necessary (Weintraub and Abeson, 1974, p. 528).

A similar set of requirements was contained in the *Mills* order. In addition to the litigation, due process requirements also became assimilated into state and federal public policy. A 1974 survey conducted by the State-Federal Information Clearinghouse for Exceptional Children revealed that twelve states were required by statute to provide such procedures and thirteen were similarly required by regulation (Bolick, 1974). The constitutional responsibility of each state to provide its residents with due process procedures was further affirmed by P.L. 93-380, in which Congress ordered assurances from the states that proper due process procedural safeguards would be adhered to in all decisions regarding the identification, evaluation, and placement of children with handicaps.

THE EDUCATION FOR ALL HANDICAPPED CHILDREN ACT OF 1975, P.L. 94-142

By April 1975, when the Subcommittee on Select Education and the Subcommittee on the Handicapped began a series of legislative hearings in both Washington, D.C., and elsewhere across the country to extend and amend the Education of the Handicapped Amendments of 1974 (Public Law 93-380), the quiet revolution to win for every handicapped child an appropriate education had reached something of a crescendo. Over half of the states by that time had either been through or were in the process of going through litigation. Increasingly, parents of handicapped children and professionals were forming statewide coalitions to file and maintain lawsuits, to advance state and local policy, and to implement newly won policy directives.

Despite this momentum, however, these congressional committees learned:

- Over 1.75 million children with handicaps in the United States were being excluded entirely from receiving a public education solely on the basis of their handicap.

- Over half of the estimated 8 million handicapped children in this country were not receiving the appropriate educational services they needed and/or were entitled to.
- Many other children with handicaps were still being placed in inappropriate educational settings because their handicaps were undetected or because of a violation of their individual rights.

It became clear that, although federal and state judicial and legislative actions had brought about progress since 1970 toward providing appropriate educational services for children with handicaps, there remained a need for greater effort. The Congress decided this effort should take the form of legislation that would later be referred to as the "Bill of Rights for Handicapped Children." Approved by an 83 to 10 vote of the Senate on June 18, 1975, and a subsequent 375 to 44 affirmation of the House of Representatives on July 29, President Gerald Ford signed this historic bill on November 29, 1975. P.L. 94-142, the Education for All Handicapped Children Act, had become law, and thus the quiet revolution to achieve the basic educational right of all children with handicaps began to conclude.

Descriptions of this comprehensive law can take many forms. One approach is to consider it from the basic perspective of the history of circumstances described earlier. While this treatment may be effective in the context of this article, it must be clear at the outset that the Act also included extensive management and finance aspects that will be addressed here in only a limited fashion.

Right to Education

The intent of the Congress to insure that this Act will provide for the education of all children with handicaps is reflected in its statement of purpose:

> It is the purpose of this Act to assure that all handicapped children have available to them, within the time periods specified, a free appropriate public education which emphasizes special education and related services designed to meet their unique needs. (Public Law 94-142, 1975, Sec. 3, c)

The time periods specified are that beginning in September 1978 all handicapped children aged three to eighteen shall receive a free appropriate public education. The law further orders that by September 1, 1980, such an education shall be available to all handicapped children aged three to twenty-one (except in instances where the education of the three to five and eighteen to twenty-one age ranges would be inconsistent with state law or practice or any court decree).

Inclusion of this right in P.L. 94-142 makes abundantly clear that it is, as the National Advisory Committee stated, national policy. After the dates specified occur, there simply will not be any grounds for depriving a handicapped child who, because of that handicap, possesses unique learning needs requiring special education. No longer will it be permissible for school persons to exclude or postpone the education of such handicapped children on the grounds that they cannot learn, their handicap is too severe, programs do not exist, or for any other reason.

This civil rights principle can also be clearly expressed in educational terms that were in fact recognized by the Nation's courts and legislators during the period prior to P.L. 94-142. First, it means that no child is uneducable or stated in another way, all children can learn. Closely related to this statement is that education cannot be defined traditionally but rather must be considered as a continuous process by which individuals learn to cope and function within their environment, regardless of their environment. It was this definition that emerged from *PARC*, specifically from testimony presented by Dr. Ignacy Goldberg. Translated to curriculum planning, it means that to provide mobility training for blind children, adaptive physical education for physically handicapped children, or instruction in bodily functioning for some mentally retarded children is no different than teaching driver education, physical education, or health and hygiene to nonhandicapped children.

The right to education also means that children with handicaps are eligible for participation in all programs and activities provided or sponsored by the schools as all other children are eligible. The presence of a handicap no longer can mean automatic ineligibility for music, athletics, cheerleading, or other extracurricular activities. By the same standard, children with handicaps may no longer be considered for noninclusion in all course offerings, most notably vocational education. Similarly, if the presence of a handicap and related special learning needs leads to the provision of special education, it does not render the child ineligible for other special services.

Included within the mandate of the right to education for all children with handicaps are those children who possess learning needs that require program delivery in public or private day or residential settings that operate on a tuition basis. In the past, some or all of these costs were, because of various state statutory approaches, partially or totally a family responsibility. Trudeau and Nye (1973) indicated that policies for partial or total tuition reimbursement for children in this situation existed in forty states. Frequently, families were simply unable to bear these costs.

To rectify this situation, the Congress in P.L. 94-142 requires that every handicapped child be provided a free appropriate public education at no additional expense to that child's parents or guardians. Furthermore, when it is determined that the child's appropriate education should be provided in a tuition based school program, the cost for receiving such services, including tuition, transportation, and room and board where necessary, must also not be automatically assigned to the parents. Misunderstanding of this mandate must not occur. Placement in tuition based programs at public cost does not occur as a function of parental option. It is only when it has been determined either through public school recommendation or as the result of due process that a tuition based setting is required to provide a child with an appropriate education that the parents shall not be required to bear the cost.

Right to Nondiscriminatory Evaluation

P.L. 94-142 addresses the well-documented and researched problem of discriminatory evaluation activities as did its predecessor, P.L. 93-380. The policy directives contained in P.L. 94-142 are straightforward and clear in their intent to remedy these negative practices that have had impact not only upon minority group children but also upon some handicapped children.

Essentially, the Act requires that the testing and evaluation materials and procedures that are used for the purposes of evaluation of children with handicaps will be selected and administered so as not to be culturally discriminatory. Further, the law specifies that such materials and procedures are to be provided in the child's native language or mode of communication. Finally, no single procedure or test can be the sole criterion for determining the appropriate educational program for a child. This last requirement clearly builds upon the maxim that standardized procedures including tests are not in themselves evil but, rather, become so if inappropriately used.

After passage of P.L. 93-380, the Bureau of Education for the Handicapped (1974) issued "advisories," which are interpretative statements designed to assist in understanding and implementing the Act. Throughout the area of nondiscriminatory evaluation in which, although a well-recognized problem, few easy solutions exist, the advisories recommended to education agencies:

> A procedure also should be included in terms of a move toward the development of diagnostic-prescriptive techniques to be utilized when for reasons of language differences of deficiencies, non-adaptive behavior, or extreme cultural differences a child cannot be evaluated by the instrumentation of tests. Such procedures should insure that no assessment will be attempted when a child is unable to respond to the tasks or behavior required by a test because of linguistic or cultural differences unless culturally and linguistically appropriate measures are administered by qualified persons. In those cases in which appropriate measures and/or qualified persons are not available, diagnostic-prescriptive educational programs should be used until the child has acquired sufficient familiarity with the language and culture of the school for more formal assessment. These evaluation procedures should also assure that persons interpreting assessment information and making educational decisions are qualified to administer the various measures and qualified to take cultural differences into account in interpreting the meaning of multiple sets of data from both the home and the school. (P. 29)

Inclusion in P.L. 94-142 of the "mode of communication" requirement is an important addition to the nondiscriminatory policy requirements. While the culturally and lingustically discriminating attributes have been recognized, no attention has been directed to the problems of children with handicaps who, because of the manifestation of their handicap, are in evaluation activities, particularly testing, and thus are also victims of discrimination. At issue is the point that the activities evaluate what is intended to be evaluated. Illustrative of these problems are children who possess motor difficulties in their arms and hands and are unable to adequately carry out various performance tasks that are common to many types of standardized tests not intended to measure motor functioning. Because a youngster can not stack or rearrange the blocks does not mean the child does not know what is required or how to do it. Consequently, evaluators under P.L. 94-142 must consider the child's mode of communication.

Right to An Appropriate Education

To deal with the past problems of inappropriate educational services being provided to children who have handicaps, the Congress included as a major component of P.L. 94-142 a requirement that each child be provided with a written individualized education program known as the IEP. The IEP required for each handicapped child is the central building block to understanding and effectively complying with the Act. In order to understand the IEP, it is important that the following progression, as described by Weintraub (1977), be understood.

> Handicapped children are defined by the Act as children who are "mentally retarded, hard of hearing, deaf, orthopedically impaired, other health impaired, speech impaired, visually handicapped, seriously emotionally disturbed, or children with specific learning disabilities who by reason thereof require special education and related services" [Sec. 4 (a)(1)]. This definition establishes a two-pronged criteria for determining child eligibility under the Act. The first criteria is whether the child has one or more of the disabilities listed in the definition. The second is whether the child requires special education and related services. Not all children who have a disability require special education, many can and should attend school without any program modification.
>
> Special education is defined in P.L. 94-142 as ". . . specially designed instruction, at no cost to parents or guardians, to meet the unique needs of a handicapped child, including classroom instruction, instruction in physical education, home instruction, and instruction in hospitals and institutions" [Sec. 4 (16)].

The key phrases in the above definition of special education that impinge upon the IEP are "specially designed instruction . . . to meet the unique needs of a handicapped child." Again, by definition, then, special education is special and only involves that instruction which is specially designed and directed to meet the unique needs of a handicapped child. Thus, for many children special education will not be the totality of their education. Furthermore, this definition clearly implies that special proceeds from the basic goals and expected outcomes of general education. Thus, for example, intervention with a child does not occur because he is mentally retarded but because he has a unique educational need that requires specially designed instruction.

Equally important to understand is the concept of related services which are defined in the Act as: "transportation, and such developmental, corrective, and other supportive services (including speech pathology and audiology, psychological services, physical and occupational therapy, recreation, and medical and counseling services, except that such medical services shall be for diagnostic and evaluation purposes only) as may be required to assist a handicapped child to benefit from special education, and includes the early identification and assessment of handicapping conditions in children" [Sec. 4(a) (17)].

The key phrase here is "as required to assist the handicapped child to benefit from special education." This leads to a clear progression: a child is handicapped because he or she requires special education and related services; special education is the specially designed instruction to meet the child's unique needs; and related services are those additional services necessary in order for the child to benefit from special educational instruction.

The term "individualized educational program" itself conveys important concepts that need to be specified. First, "individualized" means that the IEP must be addressed to the educational needs of a single child rather than a class or group of children. Second, "education" means that the IEP is limited to those elements of the child's education that are more specifically special education and related services as defined by the Act. Third, "program" means that the IEP is a statement of what will actually be provided to the child, as distinct from a plan which provides guidelines from which a program must subsequently be developed. (P. 27)

Finally, a specific definition describing the components of an IEP is included within the Act:

A written statement for each handicapped child developed in any meeting by a representative of the local educational agency or an intermediate educational unit who shall be qualified to provide, or supervise the provision of, specially designed instruction to meet the unique needs of handicapped children, the teacher, the parents or guardians of such child, and, whenever appropriate, such child, which statement shall include (A) a statement of the present levels of educational performance of such child, (B) a statement of annual goals, including short-term instructional objectives, (C) a statement of the specific educational services to be provided to such child, and the extent to which such child will be able to participate in regular educational programs, (D) the projected date for initiation and anticipated duration of such services, and appropriate objective criteria and evaluation procedures and schedules for determining, on at least an annual basis, whether instructional objectives are being achieved. (Public Law 94-142, 1975, Sec. 4, a, 19)

The IEP requirement of P.L. 94-142 has received much attention in terms of its potential for achieving the goal of the Act—appropriately educating every handicapped child. Inclusion of the teacher, for example, in the development of the IEP is designed to insure that realistic teacher concerns and needs will be considered as part of the IEP development process. It is appropriate that teachers have a major voice in program planning since they have major responsibility for program provision. Similarly, parent participation is designed to insure that the extensive amounts of information parents possess about their children and their judgments as to the education program needed will be considered. Establishment of jointly determined expectations for individual children that are known to all involved and interested in the form of goals and objectives is highly regarded because with such specificity comes a clear basis for assessing a child's progress so that inappropriate programs do not continue and necessary program changes will occur.

The importance of the total IEP provision cannot be overemphasized, nor can it be misinterpreted. It should be emphasized that the IEP is an agreement between all parties and that, while it is not a contract, it is clearly a statement setting forth what will be provided to the child. School systems, however, are legally responsible for provision of the "specific educational services" set forth in the IEP. Related then is that the IEP is a management device, not an instructional plan specifying daily teacher-child activities. Finally, the IEP serves to define for each handicapped child in need of special education services what is appropriate for that child.

No discussion of appropriate education for children who have handicaps is complete without consideration of the least restrictive placement principle. As noted, the statutory definition of the IEP itself requires consideration of "the extent to which such child will be able to participate in regular educational programs." In addition, each state must establish

> procedures to insure that, to the maximum extent appropriate, handicapped children, including children in public and private institutions or other care facilities, are educated with children who are not handicapped and that special classes, separate schooling, or the removal of handicapped children from the regular education environment occurs only when the nature or severity of the handicap is such that education in regular classes with the use of supplementary aids and services cannot be achieved satisfactorily. (Public Law 94-142, 1975, Sec. 612, 5, B)

Implementation of this portion of the appropriate requirement has been interpreted by some to mean that all handicapped children, regardless of the severity of their handicap, are to be placed in regular classroom programs. To others, these mandates mean that all handicapped children are to be placed in self-contained special education classes. Neither of these is correct. What must exist is school system capacity to provide programs that are appropriate for individual children in the least restrictive alternative setting. Conceptualizing the requirement in this manner indicates that, although placement decisions must be indicated in the child's IEP, it must follow determination of the child's learning needs and programs. Available placement options no longer can dictate placement decisions for individual children.

Right to Due Process of Law

During the revolution, the manner in which identification, evaluation, and placement decisions were made about children with handicaps were reviewed virtually throughout the country. To solve these problems, the courts ordered adherence to procedural due process. It was this solution that was also selected by the Congress as part of P.L. 94-142. Like most of the elements of this law, due process has received wide attention and discussion. It is included in the Act to insure that all of the rights created by the Act are in fact made available to children who have handicaps, their families, and the public schools. One way of expressing this intent is to suggest that the presence of due process is designed to allow for equal consideration of the interests of all who are involved in the education of a handicapped child—the child, the family, the schools.

The specific elements of due process the Congress included in the law are as follows:

1. Written notification before evaluation. In addition, the right to an interpreter/translator if the family's native language is not English (unless it is clearly not feasible to do so).
2. Written notification when initiating or refusing to initiate a change in educational placement.
3. Opportunity to present complaints regarding the identification, evaluation, placement, or the provision of a free appropriate education.
4. Opportunity to obtain an independent educational evaluation of the child.
5. Access to all relevant records.
6. Opportunity for an impartial due process hearing including the right to:
   a. Receive timely and specific notice of the hearing.
   b. Be accompanied and advised by counsel and by individuals with special knowledge or training with respect to the problems of children with handicaps.
   c. Confront, cross examine, and compel the attendance of witnesses.
   d. Present evidence:
      (1) Written or electronic verbatim record of the hearing.
      (2) Written findings of fact and decisions.
7. The right to appeal the findings and decisions of the hearing.

The procedural safeguards section of the Act includes two provisions that are of special importance. First is the requirement that for children whose parents or guardian "are unknown, unavailable or the child is a ward of the state" and who are being considered for service under this Act, procedures must be established to assign an individual "who shall not be an employee of the State educational agency, local educational agency, or intermediate educational unit involved in the education or care of the child to act as a surrogate for the parents or guardian" (Public Law 94-142, 1975, Sec. 615, 6, 1, B). Without this requirement children without parents or guardians would essentially be deprived of access to their rights of due process.

Until P.L. 94-142 was enacted, the circumstances under which due process could be invoked were limited to identification, evaluation, and placement. Under this Act, however, the Congress has extended the due process opportunity by providing "an opportunity to present complaints with respect to any matter relating to the identification, evaluation, or educational placement of the child, or the provision of a free appropriate public education to such child" (Sec. 615, b, 1, E). What is intended is to provide, as indicated earlier, a mechanism for review and rectification of inappropriate practice.

Many school systems operating under well-established and understood due process systems have found that it can provide an effective means of guiding communications with the families of children with handicaps. It sets out a series of procedures for communication that allow all interested parties to be informed as to the educational status of a handicapped child. In the vast majority of situations, the communication is what has been missing and is what is sought. When, however, there is disagreement as to the status or what is in the appropriate interest of the child, the more extensive procedures can be used. School personnel as well as parents can use these procedures to insure that what is required—the appropriate education of the child—is achieved.

THE FUTURE

Throughout this article, reference has been made to the end of the quiet revolution. Beginning in 1970 and continuing until the opening of school in September 1978, the quiet revolution effectively established in policy the educational rights of all handicapped children. With the conclusion of this revolution or at least one aspect of it, the efforts of all educators and particularly those in special education who have long worked to establish these rights must shift to achieve implementation of

these rights. P.L. 94-142 is the national policy—it is specific as
to what is to occur and it appropriates some funds to assist state,
intermediate, and local education agencies in carrying out their
state mandated responsibilities of providing for the education of
all the children residing within each state. Clearly that mandate
now applies equally to children who have handicaps.

Reference to individual state responsibilities for the education
of its resident children is appropriate. For too long in many
states, their own mandatory requirements for educating children
with handicaps were insufficiently implemented. In part, P.L.
94-142 can provide the leverage for the states to carry out their
own mandates and provide for the education of all handicapped
children. P.L. 94-142 in fact is designed to effectively join local,
state, and federal resources to achieve the full service goal.

Of crucial importance in undertaking the implementation task
is for all elements of the education community to correctly understand the Act and the reasons for its creation. Misinterpretation
and misinformation are critical dangers. Citizen voters, legislators, school board members, administrators, teachers, support
personnel, and parents of children with handicaps must be aware
of what the law does say, not what someone thinks it says. What
will happen inside the schoolhouse door will largely depend upon
members of this population who have had little or no exposure
or knowledge about children with handicaps. Above all, the
entire school community needs to become sensitized to the fact
that handicapped children are first children, and second children
with special learning needs. In large measure, the responsibility
for conveying correct information rests with those who know—
special educators.

The difficulties of implementation for even those children
who are well recognized as having handicaps and possessing
unique learning needs is only a portion of the future. Special
attention must be directed to insure that an unknown number
of such children in special circumstances also receive the benefits
of the Act. Included are American Indian handicapped children
who are located on or near Indian reservations across the country
as well as in usual educational communities; abused and neglected children who because of their mistreatment become
handicapped children possessing unique learning needs requiring

special education; and a long neglected population of handicapped children that are in the nation's foster care and juvenile corrections programs. Not to be forgotten as well are children with handicaps who, although identified, are inappropriately served in institutions and those who reside in the acutely educationally difficult inner city or sparsely populated areas.

When all is said and done and historians examine the quiet revolution, they may well determine that, while P.L. 94-142 is the premier educational policy attainment for the handicapped, the most notable overall policy for this group is Section 504 of the Vocational Rehabilitation Act of 1973 (Public Law 93-112). This small section of law prescribes that:

> no otherwise qualified handicapped individual in the United States . . . which solely by reason of handicap be excluded in the participation in, be denied the benefit of, or be subjected to discrimination under any program or activity receiving Federal financial assistance.

While this law requires that virtually the total society must provide handicapped persons with equal rights, it is of special importance in the implementation of P.L. 94-142. The regulations that accompany Section 504 contain a portion devoted totally to preschool, elementary, secondary, and postsecondary education. These regulations, which to a large degree conform to many of the P.L. 94-142 requirements, will enhance the implementation process because virtually every education agency receives federal financial assistance. To be in violation of P.L. 94-142, in most situations, also will mean a violation of Section 504, which in its finality can mean the withholding of all federal funds. This is particularly true in relation to the basic educational rights of children who have handicaps. Section 504 in concert with P.L. 94-142 will be the substance of implementation. How well that effort occurs will determine if there will be need for another revolution, and if so, the magnitude of its volume.

REFERENCES

Abeson, A.: Movement and momentum: Government and the education of handicapped children. *Exceptional Children*, 39:63-66, 1972.

Abeson, A.; Bolick, N., and Hass, J.: *A Primer on Due Process: Education Decision for Handicapped Children*. Reston, Va., The Council for Exceptional Children, 1975.

Bolick, N. (Ed.): *Digest of State and Federal Laws: Education of Handi-capped Children* (3rd ed.). Reston, Va., The Council for Exceptional Children, 1974.

Brown v. Board of Education. 1954, 347 U.S. 483, 74 S.Ct. 686, 98L.Ed. 873.

Bureau of Education for the Handicapped, U.S. Department of Health, Education, and Welfare, Office of Education. *State Plan Amendment for Fiscal Year 1975 Under Part B, Education of the Handicapped Act, as Amended by Section 614 of P.L. 93-380: Basic Content Areas Required by the Act and Suggested Guidelines and Principles for Inclusion Under Each Area.* Washington, D.C., Author, 1974 (draft).

Children's Defense Fund: *Children Out of School in America.* Cambridge, Mass., Author, 1974.

Dimond, P.: The constitutional right to education: The quiet revolution. *The Hastings Law Journal,* 24:1087-1127, 1973.

Diana v. State Board of Education. Civil Action No. C-70 37 R.F.P. (N.D. Cal., Jan. 7, 1970 and June 18, 1973).

Dunn, L. M.: Special education for the mildly retarded—Is much of it justifiable? *Exceptional Children,* 35:5-22, 1968.

Larry P. v. Riles. Civil Action No. 6-71-2270 343F. Supp. 1036 (N.D. Cal., 1972).

Lori Case v. State of California. Civil No. 13127, Court of Appeals, Fourth Dist. Calif., filed Dec. 14, 1973.

Mercer, J.: The ecology of mental retardation. In *The Proceedings of the First Annual Spring Conference on the Institute for the Study of Mental Retardation.* Ann Arbor, Michigan, 1970.

Mills v. Board of Education of the District of Columbia. 348F. Supp. 866 (D.D.C., 1972).

National Advisory Committee on the Education of the Handicapped. *The Unfinished Revolution:*

APPENDIX A

LIBRARY RESOURCE MATERIALS
Compiled by Eileen Heaser

SPEECH PATHOLOGY AND AUDIOLOGY:
SELECTED RESOURCES

Monographs concerned with the field of Speech Pathology and Audiology are classified in several areas of the library depending upon the specific approach emphasized. Below are classification numbers and the subjects covered in each.

HV 2353-2719	Deaf-means of communication Sign language
LB 1139	Speech development
LB 3454	Speech therapy
LC 4001-4028	Language, reading, and learning disability
P 135-136	Sign language; Children's language
P 215-222	Phonology and phonetic theory
QC 221-246	Physics-Acoustics
QP 306	Neural and acoustic mechanisms of speech
QP 460-471	Hearing physiology
RC 423-429	Speech disorders
RD 523-525	Cleft lip and palate
RF 25-51	Diseases—ENT (Ear, Nose, and Throat)

RF   Audiology-Hearing
121-516

RJ   Pediatric disorders with related speech problems
496

The card catalog can be searched for specific subjects relating to the above areas. Cards for *authors* and/or *titles* of individual works are also included in the card catalog.

REFERENCE RESOURCES

ref   *DSH Abstracts.* Washington, D.C.: Deafness, Speech, and
LCZ   Hearing Publications.
5721   Library has: v. 1-date; 1960-date.
D12   Provides summaries of literature published in all major
Index   language pertinent to deafness, speech, and hearing.
Area   Published quarterly.

ref   *Education Index.* New York: Wilson.
L   Library has: v. 1-date; 1929-date.
3   A monthly publication containing principally refer-
E42   ences to literature of the U.S.A.
Index
Area

Science   Excerpta Medica. *Oto-Rhino, Laryngology.*
Index   Amsterdam.
Area   Library has: v. 20-date; 1975-date.
               A monthly index with abstracts to the international
               journal literature concerned with oto-rhino laryn-
               gology.

ref   *LLBA; Language and Language Behavior Abstracts.*
PZ   New York: Appleton-Century-Crofts.
7003   Library has: v. 1-date; 1967-date.
L12   A quarterly index which provides access (comprehen-
Index   sive, current, and selective) to the world's literature
Area   pertinent to language and language behavior. Screens
               over 1,000 journals, progress and technical reports,
               occasional papers, monographs, and conference
               proceedings.

ref   *Psychological Abstracts.* Lancaster, Pa.: American Psy-
BF   chological Association.
1   Library has: v. 1-date; 1927-date.
P65   A monthly index to psychological and related literature
Area   (journals, reports, monographs, and documents) of
Index   the world.

PERIODICALS SPECIFIC TO SPEECH
PATHOLOGY AND AUDIOLOGY

Journal Title	Department
ASHA—Journal of the American Speech and Hearing Association	Education
Academic Therapy	Education
Journal of the Academy of Rehabilitation Audiology	Science
Journal of the Acoustical Society of America	Science
Acta Oto-laryngologica and Supplementum	Science 1
Acta Symbolica	Science
Acustica (German)	Science 1
American Annals of the Deaf	Education
Annals of Otology, Rhinology and Laryngology	Science
Archives of Otolaryngology	Science
Audiology (formerly *International Audiology*)	Science
Audiology and Hearing Education	Science
Brain	Science
Brain and Language	Science
British Journal of Disorders of Communication	Education
California Journal of Communications Disorders (ceased)	Science
Cleft Palate Journal	Science
Cortex	Science
Folia Phoniatrica	Science
Hearing and Speech News	Education
Journal of Auditory Research	Science
Journal of Communication	Education
Journal of Communication Disorders	Science
Journal of Fluency Disorders	Science
Journal of Speech and Hearing Disorders	Education
Journal of Speech and Hearing Research	Education
Journal of Verbal Learning and Verbal Behaviors	Education
Language and Speech	Science
Language, Speech, and Hearing Services in School	Science
Laryngoscope	Science
Merrill-Palmer Quarterly	Education
The Pointer	Education
Quarterly Journal of Speech Education	Education
Speech Monographs	Education
Speech Pathology Therapy (ceased)	Education
Speech Teacher	Education
Teacher of the Deaf	Education
Volta Review	Education
Word—Journal of the International Linguistics Association	Humanities

SPEECH AND LANGUAGE MATERIALS FROM
THE POINTER
Carolyn Dobbs

Students and professionals in the area of Speech Pathology need to be aware that pertinent materials concerning speech and language development appear in numerous professional journals in addition to those published by the American Speech and Hearing Association. In some issues of *Exceptional Children* (a publication of the Council for Exceptional Children) there are more articles related to speech and language than any other aspects of special education. A professional journal which includes speech and language related articles is *The Pointer*. It was developed by Carolyn Dobbs, a teacher of mentally retarded children in California. She has received numerous citations from state, national, and international groups for her pioneering work in special education.

The following articles are reprinted with permission of the editor of *The Pointer,* which is in its twenty-second year of publication.

1. LEARNING TO LISTEN

In the actual development of spoken language, there is a comparatively long time lag between learning to listen and learning to talk. Ordinarily, the infant learns to listen in close mother-proximity, in "homey" or familiar situations that are repeated frequently. When the infant fails to receive this kind of stimulation early, the environmental situation is changed by the time he is ready. He is more mobile, and his mother's voice is heard from a greater distance and probably not as often. He attends to other stimuli instead. Therefore, it is important to keep in mind the child's auditory-spatial world. Clinical tests have demonstrated that beyond 5 or 6 feet very young children do not attend auditorially. With the child who is not a good listener, admonishing or telling him to pay attention is rarely enough. Instead, if you want to capture his attention, stop what you are doing, and talk directly to him while he is not occupied or on the run. For some children "putting it" into their ear may be more successful.

Many of our listeners respond to all sensory stimuli—smell, sound, vision, touch. In other words, they are too attentive, but they are not selective. Try it yourself. Consciously alert yourself to what you see, hear, feel, and touch simultaneously. These children must be taught what we take for granted. Therefore, reduce stimuli, except for what you want him to learn.

Further processing time is different for many of these children. A failure to respond may be due to a delay between the actual request and the time the child can actually respond. Parents may demand a particular response and, if the child does not respond immediately, another request is made. This adds to the child's confusion.

If he responds, but the response is not appropriate, it may be that the child received only part of the message—either the beginning or the end. Perhaps he was so absorbed in processing the first part that he lost subsequent information. Recognition of his failure to respond satisfactorily may cause the child to withdraw, to precipitate a frustration tantrum, or to make him feel inadequate as a person. So learn to wait a reasonable length of time after giving a command.

Often when we give a command or message, we have no notion of how much the child has understood. He may have confused the meaning of words so the message made little sense to him. For example, the story is told of a child who, while crossing the street, was cautioned by his teacher to watch out for the wet tar. When he suddenly jumped back on the curb, he was questioned about this behavior, and repeated that he was warned to watch out for the white car.

Therefore, when you give a command, observe the child's response closely—is it inappropriate, does he appear confused, is the execution vague? If the performance is unsatisfactory, stop the child and ask (with a smile) "What did I tell you to do?" His answer may give you the information you need to know about the failure to perform properly, as well as to help him organize his thoughts and prepare for action.

The following recommendations are designed to help the child to listen, to retain, and to recall auditory information.

Listening to Interesting Sounds

1. Blow a whistle.
2. Present a recording of thunder. Fill the bladder of a basketball or beach ball with pebbles and inflate. Shake it to get the proper rumble.
3. Use one half of a rubber ball and beat out a rhythm in a box of dirt.
4. Use an assortment of chimes. Tap with a stick on pipes, glass, clay pot, etc.
5. Crackle cellophane.

Sound Discrimination

1. Match animal sounds with pictures and objects.
2. Match familiar sounds (clock, bell, washer, etc.) with pictures and objects.
3. Play games like "Simon Says" where the child must imitate your speech sounds, volume changes, rhythm alterations, etc.
4. Have the child identify without visual clues the voices of members of the family or friends.
5. Teach the child to distinguish which of two sounds is the louder. Use any instrument and have him raise his hand or clap for the louder.
6. Select simple pairs of common words where only a single sound element differs. Prepare a list (coat, boat, king, ring, hat, hot, tea, key) and randomly scatter within the list a few pairs that are alike. The child is to indicate which is the same or different. Graduate to words that require discrimination, e.g. pig, big, chip, ship, beats, beads, deer, door.

Auditory Memory

1. Non-verbal Response
   a. Place three or four simple, familiar picture cards propped up on a tabletop or in the chalkboard tray. Seat yourself and the child about 4 feet away. Ask the child to get up

and bring you a particular picture. When he can select each one correctly, substitute new pictures. Gradually, add more pictures to the group.

b. Increase the distance between the child and the pictures to 8 feet. Repeat the above process.

c. Increase the number of pictures you request at one time by starting with two.

d. Next, remove the visual clues and have him remember the command auditorally. Seat him about 8 feet from the cards and facing away from them. Repeat steps (a) and (c).

e. Place the cards in an adjacent room and repeat steps (a) and (c).

f. Increase the complexity further.

  1. Make a sequence command, e.g. "Get the car and put it under the table."

  2. Increase the time between your command and his execution of the task, e.g. "Jump, then get the car and put it on the chair."

2. Word and Number Sequencing

a. Have the child repeat unrelated words.

b. Have him repeat digits and/or letters after you. In order not to expect too much of him, norms (according to Robbins) are provided for auditory span.

Age 3	3 digits
4	4 digits
7	5 digits
10	6 digits

Increase the length of time between naming the digits as he demonstrates his competence. Repetition of digits backwards is a more difficult task and is the final step.

3. You read or tell a short, simple story containing two or more elements in a sequence, e.g. mother makes breakfast. John sets the table. Then he eats eggs.

a. Ask the child to retell the story. We are not interested in the refinements of sentence structure, but rather in the details presented in the same sequential order.

b. Ask the child, "What did I say first—last?" Vary the story.

4. Play "Going to California" (and I shall take ——). Start with two players and two items and increase the complexity as he becomes competent in handling each.

5. Sound Sequencing

a. Tell the child to say some nonsense syllables, such as *an* or *at* just after you have pronounced another sound, e.g., You say *ppp*, the child says *at*. You ask what the word is that you have both made (*pat*). Then go on to use other combinations, *mat, cat,* etc.

    b. Select one syllable words (eyes, shoe, nose, etc.). Prolong the first sound, pause, then complete the rest of the word. Ask the child to point to, pantomime, or say the word that was just spoken. As the child becomes proficient, increase the length of the pause.

6. Carrying messages and accepting phone calls (These should be prearranged). If the child exhibits difficulty in holding a sequence or two, try either

    a. separating the two events emphatically by pausing between the instructions, or

    b. asking him to repeat the message to you before carrying it to another.

7. Recommended music
"Bozo At The Circus"
"The Little Engine That Could"
"I Think I Can"
"Put Your Finger In the Air," Columbia Records J-4-187
Babbling Record, "Bye Bye Baby Talk," Pacific Record Company, Children's Music Center, 2858 W. Pico Blvd., Los Angeles, Calif.
"Babes in Toyland," Little Golden Records

8. Recommended Stories
Dr. Seuss Stories
"Read to Me Storybook" (Child Study Association of America)
"Rhymes for Children" (Expression Co., Magnolia, Mass.)
"Jack In The Box" (Expression Co., Magnolia, Mass.)
"The Three Bears"
"The Three Little Kittens"
"The Three Pigs"
"Busy Timmy"
"Monkey See—Monkey Do"
"Mother Goose"

(Sylvia B. Kottler, Learning to Listen. *The Pointer*, Vol. 14, No. 2, Winter, 1969, pp. 15-18.)

2. IMPLICATIONS OF LEARNING DISABILITY

In 1966, the United States Department of Health, Education, and Welfare began a series of research studies known as the National Research Committee Reports concerning special education. Three summaries, Task Force I, Task Force II and Task Force III, concerned learning disabilities.

Task Force I (1966) defined children with learning disabilities as being those who had average or higher IQ who were not succeeding in school in some area and whose "brains were not functioning properly." The definition selected tended to be universal, and the emphasis was on early identification.

Task Force II (1969) decided that there should be a definition set for learning disabled children because they differed so much from school to school and from state to state. It was then decided that teachers must ask themselves what each individual child is like in their area and get the definition from that.

The most recent explanation of learning disabilities comes from the findings of Task Force III (1969) and was passed in the Senate so that it would be possible for Learning Disability programs to have their own fundings. It was worded as follows:

> Children with special learning disabilities exhibit a disorder in one or more of the basic psychological processes involved in understanding or in using the spoken or written languages. These may be manifested in disorders of listening, thinking, talking, reading, writing, spelling, or arithmetic.
>
> They include conditions which have been referred to as perceptual handicaps, brain injury, minimal brain dysfunction, dyslexia, developmental aphasia, etc.
>
> They do not include learning problems which are due primarily to visual, hearing, or motor handicaps, to mental retardation, emotional disturbance, or to environmental disadvantage. (Task Force III, 1969, P. 148)

Children with special learning disabilities are those who are meeting failure in the schools. They are not being taught by the techniques and methods which have been common in many classrooms over the past several years (Task Force III, 1969, pp. 1-5).

According to the literature, the types of problems children with learning disabilities have could be grouped into four categories:

1. Perceptual-motor problems: poor balance and posture, inadequate body image concept, poor perceptual-motor match or visual motor difficulties, unstable oscular control and faulty form perception.

2. Language problems: reception, integration, and expressions of aural-oral language, including poor memory, evidence of poor grammar and closure difficulties.
3. Remedial academics: higher level language difficulties in reading, spelling, writing and arithmetic.
4. Behavioral management difficulties: the Strauss syndrome child, aggressive and passive behavior and general lack of response to classroom control. (Task Force III, 1969)

Children with learning disabilities come to the attention of the schools for a number of reasons. Sam Clements listed more than 100 specific behaviors under sixteen general categories from recent publications alone. James and Joan McCarthy list the ten most frequently noticed characteristics of a learning disabled child as follows:

1. Hyperactivity
2. Perceptual-motor impairment
3. General orientation defects
4. Emotional lability
5. Disorders of attention (e.g. short attention span, distractibility)
6. Impulsivity
7. Disorders of memory and thinking
8. Specific learning disabilities in reading, arithmetic, writing and spelling
9. Disorders of speech and hearing
10. Equivocal neurological signs and electroencephalographic irregularities. (McCarthy & McCarthy, 1968, P. 8)

It is important to note that all children do not have all ten signs and some who are normal may show some of them.

The primary difficulty in the public schools is that the learning disabled child is often incorrectly labeled as mentally retarded, which is seldom the case. This results in placement in classes that are not designed to rehabilitate those with specific learning disabilities.

It is hoped that the results of Task Force III will enable the school personnel to become more aware of the individual needs of children and will give them the opportunity to become well acquainted with new teaching methods specifically designed to meet those needs.

Bibliography

Chalfant, James and Schefflen, Margaret. Central Processing Dysfunctions in Children. Task Force III. Washington, D.C.: U.S. Department of Health, Education, and Welfare, 1969.

Clements, Sam D. Minimal Brain Dysfunction in Children: Terminology and Identification. Task Force I. Washington, D.C.: U.S. Department of Health, Education, and Welfare, 1966.

McCarthy, James and McCarthy, Joan. Learning Disabilities. Boston: Allyn and Bacon, Inc., 1969.

Magary, J. F., Ph.D. Preface Sequential Perceptual-Motor Exercises. Duboff School Program, Level I. Boston: New York Teaching Resources Corporation, 1967.

U.S. Department of Health, Education, and Welfare: Public Health Service. Minimal Brain Dysfunction in Children. Task Force II. Washington, D.C.: Department of Health, Education, and Welfare, 1969.

(Susan Lockhart, Implications of Learning Disability. *The Pointer,* Vol. 16, No. 2, Winter, 1971, Pp. 150-151)

3. SPEECH DEVELOPMENT FOR THE TMR CHILD

The speech characteristics which typify trainable mentally retarded children extend from inability to utter an intelligible word to ability to speak with a limited vocabulary of phrases and short sentences. Concomitant with this delayed or limited speech are a number of more specific qualitative speech defects, such as problems in articulation, voice and rhythm. The primary focus here is on the young trainable child, with a quantitative approach to speech therapy and training.

As a general rule, there has been, and for the most part there still is, much neglect in speech therapy and training programs for the trainable. However, with the accumulation of research data and promising habilitation programs, we are experiencing a change in the attitudes of speech clinicians and educators toward speech communication therapy and training for such children.

On the basis of research and program development, the following factors are presented as being important, if not essential, to an effective plan for adequate speech communication improvement:

1. The initiation of early therapy and training (2-4 years).
2. A program of parental guidance and assistance.
3. A coordinated working relationship between the speech clinician and the classroom teacher.
4. A structured classroom program in speech communication training which fits the needs and developmental level of each child.

The Initiation of Early Therapy and Training

Early speech therapy and training are dependent on early presentation of the child to the clinicians and educators. In the majority of the cases, the moderately and severely retarded children will have other symptoms concomitant with the delayed or limited speech. These other symptoms aid in the diagnosis of moderate or severe mental retardation.

Early therapy and training will give each child a much needed head start in acquiring verbal skills. Once the child begins to learn to speak, he tends to show growth in social skills, IQ scores, the ability to comprehend directions, and the ability to relate better to his environment.

A Program of Parental Guidance and Assistance

The two following studies suggest that parents have difficulties adjusting emotionally to the problems of having a delayed-speech child. In neither of these studies was it stipulated that a mental handicap was the cause of the delayed speech. However, we can generalize from these accumulated facts that the majority of cases of delayed speech are the result of mental retardation.

In the first study, half of the twenty mothers who participated in the study showed evidence of anxiety, and six mothers spoke of guilt feelings. Another six mothers stated that the handicap made them feel inadequate. In summing up his results, the author states:

> There may be a complex of interrelationships among the goodness and quietness described by most of the mothers: The possible excessive closeness of the mother-child tie, the anxiety and guilt expressed by the mothers, and the children's language development beyond that attributable to the basic etiology of the problem.

The second investigation showed that parents of delayed-speech children are frequently unrealistic in their expectations. It appears clinically to be a tendency on the part of some parents to attempt to push the seriously retarded child beyond his capabilities. In other cases there is the tendency to overprotect and understimulate.

It takes much longer for the TMR child to move from one level of speech development to the next, and unless the parents understand their child's development patterns, they may become discouraged from lack of adequate feedback. They may react either by giving up altogether or by moving to a higher level of stimulation, which may make it impossible for the retarded child to respond.

It is important, then, from an emotional point of view, that the parents have some kind of guidance available to help them overcome some of their feelings of guilt, frustration, and anxiety.

Another important function of the parent guidance program should be to provide the parents with actual information about their child's speech development. In the case of the parent with a prelinguistic TMR child, it would be wise to discuss Goda's five "prelinguistic speech levels." These levels are:

1. Syllabic chain utterances without auditory awareness
2. Auditory awareness of self-produced sounds with frequent repetition of favored sounds
3. Auditory awareness of the sounds of others
4. Imitations of the sounds of others
5. The acquisition of one or several meaningful words

The therapeutical importance of these prelinguistic levels becomes apparent with Goda's suggestion for the therapy of the prelingual retardates.

First, he states that if the child makes no observable vocalizations in four to eight months of "intensive" language therapy, the prognosis might be considered poor. Second, if the child makes "kinesthetic pleasure sounds" only, the clinician should attempt to involve the child into hearing the sounds that he makes. Third, if the child is at the "lalling" stage of development, someone (teacher, clinician, or parent) needs to repeat the sounds of the child, pausing to allow the child time to repeat.

Finally, when the child reaches the state of repeating his own utterances, the attempt should be to assist him to derive "linguistic meaning" from the imitative speech. For example, the clinician, teacher, or parent might use any one of the child's cherished possessions, showing or giving it to the child as his utterance is repeated.

If the child repeats this same utterance again, an effort should be made to present the same possession to the child. It is hoped that linguistic meaning may be derived from associating the possession with the utterance.

If parents of a TMR child were to receive information about normal speech acquisition and were assisted in relating that information to their own child's speech development pattern, then they would be in a better position to make a realistic adjustment to their child's speech acquisition progress. Also, with this information and assistance, the parents would be in a better position to help with the training of their child.

Coordination Between the Speech Clinician and the Classroom Teacher

Even if there were enough speech clinicians available to meet the needs of the TMR children, the school districts would not, by any stretch of the imagination, be willing to hire an adequate number. Therefore, teachers of such pupils must be prepared to do most of the training of speech communication in the classrooms.

This does not mean that the teacher is qualified to remediate specific speech defects. However, with guidance from qualified speech clinicians, the teacher can adequately carry on a program of speech development in the classroom situation.

The effectiveness of a program such as this is suggested in the results of an interim report by Doug Guess et al. In this project, they used two sub-professional personnel in a classroom setting. With very little training, the two "language developmentalists" were able to carry on a very adequate program of language development.

Structured Classroom Program

In order to provide an effective speech training program for the TMR, we must first have some knowledge of their intellectual characteristics. Ruth Arnold offers nine mental characteristics which may be considered unique to the mentally retarded:

1. The mentally handicapped show a tendency to stereotyped answers by repeating the same responses to different queries.
2. They lack powers of self-criticism.
3. They have limited power for the association of ideas.
4. They have a comparatively short auditory span.
5. They are inclined to be easily distracted.
6. They usually fail to detect absurdities in commonplace situations.
7. They tend to have greater ability in dealing with the concrete idea rather than with the abstract.
8. They have limited powers of reasoning, visualization, and similar mental traits.
9. In numerous instances, their diadochokinetic rate is slow, one of the signs of poor neuromuscular coordination.

The author goes on to stress a number of procedures of speech and language training which take into account the above characteristics:

Constant, but meaningful repetition; short periods of therapy; reliance upon concrete examples and simple motor skills; a frame of reference closely allied with the child's experiences; opportunities for frequent relaxation; complete acceptance and understanding of the child's limitations; constant observances of the child's physical well-being; and finally, the wise, but generous use of approval and praise of the child's every attempt in the rehabilitation of his speech.

Lillywhite and Bradley stress the importance of simplifying instruction and conversing "with the retarded at his current level of language function;" ". . . often the retardate individual is confused by too much verbal instruction and too little opportunity to practice skills himself."

Expectations which are within the capacities of the child and rewards for achieving the expected goals will do much to enhance a willingness to try new and more complex tasks.

In summary, four factors have been presented as essential to an effective plan for adequate speech communication development. I am optimistic about the future of speech communication therapy and classroom training for the TMR. (Larry Sumner, Speech Development for the TMR Child. *The Pointer*, Vol. 15, No. 3, Spring, 1971, pp. 55-57)

4. WHY HAVE LANGUAGE TRAINING FOR
TRAINABLE CHILDREN?

Because of Craig

Today, Craig said "Hi." He did it on his own with no prompting, even seeking out the person. For one whole year we have been working and hoping with Craig, and today we made it. He likes people; he will talk to us. We have found one of the many keys he needs to start the long hard road to normality, a road that probably is much too long and too hard for Craig. But we are going to try.

A high "EEEEEE" and machine-gun "uh, uh, uh" were the extent of Craig's vocabulary a year ago, although, once, under extreme stress, he had uttered a few words and the sentence, "I am Craig."

While he accepted people, he really concentrated on things, especially rocks. We had to use a language board with reading to help him talk. Though he has perfect hearing, he still does not learn well by listening and must be taught visually or with tactile stimuli.

He is slowly learning to ask for his needs and wants. His voice is getting louder and his speech clearer. He needs a special reading program which will teach him language concepts at the same time. But so far we have not found one already developed. The school says he is trainable yet if we must have labels, a more appropriate one might be aphasia.

Because of Clarence

Clarence played on the slide yesterday and on the climbing bars. He did it all by himself with no prompting and in spite of the fact that there were many other children on the equipment. One may ask him, "What's that?" and he will tell about thirty items. He can match printed words and take your hand to go with him to the speech room.

A year ago, Clarence screamed and ran from any human contact. He shook violently if one tried to hold him. Even lying on a shag rug frightened him terribly. None of his sounds resembled a word, and he did not cry or laugh. Now he cries and laughs, not always in response to external stimuli, but

enough so that we know he likes our world and maybe, with a little more help, he will decide to stay in it.

It has not been easy, working with Clarence. Progress seems terribly slow. He still covers his ears with his hands because sound interferes with his very own private world. When he is given a command he does not like, he closes his eyes. A repetition of the command brings his hands to his ears. A forceful, loud, much closer repetition brings the legs into a fetal position. It was not until we withheld food that he decided to operate in our world.

The words Clarence does say now are clear, although they need to be louder.

Holding him took a solid week of just sitting and stroking him while he screamed, went rigid, and even shook. Now he gestures and pulls a person to hold him.

In spite of the frustrations, we see a bright glimmer here and there. It is enough to make us determined to keep trying, even though normality seems out of reach. The school and some medical reports say Clarence is trainable, but perhaps another label, autism, should be considered.

Because of Anabel

Anabel has a small hearing and vision loss, a cleft palate, a harelip, five siblings and no father, as well as numerous other problems of lesser magnitude. Her speech is slightly blurred by the cleft but quite intelligible, and her sentences are complete, though simple. She seems to understand most directions and requests, but does not differentiate between paired opposites.

In addition, she is not able to manipulate concepts in new situations. She is quite sweet and seems to need much physical affection, but is easily distracted from the task at hand. She writes her own name and spells the letters in it. She seems much more like a deprived child than a TMR child. We hope by language training to make her eligible for an educable mentally retarded, if not a multihandicapped, class.

Because of Crystal

Crystal is a Down's syndrome child. Her parents are very sensible and encourage her to be as normal as possible. She talks in complete sentences, draws well, and is advancing rapidly in the Distar Language Program.

Many Down's syndrome children seem excessively shy, hide their faces, and refuse to talk to new people. Crystal is no exception. She is also bright enough to say, "Mommy doesn't want me to," when she does not want to do a task. She has much potential in a trainable program, even perhaps, in an educable class.

Because of Harry

Harry said, "Throw da ball," for the first time last week. He does not drool anymore, and his fat, thick tongue stays inside his closed mouth. He is asking for his needs almost daily now, compared to last year when he giggled, drooled, and said, "guh." He no longer hits, pinches, or kicks other children when they have something he wants, and he obeys commands.

Behavior modification, with the rewards of food and a special place to play when he has earned points, has made the difference. A technique used with cerebral palsied children, called "icing and brushing," stopped the drooling, although a toothpaste called Sensodyne® has been successful with other trainable children.

There Are Others

Bright little Carla, whose mother was a drug addict; Belle, who had meningitis at two years old and now has severe motor problems including disarthria; Freddie, who converses beautifully in social situations but is terribly hyperactive even with heavy medication; and Luigi, who just barely moves anytime, despite all our techniques, devices, and blandishments.

These are all designated as trainable children. They all desperately need language training to allow them to pursue even part of the "life, liberty, and happiness," the rest of us take for granted. (Kathy Thornton, Why Have Language Training for Trainable Children? *The Pointer,* Vol. 16, No. 3, Spring, 1972, pp. 219-220)

5.   A READING CLUB SERVES AS A REINFORCER

A reading club is an excellent means of developing and demonstrating appropriate behavior models for handicapped children. Their peers can provide positive social reinforcement when the children achieve some approximation of the model. In many instances, the peers serve as teacher surrogates. By replacing the teacher in this capacity, they free her to work on other activities and needs. And a club, as a social vehicle, can command the children's loyalty and performance because they like the identification of "belonging."

The Club ILOR

Club ILOR (I Love Reading) was developed with a group of children who attended a reading resource room. They required special help in developing both reading skills and an appreciation for the reading process as a vital tool for learning and success. The key character in the club was The Book Worm, who served as the club president and issued a Club ILOR membership card as illustrated in Figure A-1.

As indicated on the membership card, the name of The Book Worm was ILOR. Since young children like to have secrets, the meaning of ILOR was to be kept a secret from students not attending the special resource room (Club ILOR). While some students made every effort to keep the secret, after a few years it was common knowledge to the general school population.

CLUB ILOR

Membership Card — 1975-76

I, _____

       first name   last name

promise to be an active member of the club. I will try to read as many books and magazines as time will allow. Our club members learn to read in order to know, to do interesting projects, to travel, and for fun.

Recommended by: Approved:

Mrs. Patricia E. Lazar   ILOR
                                   The Book Worm

Figure A-1.

One minor problem was that children not requiring special help would want to join. When they were denied the opportunity, they often reacted with frustration and anger. To prevent such behavior from developing, visitors' periods were established. A child was allowed on a regular basis to invite a friend not normally assigned for remedial help. Regular class teachers supported this move because they found this made an excellent reward for good work with their own students. Before a child was permitted to accept an invitation, he had to meet certain class requirements regarding his own work.

ILOR also had a bulletin board with a picture of himself, and envelopes where children placed and received their contracts. This allowed the teacher to deliver notes to the children about their progress and club members to exchange secret messages. During conferences parents reported their children displaying a strong positive attitude toward Club ILOR because it afforded positive status.

In summary, a club, if properly organized, can serve as an excellent vehicle for the special class teacher or resource specialist to make use of the principles of applied behavior analysis. Especially useful will be the opportunity of using appropriate peer models and positive social reinforcement. It also will allow the teacher time and energy for other activities. (Alfred L. Lazar and Patricia E. Lazar, A Reading Club Serves as a Reinforcer. *The Pointer*, Vol. 20, No. 3, Spring, 1976, pp. 48-49)

6.   LET'S DO DRAMA!

Drama can have a significant part in the growth of the child with learning disorders. It exercises essential skills in an enjoyable way. The children participate enthusiastically, and they learn effectively, if the conditions are right.

But their very enthusiasm can lead to problems. Disorganization and poor control of impulses cause overstimulation, confusion, and failure unless the drama experience is tailored to their needs. It must be carefully planned for order, concentration, and success.

Books on creative dramatics or on drama for the regular school classroom may not offer much immediate help to teachers of LD children. The suggested activities offer too many choices for the children, too few controls, and goals which are not sufficiently concrete.

Instructions for drama activities in the LD classroom need to be given in detail: each step must be planned and must have a clear beginning and ending. The space must be limited and its use organized. The children's choices must be simplified and enumerated. A firm structure ensures both order and success.

Getting Ready

Certain simple preparations make this easier than it sounds.
1. Plan the space exactly. Show the children—and mark with tape or chalk—exactly where they are to stand or sit for any activity. If they will be moving from one place to another, mark the pathway of the movement and insist that it be used.
2. Set up signals for beginning and ending an activity. The teacher can simply say "start" and "stop." A gong, a drum, or a light are also effective. Practice the signal with the children and then use it consistently.
3. At first, when the students are asked to contribute sounds, movements, or ideas, they should choose from a limited number of possibilities. A list of choices can be written on the board for readers, but pictures or real objects are often better and more fun. If the choices are clear and concrete, no one will be at a loss for an appropriate response. There will be less tendency to silliness.
4. Let the children first watch a demonstration of what they are expected to do. The more exact and exaggerated the demonstration, the clearer it will be in their minds and, therefore, the more clearly they will do it.

What kinds of drama work best? It is wise to begin very simply. Try stories which incorporate sound effects, hand movements, or elementary pantomime by the children. Try paper puppets to illustrate a simple rhyme or tale. Acting out whole scenes or stories should come later. Role-playing or improvisation should only be started after a lot of work together. Performing for an audience should never be undertaken without careful consideration of the pros and cons. Some groups of LD children may benefit greatly from success in performing, while others may suffer too much from the inevitable pressures.

Stories and Sound Effects

Here is a simple beginning activity which works well. The concept can be adapted for various age groups and various subjects. Use any story which involves sounds the children can imitate, or make up a story, like the following, to fit the needs of the group.

> One day I was out walking. I saw an old empty house. I wondered if it were haunted. I walked up the steps (1). I rang the doorbell (2) and then I knocked on the door (3). No one answered so I opened the creaky door (4) and went in.
>
> The house was very quiet. All I could hear was a fly buzzing in the hall (5) and the wind blowing outside (6).
>
> I tiptoed though the big empty rooms. Everything was absolutely silent (7). Then suddenly I thought I heard a whistling sound (8) . . . then a bump (9) . . . and a groan (10).
>
> I was so scared that I ran out of the house and home as fast as I could go. Was it all in my imagination? Well, maybe it was.

First tell the story with no sound effects. Then give the children numbers from 1 to 10. Tell the story again slowly, stopping for each child to contribute his/her sound in the correct place. (On #7—silence—everyone must help)

After the group has worked this out so that it goes smoothly, repeat the story with the numbers backwards, #10 making the first sound, #9 next, and so forth. The result is usually funny.

Pantomime

Large, simple pantomime is valuable for children who are developing further in motor control. Make a poster with pictures of objects which are easy to pantomime. The pictures can be selected at random or with relation to the curriculum. Some easy categories for pantomime are: objects that belong in the kitchen or in the yard; things that are used in the morning or the afternoon; articles that begin with a given letter of the alphabet; things used in sports.

First, have the group look at each picture and name the object. Next demonstrate the game: pantomime one of the pictures without naming it and let them identify which picture you are pantomiming. It is important to make this demonstration-pantomime as large and as precise as possible. For example, if the pictures are of food and you demonstrate eating soup, be sure to pick up an imaginary spoon and to take each spoonful clearly and carefully. A teacher needn't be an artist in mime to demonstrate pantomime; it is only necessary to think of each move, step by step, and to exaggerate it. The children will quickly identify the action. They will also imitate the exaggeration when they do the action.

The children then take turns pantomiming and identifying the pictures. Remind the group that their objective is to *show* what they have in mind. They are not trying to trick anyone or to keep him guessing. The more quickly the audience knows what is being pantomimed, the more successful the actor has been. Insist on silence during each turn; no one is to say the word until the pantomime is finished.

Speech Without Words

Youngsters with greater self-control will be ready for more spontaneous activity. The work still needs careful organization to minimize self-consciousness and distractions. Since the perceptual problems of many LD children cause them to misread the behavior of others, a good plan might begin with the concept of speech without words. The objective is to increase awareness of how we communicate through "body language."

Make a list of some common nonverbal signals, such as yes (nod the head), no (shake the head), stop (hand up, palm out, like a policeman), and shhh (finger to lips). Use one or two of these as a demonstration: make the signal and let the class identify its meaning. Then write the list on the board. Write only the words and let the children take turns demonstrating a signal to match each word.

Let volunteers in pairs choose a signal and invent a short pantomimed scene using it. No talking is allowed in the scene, only gestures. Perhaps one person enacts a librarian checking out books, while the second enacts a noisy patron. This could lead to the use of the shhh signal.

Role-Playing

Speech without words may lead directly into role-playing or problem solving. Invent situations around the nonverbal signals. For example, if you saw a friend take someone's quarter and your friend signalled "shhh," what would you do? Groups of three can act out the scene inventing their own endings.

After a while the group begins to realize how much can be expressed nonverbally. They can relate this to what happens in the classroom. "I know John is cold by the way he huddles up." "I know Mary doesn't want to talk to me because she turns away." "I know you don't like the taste because you made a face."

Speech should be added to scenes last of all. Emphasize that every word spoken must be relevant to what is happening in the scene. Some verbal children will let speech run away with them and distract them from the point.

Once the group begins to show clearly what they are doing in each scene, they can begin to invent their own material more freely. They have a base from which to work. Now they can use drama from many sources: history, the news, literature, family and community life. They can explore value judgements and human relationships. Insist that they continue to follow the guidelines set up for acting: exact location of places; how to begin and end; when to be audience; clear communication of ideas to others.

Used in this way, drama is an invaluable tool for learning. The children first grow in their ability to work in a group, listening and watching more carefully, following directions more exactly. They develop an awareness of the need to communicate clearly and appropriately. They develop new ways to do so.

Children, even those with memory difficulties, remember much of what is done in drama and remember it a long time. Concentration expands when groups are working well together and concentration leads to greater poise and confidence in front of others. A great many mental skills are also being practiced and integrated along the way.

The amount of the learning depends, of course, on how much time can be given to doing drama. If it is done often enough, children will make visible progress in a wide range of skills. Once a month or even once a week may not be enough to achieve this. If drama can be done regularly for half an hour two or three times a week, results will be evident. Drama then proves to be as rich in learning as it is in fun. (Alice B. Snyder, Let's Do Drama! *The Pointer*, Vol. 21, No. 3, Spring, 1977, pp. 36-40)

101 BOOKS FOR THE SPEECH AND LANGUAGE CLINICIAN

Compiled by Morris Val Jones, Ph.D.

To maintain an up-to-date and balanced personal professional library is both time consuming and expensive. This bibliography, revised annually, attempts to provide some guidance in the task. Hopefully, it will help in selecting books for keeping up in the fields of speech, hearing, and language. Suggestions for future revisions of the list (limited to 101) are requested from the consumers.

25th Revision, 1977

1. Anderson, Virgil A. and Newby, Hayes: *Improving the Child's Speech.* Oxford U. Press, 1973.
2. Aukerman, Robert C.: *Approaches to Beginning Reading.* John Wiley & Sons, 1971.
3. Bentley, R. H. and Crawford, S. D.: *Black Language Reader.* Scott-Foresman, 1973.
4. Berger, Kenneth W.: *The Hearing Aid: Its Operation and Development.* Charles C Thomas, 1974.
5. Bigge, June and O'Donnell, Patrick: *Teaching Individuals with Physical and Multiple Disabilities.* Charles Merrill Publishers, 1976.
6. Bloodstein, Oliver: *A Handbook of Stuttering.* Society for Crippled Children and Adults, 1969.
7. Bloom, Lois: *Language Development: Form and Function in Emerging Grammars.* The MIT Press, 1970.
8. Boone, Daniel: *Voice and Voice Therapy.* Prentice-Hall, 1970.
9. Bower, Eli: *Early Identification of Emotionally Disturbed Children in School.* Scott, Foresman and Co., 1970.
10. Bradfield, Robert H.: *Behavior Modification of Learning Disabilities.* San Rafael, CA, Academic Therapy Publishers, 1971.
11. Brookshire, R. H.: *An Introduction to Aphasia.* Minneapolis, BRK, 1973.

12. Brown, Roger: *A First Language*. Harvard H. Press, 1973.
13. Bzoch, Kenneth (Ed.): *Communicative Disorders Related to Cleft Lip and Palate*. Little Brown, 1972.
14. Calvert, Donald and Silverman, S. Richard: *Speech and Deafness*. Alexander Graham Bell, 1975.
15. Cazden, Courtney: *Child Language and Education*. Holt, Rinehart and Winston, 1972.
16. Cratty, Bryant J.: *Perceptual-Motor Behavior and Educational Processes*. Charles C Thomas, 1972.
17. Crawley, John and Goodstein, Henry A.: *The Slow Reader and the Reading Problem*. Charles C Thomas, 1972.
18. Cronbach, Lee J.: *Essentials of Psychological Testing* (3rd ed.). Harper and Row, 1970.
19. Cooper, Morton: *Modern Techniqes of Voice Rehabilitation*. Charles C Thomas, 1973.
20. Crickmay, Marie: *Help the Stroke Patient to Talk*. Charles C Thomas, 1977.
21. Cruickshank, William: *Cerebral Palsy, a Developmental Disorder* (3rd ed.). Syracuse U. Press, 1976.
22. Dale, Philip: *Language Development: Structure and Function*. Dryden Press, 1972.
23. Dale, D. M. C.: *Applied Audiology for Children*. Charles C Thomas, 1974.
24. Darley, Frederick; Aronson, Arnold, and Brown, Joe R.: *Motor Speech Disorders*. Saunders, 1975.
25. Davis, Hallowell and Silverman, S. Richard: *Hearing and Deafness* (3rd ed.). Holt, Rinehart and Winston, 1970.
26. Devito, J. A.: *The Psychology of Speech and Language, an Introduction to Psycholinguistics*. Random House, 1970.
27. Dickson, Stanley (Ed.): *Communication Disorders Remedial Principles and Practices*. Glenview, Illinois, Scott, Foresman and Company, 1974.
28. Dunn, Lloyd (Ed.): *Exceptional Children in the Schools* (2nd ed.). Holt, Rinehart and Winston, 1973.
29. Eisenson, Jon: *Aphasia in Children*. Harper and Row, 1972.
30. Eisenson, Jon: *Adult Aphasia*. Appleton-Century-Crofts, 1973.
31. Emerick, Lon L. and Hatton, John T.: *Diagnosis and Evaluation in Speech Pathology*. Prentice-Hall, 1974.
32. Evans, Richard: *Jean Piaget, The Man & His Ideas*. E. L. Dutton, 1973.
33. Faas, Larry A.: *Learning Disabilities: A Book of Readings*, Thomas, 1972. *Learning Disabilities: A Competency Based Approach*. Houghton Mifflin, Boston, 1976.
34. Frostig, Marianne and Maslow, Phyllis: *Learning Problems in the Classroom*. New York, Grune & Stratton, 1973.

35. Gallagher, James J. (Ed.): *Application of Child Development Research to Exceptional Children.* Rector, Virginia, The Council for Exceptional Children, 1975.
36. Gardner, Warren H.: *Laryngectomee Speech and Rehabilitation.* Charles C Thomas, 1971.
37. Gardner, William: *Behavior Modification in Mental Retardation.* Chicago, Illinois, Aldene-Atherton, 1970.
38. Gray, Burl and Ryan, Bruce: *A Language Program for the Non-language Child.* Research Press, 1972.
39. Greene, Margaret C. L.: *The Voice and Its Disorders* (3rd ed.). Philadelphia, Lippincott, 1973.
40. Halpern, Harvey (Ed.): Bobbs-Merrill Series in Communication Disorders, 1972.
    Psycholinguistics, by Joseph A. DeVito
    Disorders of Voice, by Margaret C. L. Greene
    Disorders of Articulation, by John Irwin
    Speech Acoustics and Perception, by Phillip Lieberman
    Clinical Audiometry and Masking, by Frederick N. Martin
    The Development of Speech, by Paula Menyuk
    Principles of Aural Rehabilitation, by Mark Ross
    Cerebral Palsy, by Daniel Boone
    Speech Therapy in the Public Schools, by Martha E. Black
    Disorders of Hearing, by Victor Goodhill
    Stuttering: Differential Evaluation and Therapy, by Hugo Gregory
    Adult Aphasia, by Harvey Halpern
    Anatomy and Physiology, by Irving Hockberg
    Language Disorders in Children, by Frank R. Kleffner
    Hearing Aids, by Maureice Miller
    Cleft Palate, by Gene R. Powers
    The Historical Roots of Communicative Disorders, by Robert Rieber
    Mental Retardation, by Bernard Schlanger
41. Hurley, R. and Ingram, E.: *Language Acquisition: Models and Methods.* New York, Academic Press, 1971.
42. Irwin, John and Marge, Michael (Eds.): *Principles of Childhood Language Disabilities.* Appleton-Century-Crofts, 1972.
43. Jeffers, Janet and Barley, Margaret: *Speechreading (Lipreading).* Charles C Thomas, 1971.
44. Kanner, Leo: *Childhood Psychosis* (4th ed.). Wiley, 1972.
45. Jones, Morris Val (Ed.). *Language Development: The Key to Learning.* Charles C Thomas, 1972.
46. Jenkins, James J.; Jimenz-Pabon, Edward; Shaw, Robert E., and Sefer, Joyce W.: *Schuell's Aphasia in Adults.* Harper & Row, 1975.

47. Jerger, James (Ed.): *Modern Developments in Audiology.* Academic Press, 1973.

48. Katz, Jack (Ed.): *Handbook of Clinical Audiology.* Williams and Wilkins, 1972.

49. Kirk, Samuel and Kirk, Winifred D.: *Psycholinguistic Learning Disabilities.* Urbana, Illinois, U. of Illinois Press, 1971.

50. Koth, Richard, and de la Cruz, Felix F. (Eds.): *Down's Syndrome* (Mongolism), New York, Brunner/Mazel, 1975.

51. Krusen, Frank H. (Ed.): *Handbook of Physical Medicine and Rehabilitation* (2nd ed). Philadelphia, V. R. Saunders and Co., 1971.

52. Lee, Laura: *Developmental Sentence Analysis.* Evanston, Illinois, Northwestern University Press, 1974.

53. Lee, Laura; Koenigsknecht, Roy A., and Mulhern, Susan T.: *Interacting Language Development Teaching.* Northwestern University Press, 1974.

54. Lerner, Janet W.: *Children with Learning Disabilities* (2nd ed.). Houghton Mifflin Co., Boston, 1976.

55. Licht, Sidney (Ed.): *Stroke and Its Rehabilitation.* Baltimore, Md., Waverly Press, Inc., 1975.

56. Lloyd, Lyle L. (Ed.): *Communication Assessment and Intervention Strategies.* Baltimore University Park Press, 1976.

57. Lovaas, Ivar O. and Bucher, Bradley D. (Eds.): *Perspectives in Behavior Modification with Deviant Children.* Prentice-Hall, 1974.

58. McCandless, Boyd R. and Evans, Ellis D.: *Children and Youth: Psychosocial Development.* Hinsdale, Illinois, Dryden Press, 1973.

59. McKee, Bob J.: *Speech Workbooks for Articulation,* 1976. 3415 Ione Drive, Los Angeles, CA 90068.

60. McLean, J. E.; Yoder, D. E., and Schiefelbusch, R. L. (Eds.): *Language Intervention with the Retarded.* Baltimore, Md., University Park Press, 1972.

61. Medlin, Lunn and Quattrock, Judy: *Activities for Renovation of Auditory Disabilities.* Jackson, Miss. (P.O. Box 3171), Education Innovations, Inc., 1972.

62. Moore, G. Paul: *Organic Voice Disorders.* Prentice-Hall, 1971.

63. Morehead, Donald M. and Anne E.: *Normal and Deficient Child Language.* University Park Press, 1976.

64. Morley, Muriel: *The Development and Disorders of Speech in Childhood* (3rd ed.). London, Churchill Livingston, 1972.

65. Nation, J. E. and Aram, D. M.: *Diagnosis of Speech and Language Disorders.* St. Louis, C. V. Mosby Co., 1977.

66. Netter, Frank H.: *Nervous System,* Vol. I. 556 Summitt, N.J., The Ciba Collection of Medical Illustrations.

67. Northern, Jerry and Downs, Marian: *Hearing in Children.* Williams & Wilkins, 1974.
68. Musser, Paul H.: *Carmichael's Manual of Child Psychology.* John Wiley, 1970.
69. Myklebust, Helmer: *Development and Disorders of Written Language,* Volume I (1965), Volume II (1973). Grune and Stratton.
70. Myklebust, Helmer (Ed.): *Progress in Learning Disabilities,* Volume I (1968), Volume II (1971), Volume III (1975). Grune and Stratton.
71. Mysak, Edward D.: *Pathologies of Speech Systems.* Williams & Wilkins, 1976.
72. O'Rourks, T. J. (Ed.): *Psycholinguistics and Total Communication: The State of the Art.* American Annals of the Deaf, 1972.
73. Palmer, James O.: *The Psychological Assessment of Children.* John Wiley, 1970.
74. Pearson, Paul R.; Williams, Carol, and Green, Leila: *Physical Therapy Services in the Developmental Disabilities.* Charles C Thomas, 1972.
75. Perkins, William H.: *Speech Pathology and the Applied Behavior Science* (2nd ed.). St. Louis, C. V. Mosby Co., 1977.
76. Pollock, Michael C.: *Amplification for the Hearing-Impaired.* Grune and Stratton, 1975.
77. Polow, Nancy: *An Articulation Curriculum for the /s/ Sound* and *A Stuttering Manual for the Speech Therapist.* Charles C Thomas, 1975.
78. Ross, Robert B. and Johnston, Malcolm C.: *Cleft Lip and Palate.* Williams and Wilkins, 1972.
79. Rutter, Michael and Martin, J. A.: *The Child with Delayed Speech.* London, Heineman Books, 1972.
80. Ryan, Bruce P.: *Programmed Therapy for Stuttering in Children and Adults.* Charles C Thomas, 1974.
81. Sanders, Derek: *Aural Rehabilitation.* Prentice-Hall, 1971.
82. Sarno, Martha Taylor: *Aphasia: Selected Readings.* Appleton-Century-Crofts, 1972.
83. Schiefelbusch, Richard and Lloyd, Lyle L. (Eds.): *Language Perspectives.* Baltimore, University Park Press, 1974.
84. Schreiber, Flora R.: *Young Child's Speech.* New York, Hash-Marc/Ballatine, 1973.
85. Sheehan, Joseph: *Stuttering, Research and Therapy.* Harper and Row, 1970.
86. Silverman, Franklin H.: *Research Design in Speech Pathology and Audiology.* Prentice-Hall, Inc., 1977.
87. Simoes, Antonio, Jr.: *The Bilingual Child.* New York, Academic Press, 1976.

88. Snidecor, Joseph C.: *Speech Rehabilitation of the Laryngectomized* (2nd ed.), Charles C Thomas, 1968.
89. Strickland, Ruth G.: *The Language Arts in the Elementary School* (3rd ed.). Lexington, Mass., D.C. Heath and Co., 1969.
90. Tinker, Miles and McCullough, Constance: *Teaching Elementary Reading* (2nd ed.). Appleton-Century-Crofts, 1971.
91. Tjossern, T. D. (Ed.): *Intervention Strategies for High Risk Infants and Young Children.* University Park Press, 1976.
92. Travis, Lee E. (Ed.): *Handbook of Speech Pathology and Audiology.* Appleton-Century-Crofts, 1971.
93. Van Riper, Charles: *The Nature of Stuttering.* Prentice-Hall, 1971.
94. Van Riper, Charles: *Speech Correction: Principles and Methods* (5th ed.). Prentice-Hall, 1972.
95. Weiner, Irving B. and Elkind, David: *Readings in Child Development.* John Wiley, 1972.
96. Wells, Charlotte G.: *Cleft Palate and Its Associated Speech Disorders.* New York, McGraw, 1971.
97. Weston, Alan: *Communicative Disorders.* Charles C Thomas, 1972.
98. Wiig, Elizabeth and Semel, Eleanor Messing: *Language Disabilities in Children and Adolescents.* Columbus, Ohio, Charles E. Merrill, 1976.
99. Wilson, D. Kenneth: *Voice Problems in Children.* Williams and Wilkins, 1972.
100. Winitz, Harris: *Articulatory Acquisition and Behavior.* Appleton-Century-Crofts, 1969.
101. Zemlin, Willard R.: *Speech and Hearing Science—Anatomy and Physiology.* Prentice-Hall, 1968.

GLOSSARY

The content of the glossary was selected by a ten-member committee from Speech Pathology 120 (a beginning survey course) at California State University, Sacramento, California (chairperson: Lore Young).

abnormal: Deviating significantly from the normal; contrary to the usual size, location, condition or system to such a degree so as not to be "within normal limits."

acalculia: Inability to solve mathematical problems or to do calculations; loss of ability in using mathematical symbols due to central nervous system dysfunction.

ACLC: *Assessment of Children's Language Comprehension,* a test used to study the language development of children.

adjunct: Joined or added to another object but not necessarily a part of it. Appendage, appurtenance, accessory.

adventitious: Accidently acquired after birth, as opposed to congenital.

afferent system: A system which carries impulses toward a center, i.e. nerves that transmit impulses from the periphery toward the central nervous system.

affricatives: A stop consonant with a fricative release; the group of two sounds, /ch/ and /j/, which are combinations of one plosive and one fricative to form a voiced-voiceless pair.

agraphia: A loss of ability to express oneself in writing due to a central lesion and/or muscular incoordination.

alae pinching: Spontaneous pinching together of the nostrils in an attempt to diminish nasal emission; may lead to facial grimaces in relation to cleft palate.

alexia: Inability to read due to central nervous system dysfunction. Partial loss is known as dyslexia.

alveolar ridge: Area or crest just behind the teeth.

ambidexterity: Ability to work effectively with either hand.

amplification: Make larger or louder. Hearing aids are used for amplification of the auditory stimulus.

375

anomaly: An organ or structure which is abnormal with reference to form, structure, or position; a malformation.

anoxia: Oxygen deficiency; reduction of oxygen in body tissues below normal physiologic levels.

aphasia: Inability to express oneself properly through speech and/or loss of ability to comprehend oral language; impairment in the use of meaningful symbols due to central nervous system dysfunction.

aspirate voice: An excess of air passing through the glottis during phonation to result in breathiness. A whispered voice.

assessment: Evaluation; a determination of the present level of functioning.

ataxia: A type of cerebral palsy as a result of injury to the cerebellum characterized by lack of balance and muscular incoordination.

athetosis: A type of cerebral palsy characteriezd by slow, irregular, twisting, snakelike muscular movements, seen mostly in the upper extremities. The symptoms may be due to various diseases of the central nervous system, with the primary site of lesion in the basal ganglia.

atonia: Absence or lack of normal muscular tonus. A lesser degree is known as dystonia.

audiogram: The graphic record drawn from the results of hearing testing with an audiometer.

audiologist: A professional who studies the science concerned with the sense of hearing.

audiology: Science concerned with the sense of hearing.

audiometer: An electrical instrument for measuring the threshold of hearing for pure tones of frequencies from 125 to 8,000 cycles per second.

auditory memory: The ability to recall a series of test sounds, syllables, or words.

auditory nerve: The 8th cranial nerve; it is a sensory nerve with two sets of fibers: cochlear (hearing) and vestibular (equilibrium).

auditory perception: Involves detection, discrimination, identification and association of incoming auditory stimuli.

aural rehabilitation: Retraining in the interpretation of speech sounds for individuals whose residual hearing has become less serviceable through disuse or failure to listen. Those who have had prior oral language and speech experience may be taught either to retain the present ability or to improve upon their communication ability. Three areas are usually emphasized: speech reading, auditory training and counseling.

auricle: The visible outer ear; the protruding portion of the external ear which surrounds the opening of the external acoustic meatus; the pinna.

autism: An emotional disturbance in children resulting in a detachment from their environmental surroundings; almost complete withdrawal from social interaction; a self-centered state from which reality tends to be excluded.

babbling: A prelinguistic stage of vocalization in which the infant plays with sounds.

babinski: A type of reflex which consists of the extension of the big toe upon stimulation of the sole of the foot (positive Babinski).

basilar membrane: Base covering on the cochlea of the inner ear.

behaviorists: Persons who believe that the thoughts, impulses, and actions of man are purely mechanical results of training.

bibliotherapy: Use of selected reading material to influence total behavior; a process of interaction between reader and literature which is used for personality assessment, adjustment, and growth.

bilabial: A consonant classification in which speech sounds are made by the approximation of both lips.

bilingualism: The ability to speak two languages; an environment where two languages are used.

breathiness: A voice quality resulting from an excess of air being emitted between the vocal folds during phonation.

Broca's area: An area of the frontal lobe of the cerebrum associated with oral expression.

carcinoma: Any of several kinds of cancer.

carryover: The ability to retain new-learned behavior beyond the clinical setting.

cerebellum: The section of the brain behind and below the cerebrum; also known as the "little brain."

cerebral palsy: Defect of motor power and coordination related to damage to the central nervous system, which may occur before, during, or soon after birth.

cerebrum: The main part of the brain, which is divided into four lobes in each hemisphere.

cineflurography: X-ray radiography combined with motion picture photography.

cleft palate: A congenital malformation in which the palate fails to fuse at the midline.

cochlea: The essential organ of hearing in the inner ear, curled upon itself around a bony central axis and surrounded by a fluid.

cognition: The process of acquiring a mental image; perception, thinking, knowing.

conceptualizaton: To form a concept or to get a general idea.

congenital: Relating to existing characteristics dating from birth.

"cul-de-sac" resonance: The intensification of a sound produced by the communication of a vibration to an external sound in a saclike cavity or tube open only at one end.

deaf: Lacking the sense of hearing to the degree that the auditory modality is ineffective for language or learning. (Loss above 85 dB.)

decibels (dB):   1/10 of a bel; the common unit of power ratio; a measure of sound intensity.

delayed language: A condition in which the child's language development is significantly below normal for his or her chronological age.

denasal: Lack of adequate nasal resonance.

developmental aphasia: Inability to develop speech patterns as a result of injury or immaturity of the central nervous system.

diagnosis: Identification of diseases or disorders by their distinctive symptoms; the conclusion reached.

diphthong: A continuous monosyllabic speech sound made by gliding from the articulatory position for one vowel toward that for another.

diplegia: Paralysis of corresponding parts on both sides of the body.

distinctive features: Characteristics which differentiate one speech sound from another; a system for identifying speech sounds.

distortion: A type of articulatory error in which the speech sound is attempted but not made correctly; the approximation is near enough so that it cannot be classified as a sound substitution.

Down's syndrome: Mongolism; a congenital condition characterized by obliquely set eyes, open mouth, flabby muscles, soft skin, and a broad face. There is usually mental retardation.

dysarthria: Misarticulation due to paralysis or incoordination of the muscles used for speaking.

dysdiadochokinesis: Impairment of the power to move opposing sets of muscles as for flexion and extension.

dysfluency: Lack of rhythm in speaking, the chief form of which is stuttering.

dyskinesia: Difficulty in performing voluntary muscular movements.

dysphonia: Abnormality of speech sound production in terms of pitch, volume, or quality; a voice problem.

dyspraxia: Inability to move the muscles of articulation voluntarily, even though they function adequately for nonspeech activities, such as chewing.

dystonia: A state of abnormal tonicity of the muscles, either hypertonia or hypotonia.

echolalia: The production of sounds as specific imitative responses to specific stimuli.

eclectic: The selection of the better features of several systems or methods.

egocentric: Self-centered; viewing matters in their relationship to oneself.

electroencephalogram: A tracing or linear record of the electric currents generated by the brain.

embryology: The science which deals with embryos, their development and formation.

encephalitis: Inflammation of the brain.

encoding: The comprehension of incoming stimuli.

esophageal speech: Speech coming from the esophagus, used

by a person whose larynx has been removed, usually because of cancer.

etiology: Study of the causes of any disease or condition.

eustachian tube: A passage leading from the nasopharynx to the middle ear, essential for equalization of air pressure on both sides of the eardrum.

expressive vocabulary: The words used by an individual in oral or written communication.

external auditory canal: The passage leading from the external ear to the tympanic membrane (eardrum), by which sounds reach the middle and inner ears; also called external auditory meatus.

falsetto: A tone of voice pitched higher than the normal voice, produced by reduction of the vocal fold mass that vibrates.

fricatives: Consonant sounds which depend for their characteristics upon the passing of air through a narrow opening between the articulators, such as the teeth and the lips for /f/.

gastrointestinal tract: Relating to both the stomach and the intestines.

glottal: A sound, such as /h/, is made by the air stream coming through the opening between the vocal folds without modification by other articulators.

hearing threshold level (HTL): The number of decibels needed before the individual hears a sound at a specified frequency relative to standard audiometric thresholds which have been based on normal hearing young adults. Hearing thresholds are plotted on the audiogram.

heredity predisposition: A condition of special susceptibility derived from ancestry to a disease which is transmitted from parent to offspring through the genes.

hemiplegia: Paralysis of one side of the body.

Hertz (Hz): In recognition of Heinrich Hertz and his work with electromagnetic waves, the term was adopted for cycles per second.

H.E.W.: The Department of Health, Education and Welfare.

holistic: The consideration of man functioning as a complete integrated unit.

holophrastic stage: A stage of language development in which one word utterances are used to express various meanings.

hot cautery: An agent used for scarring or burning the skin or tissues by means of heat.

hyperactive: Excessively or pathologically active.

hyperfunction: Characterized by increasing contraction and tension of the muscles, such as in the walls of the resonating cavities or in the vocal folds.

hypernasality: A vowel quality characterized by presence of excessive resonance of the voice in the nasal cavity, usually due to varying degrees of functional or structural inadequacy of the velopharyngeal mechanism.

hyponasality: Disorder of speech resulting from diminished nasal resonance of the three nasal consonants, /m/ /n/ /ng/.

hypopharynx: The lowest portion of the pharynx which connects with the esophagus and the trachea.

hypotonia: A condition of diminished tone or firmness, as of a muscle.

idioglossia: A special oral communication system which is developed by young children, especially twins; it seems to convey meaning to the participants but remains unintelligible to others.

implants: Material inserted or grafted into intact tissues; they may be used in the pharyngeal wall to assist in obtaining velopharyngeal closure; in hearing, the still experimental implantable hearing aid.

incus: The middle bone of the three ossicles in the middle ear.

innate capacity: An inborn ability.

innervation: Activation of muscles by efferent nerves.

intraoral pressure: Air pressure within the mouth; varying degrees of such pressure are required for the production of the plosives and fricatives.

IPA: International phonetic alphabet, an international system used to represent speech sounds.

jargon: A stage of prelinguistic development in which the child uses speech sounds and seems to produce the melodic pattern of real oral communication, but the resulting product is unintelligible.

juvenile perseveration (*Voice*): Retention of a preadolescent quality and pitch of voice into adulthood, more noticeable in males.

juxtaposition: Side by side; contiguous.

kernal sentence: A simple, active, declarative sentence which in transformational grammar is the deep structure of every sentence.

kinesthesia: The perception of movement; the muscular sense.

labio-dental: Pertaining to the lips and teeth in speech production.

laryngectomy: Surgical removal of the larynx.

laterality: Preference in the use of homologous parts (hand, foot, eye) on one lateral half of the body over those on the other half.

lesion: A wound or injury; a pathological change in the tissues.

lingua-alveolar: Pertaining to the tongue and alveolar ridge in speech production.

lingua-palatal: Pertaining to the tongue and palate in speech production.

lingua-palatal: Pertaining to the tongue and plate in speech production.

lingua-velar: Pertaining to the tongue and soft palate (velum) in speech production.

linguistic competence: Pertaining to the degree of understanding an individual has of his native language.

linguistic-performance: Pertaining to the ability of an individual to produce his native language.

Little's disease: An early designation of cerebral palsy as described by Doctor William Little of England.

malleus: The club-shaped largest bone of the middle ear, the first of the three ossicles nearest the tympanic membrane.

malocclusion: Faulty meeting or closing, as of the upper and lower teeth.

mandible: The lower jaw bone.

medulla oblongata: The lowest part of the brain stem, narrowing down into the spinal cord.

meningitis: A disease or inflammation of the coverings of the brain, especially in the pia mater and arachnoid.

mongolism: Also known as Down's syndrome.

monoplegia: Paralysis of one extremity of the body.

morpheme: The smallest meaningful unit of a language or dialect.

morphology: The changing of meanings by the addition of morphemes, such as plurals or possessives.

nasal emission: An excessive amount of air is emitted through the nose, sometimes characteristic of the speech of individuals with cleft palate.

nasopharynx: The upper part of the throat, lying behind the nasal cavity.

neurology: The medical science which deals with the nervous system and its disorders.

nystagmus: An involuntary, rapid movement of the eyeball which may be horizontal, vertical, rotary, or mixed.

obturator: A prosthetic device which is designed to bridge an unnatural opening, such as a cleft in the velum.

occluded: Closed or obstructed (as the Eustachian tube); or brought together (as the upper and lower teeth).

olfactory: Pertaining to the sense of smell.

operant conditioning: Conditioning based on the principle of reinforcement.

oro-facial anomalies: Abnormalities in the structures of the mouth and face. In many cases these anomalies are congenital, as with cleft palate.

organ of corti: Structure attached to the basilar membrane of the cochlear portion of the inner ear; the hair cells in this structure are auditory receptors.

orifice: The entrance or outlet of any cavity of the body.

oropharynx: The central portion of the pharynx which lies between the soft palate and the upper portion of the epiglottis.

orthopedically handicapped: Those individuals handicapped with disorders involving locomotor structures of the body.

otitis media: Inflammation of the middle ear.

otologist: A professional who has specialized in that branch of medicine which deals with the anatomy, physiology, and pathology of the ear.

paraplegia: Paralysis of the lower limbs.

pedodontics: Dentists who specialize in working with children.

perception: The process of knowing objects and objective events by means of the senses.

perinatal: Occurring in the period during or immediately after birth.

perseveration: The continuation of an activity beyond its usefulness; the persistence of a trait beyond the time it would normally have disappeared.

pharyngeal flap: A tongue or lip of tissue which is cut from the pharynx, but left attached at one end. The unattached end is sutured to the velum to assist in velopharyngeal closure.

phonation: The production of sounds by the vibration of the vocal folds.

phoneme: A minimal significant contractive unit in the phonological system of a language. A group of similar sounds considered equivalent within a language.

pinna: That portion of the external ear which protrudes from the sides of the head; it functions to collect and direct sound waves toward the middle ear.

plosives: Consonant sounds which require a complete stoppage of the air stream and then a release of the air by the articulators, for example, /b/ or /k/.

postnatal: Occurring after birth.

prenatal: Prior to birth.

prognosis: An "educated" guess as to the outcome of treatment.

projection (voice):   The process of making speech intelligible in a large room; three factors are important: (1) increased volume, (2) slower rate, and (3) more precise articulation.

prosthesis: An artificial part substituted for a missing or defective part of the body.

prosthodontist: A specialist engaged in the branch of dentistry pertaining to the restoration and maintenance of oral function by the replacement of missing structures by artificial devices, such as dentures or obturators.

pseudoglottis: The opening between the false vocal folds.

psychogenic dysphonia: A psychologically induced disorder of phonation.

psychosis: A severe mental disorder characterized by disorganization of the thought processes, disturbances in emotionality, disorganization as to time, space, and person, and in some cases, hallucinations and delusions.

psycholinguistics: The study of the interrelation of psychological and linguistic behavior.

quadraplegia: Paralysis affecting all four extremities.

receptive vocabulary: A listing of the words of the language which are understood by the individual; this usually precedes expressive vocabulary by two or more months.

REEL Scale: Receptive-Expressive-Emergent-Language Scale; a scale for the measurement of language skills in children under three years of age.

residual air: The amount of air remaining in the lungs after the fullest possible expiration.

retropositioning: Posterior displacement of a structure, such as a palate or mandible.

rhinolalia: Nasal resonance; rhinolalia aperta (too much); rhinolalia clausa (not enough).

rubella: German measles, often the cause of cerebral palsy, hearing loss, or other birth deformities, especially when the mother has the disease in the first three months of pregnancy.

schizophrenia: Any of a number of psychotic conditions characterized by withdrawal from reality, with highly variable accompanying affective, behavioral, and intellectual disturbances.

self-talk: The verbal expression of thought by articulation of sounds to oneself, often used as part of therapy with non-verbal children.

smiling behavior: Smiling spontaneously by the infant, usually begins in the second month of life.

spasticity: A type of cerebral palsy in which the muscles are hypertense, characterized by the stretch reflex.

speech sound discrimination: The ability to distinguish speech sounds from each other, such as /p/ from /b/ or /s/ from /sh/.

stapedius: A small muscle in the tympanum of the middle ear, inserted into the neck of the stapes. Its primary purpose seems to be protective by contracting in the presence of loud sound.

stapes: One of the three small bones located in the middle ear, nearest the oval window.

static balance: The maintenance of equilibrium without movement.

stimulability: In articulation testing, the ability of the client to reproduce speech sounds when given the model.

subglottic pressure: Pressure built up by the exhaled air stream below the opening between the vocal folds.

submucous cleft: A failure of the palatal muscles to fuse at the midline, while the mucous tissue is intact.

substitution error: The substituting of one speech sound for another, the most common articulatory error, such as /t/ for /th/ or /w/ for /r/.

syntax: The way in which words are put together to form clauses, phrases and sentences.

tactile: Related to the sense of touch.

teratogenic: Causing congenital deformities.

tensor tympani: A muscle of the middle ear whose tendon attaches to the malleus.

trachea: The windpipe; the tube extending from the larynx to the branching off of the bronchi.

TMR: Trainable mentally retarded.

triplegia: Paralysis of three extremities.

tympanic membrane: Eardrum; a membrane which separates the external auditory canal from the tympanic cavity in the middle ear.

unilateral: Confined to one side of the body.

velar: Pertaining to the velum or soft palate.

velopharyngeal insufficiency (*VPI*):   Insufficient function of the soft palate and the posterior nasopharyngeal wall in order to produce closure between the oral and nasal cavities. The result is hypernasality and/or nasal emission.

vomer: A flat bone of trapezoidal shape forming the inferior and posterior portions of the nasal septum; the bone to which the palatal shelves attach when they fuse at the midline.

INDEX

PERSON INDEX

A

Adkins, Carol S., 228
Anderson, Virgil A., 8, 25, 35
Aronson, Arnold, 75

B

Benda, Clemens E., 237
Berger, Kenneth, 129
Berry, Mildred, 12
Bettelheim, Bruno, 255
Birch, Herbert G., 196
Bloom, Lois, 10
Bobath, Karel, 140
Boone, Daniel R., 70-81, 83, 84, 90
Bradley, Doris P., 181, 183
Broadbent, D. E., 53
Brodnitz, Friedrich, 79
Brown, Roger, 13
Bryngelson, Bryng, 97
Bzoch, Kenneth, 7, 21, 187

C

Calvert, Donald, 128
Carrell, James, 41
Carrier, J. K., Jr., 64, 241
Chisum, L., 46
Chomsky, Noam, 3, 13, 25, 36
Coccaro, Peter J., 182
Cole, Richard, 186
Cooper, Morton, 77, 83, 85
Cruickshank, William, 140
Cunningham, M. A., 253, 255
Curtis, J. F., 73-77

D

Dale, Philip, 10, 56
Darley, Frederic, 75, 199

D (cont.)

Davis, B. J., 253
de Hirsch, Katrina, 255
De Myer, Marian, 251
Denes, Peter B., 69, 70
Denhoff, Eric, 142
DiCarlo, Louis, 125

E

Eisenson, Jon, 35, 198, 200, 220, 226, 230
Emerick, Lon, 296
Erikson, Erik, 209
Evans, Kathleen, 238

F

Fay, W. H., 253
Fogh-Anderson, Poul, 172
Frankenburg, William, 5
Froeschels, Emil, 79
Frostig, Marianne, 206

G

Gardner, R. A., 64
Gardner, Warren H., 88, 90, 95
Goldberg, Ignacy, 333
Goldfarb, W., 255
Gray, B. B., 64
Green, Deborah, 94
Greene, Margaret C. L., 68-71, 76, 77
Greenfield, Patricia, 11

H

Hahn, Elise, 192
Hartman, Heinz, 208
Heber, Rick, 234
Hewett, F. M., 256

389